Register Now for Online Access to Your Book!

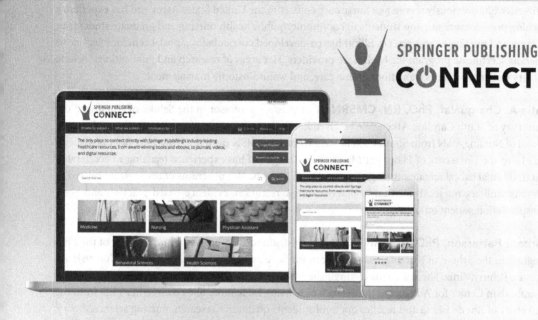

SPRINGER PUBLISHING
CONNECT™

Your print purchase of *Veteran-Centered Care in Education and Practice* **includes online access to the contents of your book**—increasing accessibility, portability, and searchability!

Access today at:
http://connect.springerpub.com/content/book/978-0-8261-3597-1
or scan the QR code at the right with your smartphone
and enter the access code below.

M1BNJDHV

Scan here for quick access.

If you are experiencing problems accessing the digital component of this product, please contact our customer service department at cs@springerpub.com

The online access with your print purchase is available at the publisher's discretion and may be removed at any time without notice.

Publisher's Note: New and used products purchased from third-party sellers are not guaranteed for quality, authenticity, or access to any included digital components.

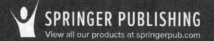

SPRINGER PUBLISHING
View all our products at springerpub.com

Brenda Elliott, PhD, RN, CNE, is an assistant professor and coordinator of MSN, CAGS, and RN-to-BSN programs in the Department of Nursing at Messiah University in Mechanicsburg, Pennsylvania. She received a BSN from Lycoming College, MSN from Bloomsburg University, and PhD from Widener University. She previously served as a nurse corps officer in the United States Army and has experience teaching pre-licensure nursing students in community/public health nursing and graduate students in research and nursing education. Dr. Elliott has co-developed curricula for a post-bachelor's Service to Veterans' Certificate program for healthcare providers. Her areas of research and publications include military nursing, veteran's transitions, home care, and wound/ostomy management.

Katie A. Chargualaf, PhD, RN, CMSRN, is an assistant professor in the School of Nursing at the University of South Carolina Aiken. She received her diploma in nursing from Bon Secours Memorial School of Nursing, BSN from South Dakota State University, MSN from the University of Phoenix, and PhD from the University of Hawaii at Mañoa. Dr. Chargualaf has experience teaching in accelerated and traditional baccalaureate nursing programs in all formats. Her programs of research are related to veterans, military nurses, transition to practice, nurse retention, evidence-based practice, and post-transplantation patient outcomes.

Barbara Patterson, PhD, RN, ANEF, FAAN, is distinguished professor and director of the PhD Program in the School of Nursing, associate dean for Scholarship and Inquiry, Widener University in Chester, Pennsylvania. She is also the distinguished scholar in the National League of Nursing (NLN)/Chamberlain Center for Advancing the Science of Nursing Education. She received her PhD from the University of Rhode Island and teaches doctoral students qualitative research, nursing science/theory, leadership, and dissertation advisement. Dr. Patterson has chaired more than 50 PhD dissertations, many investigating nursing education topics, and has presented and published extensively in the areas of evidence-based teaching, veteran transitions, and leadership in nursing education. She was faculty for the Nurse Faculty Leadership Academy of Sigma Theta Tau International, helping to develop the leadership skills of novice nurse educators, and chair of NLN's Research Review Panel (2012–2015). Dr. Patterson is the editor for Nursing Education Perspectives.

VETERAN-CENTERED CARE IN EDUCATION AND PRACTICE

An Essential Guide for Nursing Faculty

Brenda Elliott, PhD, RN, CNE

Katie A. Chargualaf, PhD, RN, CMSRN

Barbara Patterson, PhD, RN, ANEF, FAAN

Editors

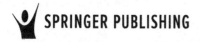 SPRINGER PUBLISHING

Springer Publishing Company, LLC
11 West 42nd Street, New York, NY 10036
www.springerpub.com
connect.springerpub.com/

Acquisitions Editor: Adrianne Brigido
Compositor: Transforma

ISBN: 978-0-8261-3596-4
ebook ISBN: 978-0-8261-3597-1
DOI: 10.1891/9780826135971

20 21 22 23 24/5 4 3 2 1

The author and the publisher of this Work have made every effort to use sources believed to be reliable to provide information that is accurate and compatible with the standards generally accepted at the time of publication. The author and publisher shall not be liable for any special, consequential, or exemplary damages resulting, in whole or in part, from the readers' use of, or reliance on, the information contained in this book. The publisher has no responsibility for the persistence or accuracy of URLs for external or third-party internet websites referred to in this publication and does not guarantee that any content on such websites is, or will remain, accurate or appropriate.

Library of Congress Cataloging-in-Publication Data
Names: Elliott, Brenda, editor. | Chargualaf, Katie A, editor. | Patterson,
    Barbara J., editor.
Title: Veteran-centered care in education and practice : an essential guide
    for nursing faculty / [edited by] Brenda Elliott, Katie A Chargualaf,
    Barbara Patterson.
Description: New York, NY : Springer Publishing Company, [2021] | Includes bibliographical references and index.
Identifiers: LCCN 2020030116 (print) | LCCN 2020030117 (ebook) | ISBN
    9780826135964 (hardback) | ISBN 9780826135971 (e-book)
Subjects: MESH: Education, Nursing--methods | Veterans Health--education |
    Veterans Health Services | Patient-Centered Care | Veterans--education |
    United States
Classification: LCC RT71 (print) | LCC RT71 (ebook) | NLM WY 18 | DDC
    610.73071--dc23
LC record available at https://lccn.loc.gov/2020030116
LC ebook record available at https://lccn.loc.gov/2020030117

Brenda Elliott ORCID: 0000-0003-2500-6508
Katie A. Chargualaf ORCID: 0000-0001-9498-2604
Barbara Patterson ORCID: 0000-0003-0386-9636

Contact us to receive discount rates on bulk purchases. We can also customize our books to meet your needs. For more information please contact: sales@springerpub.com

Publisher's Note: **New and used products purchased from third-party sellers are not guaranteed for quality, authenticity, or access to any included digital components.**

Printed in the United States of America.

*This book is dedicated to all service members, veterans,
and their family members.*

CONTENTS

SECTION III   ENHANCING CULTURAL SENSITIVITY IN PRACTICE AND ON CAMPUS

CONTRIBUTORS

Myrna L. Armstrong, EdD, RN, ANEF, FAAN
Nursing Consultant, Colonel, U.S. Army (Retired)
Professor Emerita
Texas Tech University Health Sciences Center, Marble Falls, Texas
ORCID: 0000-0002-4756-8168

Patricia L. Conard, PhD, RN
Associate Professor
University of Arkansas, Van Buren, Arkansas
ORCID: 0000-0002-7112-4380

Sean P. Convoy, DNP, RN, PMHNP-BC
Commander, Nurse Corps, U.S. Navy (Retired)
Assistant Professor
Duke University, School of Nursing, Durham, North Carolina
ORCID: 0000-0001-8911-4423

Barbara Champlin, PhD, RN
Associate Professor
University of Minnesota School of Nursing, Minneapolis, Minnesota
ORCID: 0000-0002-3488-8197

Katie A. Chargualaf, PhD, RN, CMSRN
Assistant Professor
University South Carolina Aiken, Aiken, South Carolina
ORCID: 0000-0001-9498-2604

Julie L. Decker, DNP, RN
Assistant Teaching Professor in Nursing
Penn State Altoona, Altoona, Pennsylvania

Kelly L. Dyar, EdD, RN, CNN, CNE
Assistant Professor
University of West Georgia, Douglasville, Georgia
ORCID: 0000-0003-4045-0164

Brenda Elliott, PhD, RN, CNE
Assistant Professor
Messiah University, Mechanicsburg, Pennsylvania
ORCID: 0000-0003-2500-6508

Carma Erickson-Hurt, DNP, ACHPN, LCDR, USN, RET
Adjunct Faculty
College of Nursing and Health Care Professions, Grand Canyon University, Phoenix, Arizona

Gwendolyn M. Hamid, BA, MSN, RN
Doctoral Student and Jonas Scholar for Veterans' Health
Adjunct Clinical Instructor
M. Louise Fitzpatrick College of Nursing, Villanova University, Villanova, Pennsylvania

Michael J. Keller, PhD, RN, FACHE
Colonel, U.S. Army (Retired)
Assistant Manager
Home Based Primary Care, Lubbock VA
ORCID: 0000-0001-5490-1996

Donna M. Lake, PhD, RN, NEA-BC, FAAN
Colonel, USAF Nurse Corps (Retired)
Clinical Professor
College of Nursing, East Carolina University, Greenville, North Carolina
ORCID: 0000-0001-6861-1682

Raney Linck, DNP, RN
Assistant Professor
University of Minnesota School of Nursing, Minneapolis, Minnesota
ORCID: 0000-0001-9834-700X

Edna R. Magpantay-Monroe, EdD, APRN
Professor of Nursing, Marianist Educational Associate
Chaminade University of Honolulu, Honolulu, Hawaii
ORCID: 0000-0002-8326-3150

Libba Reed McMillan, RN PhD
Associate Professor
Auburn University School of Nursing, Auburn University, Alabama
ORCID: 0000-0003-4688-8087

Helene Moriarty, PhD, RN, FAAN
Professor, Diane & Robert Moritz Jr. Endowed Chair in Nursing Research
M. Louise Fitzpatrick College of Nursing, Villanova University, Villanova, Philadelphia
Nurse Scientist
Co-Program Director, VA Interprofessional Fellowship in Patient Safety
Corporal Michael J Crescenz Veterans Medical Center, Philadelphia, Pennsylvania

Barbara Patterson, PhD, RN, ANEF, FAAN
Professor
Widener University, Chester, Pennsylvania
ORCID: 0000-0003-0386-9636

Richard J. Westphal, PhD, RN, FAAN, PMHCNS/NP-BC
Captain, Nurse Corps, U.S. Navy (Retired)
Professor
University of Virginia, School of Nursing, Charlottesville, Virginia
ORCID: 0000-0003-0716-8976

FOREWORD

This book is an essential and important read for nurses, regardless of employment in healthcare organizations or in academia. While this book is particularly applicable to nurse educators, it is useful for nurses in all settings. As a veteran and nurse educator, I greatly welcome this book and was honored when the editors asked me to write the foreword. I served for 25 years on active duty as a U.S. Air Force nurse, including several overseas assignments. Today, after many years of deployments to the wars in Iraq and Afghanistan, scores of military troops are returning to U.S. shores. Many are trading their combat boots and battle uniforms for a stethoscope and nursing scrubs as students or practicing nurses.

As I read the chapters of this book, I was transported back to my years as a military nurse, the places where I served, the military culture and lifestyle that became part of me, the strong bonds with the people I served with all over the globe, and the pride in wearing America's uniform. As a flight nurse with the 2nd Aeromedical Evacuation Squadron based in Germany, I served on temporary duty all over Europe, the Middle East, Africa, and in southeast Asia. Later, as Chief Nurse at the 48th Fighter Wing Hospital in the United Kingdom, I trained my subordinates to deploy as the first cadre of Air Force nurses and medical technicians to a hospital in the Bosnian conflict. In 1997, I hung up my uniform and embarked on transition to civilian life, a new practice milieu, and my evolution as a nurse educator. It was a transition I welcomed, but I must admit it seemed daunting at times. After retirement from active duty, I found myself in an unfamiliar environment where I felt uneasy, lacking my usual confidence, missing the "espirit de corps" I was so accustomed to, and longing for the lifestyle I left behind. My coping skills were tested as I tried to assimilate a new "academic" vocabulary, tasks like creating a syllabus, using test scoring programs, and trying to understand and adhere to academic bylaws.

After over 40 years as a nurse and educator, it has been my experience that the vast majority of nurses and society in general do not understand much about the military experience, culture, lifestyle, occupational and environmental hazards, transition obstacles and uncertainties, and physical/mental demands and stressors placed on those who serve our country in military service. Historically, nurses in practice have not been prepared academically to address the healthcare needs of this population. Further, veteran students entering nursing programs today represent an American generation who have grown to young adulthood while the United States was engaged in the Global War on Terrorism since the attacks of 9/11/2001.

Post-9/11 veterans have demonstrated some specific health and well-being concerns related to a range of occupational and environmental exposures that include toxic burn pits, depleted uranium ammunition, and the physical trauma of combat and accidents that included a high rate of limb amputations and traumatic brain injuries. The intense psychosocial stressors associated with military service in the Post-9/11 era can result in depression, excessive worry, sleep disorders, suicidal ideation, substance abuse, and post-traumatic stress disorder. The military culture bonds members closer together than most people can imagine. The loss or injury of a colleague often is as powerful as the loss of a spouse or beloved family member.

This book skillfully details what nurses and nursing educators need to know in helping veterans navigate the experience of returning to school after military service. As we know the curriculum can be challenging and most of their fellow students, faculty, and administrators will not have shared in the military experience. Some former military students may be emotionally, behaviorally and psychologically struggling to cope with the demands of transition to civilian life and the academic environment. I believe veterans have much to offer the nursing profession. I see them bringing many strengths with them as they leave military service. My experience has demonstrated that these folks are mission-oriented, goal-focused, and dedicated to a cause greater than themselves. They have lived by a moral code of conduct and are team-players. However, these very qualities may become vulnerabilities in their new environment. Academic activities, clinical experiences and assignments that engage students in recalling trauma or loss experiences can induce reverberations of the situation and bring the emotions and thoughts of the event into the academic experience.

I applaud the editors and chapter authors for their truly superb job of focusing on significant topics that nurses and nurse educators need to know in order to help veterans plot out a path to be successful in any nursing program. Additionally, clinical educators will find this book to be a valuable resource and "roadmap" in guiding practicing nurses to understand and appreciate the perspective of veterans they may have as practice colleagues or as patients.

Elizabeth Scannell-Desch, PhD, RN, FAAN
Colonel, United States Air Force, Nurse Corps (Retired)

PREFACE

Healthcare needs for our military and veterans is something that has a long history and will continue into the foreseeable future. Likewise, families who support these service members and veterans may still be reminded on a daily basis, the sacrifice of service. In response, the Department of Defense and the Department of Veterans Affairs have answered the call in many ways to enhance services and programs to meet the needs of service members, a large growing group of Post-9/11 veterans, and their families. The global war on terrorism spans decades, sparking the country into action to support returning troops. Yet, we fear that the momentum may have slowed. Initiatives from the White House to Join Forces may be less at the front and center of curricular change in nursing education as the next new hot topics emerge. However, the care of military service members, veterans, and their families is a national public health concern and as nurses we have a duty to provide care to this population in a culturally sensitive manner. More work needs to be done, and we cannot do it alone.

This book was undertaken to honor the sacrifices of our military and veteran populations and to provide all nurse educators one comprehensive resource they can turn to for ideas and suggestions incorporating care of these individuals into the courses they teach and the clinical experiences of students and practicing nurses. Nurses encounter this population every day and we know that through exposure and education, nurses can make a meaningful difference in the lives of this unique group of Americans. Not only do nurses need to understand how to care for military service members, veterans, and their families, nurse educators also need to be prepared to work with veterans in the classroom. That is why we took time to put together a book that not only addresses what every nurse should know about military culture and the unique healthcare needs of this population, but also what and how to teach the content and engage student veterans in the classroom. Readers will find that some chapters focus more on the clinical application of the content, while others focus slightly more on the veteran as a student. It is up to the reader to determine how to best utilize the information.

This book is divided into three sections. Section I: Military and Veteran Culture 101 includes four chapters, the first of which provides a context for understanding the importance of military and veteran healthcare in nursing education. The remaining three chapters focus on the basics of being in the military and becoming a veteran in the community. In this section, readers will learn about the background of military personnel, their unique culture, training, and overall way of life. The authors cover critical elements to understanding the major transitions military service members, veterans, and their families go through during service and upon reintegration after deployment. In addition, the transition and reintegration back to civilian life and into the community is highlighted. The role of veteran service organizations, ways in which nurses can advocate for this population, and social issues such as homelessness are covered.

Section II: Veteran-Specific Healthcare Issues includes four chapters on the major health issues and disabilities that are unique to the military and veteran population. Occupational and environmental exposures specific to military training and deployments are covered, as well as common physical injuries that are generally associated with military service. Men and women who serve in the military are exposed to numerous stressors through their time in uniform. Therefore, one chapter is dedicated to understanding the scope and breadth of mental health challenges they face from a stress first aid approach. Important in this chapter is understanding that not every veteran has post-traumatic stress disorder. In addition, four special populations are highlighted (women, LGBT, Reserve and National Guard, and military contractors) as they have unique needs beyond those discussed in the other chapters within this section.

Lastly, Section III: Enhancing Cultural Sensitivity in Practice and on Campus includes four chapters on teaching nursing students about the healthcare needs of this population by focusing on what should be taught and suggestions on how to do to it. Competencies for students, faculty, and practicing nurses are included, along with examples of assignments in both classroom and clinical settings. With the increase in the number of veterans in nursing school, we dedicated the last chapter to this group of students. Faculty have the power to improve the health and well-being of military service members, veterans, and their families by making curricular changes but also by facilitating student veterans' growth and development into nursing careers.

As you read the book, we want to highlight a few key points. The healthcare needs of military service members, veterans, and their families is a global issue. While this book may be U.S. centric, we believe the content and ideas are transferable to other countries and we welcome feedback from our international colleagues. Military service members refer to anyone who is currently serving, in any capacity (Reserves, National Guard, or Active Duty). A veteran refers to anyone who is no longer serving but has served in any capacity, being discharged honorably. Lastly, family members include spouses, children, and parents of these individuals. We have tried to avoid the use of military language or terms that a non-military person would not understand, although some may still exist. While some organizations use the capitalization of "veterans" we have opted not to do that in this book.

Military service members, veterans, and their families deserve culturally sensitive patient-centered care. It is our hope that this book serves not only faculty who teach nursing students, but also practicing nurses and nurse educators in hospital and community-based settings who want to enhance the quality of care delivered to this population. There is a vital need to share best practices and conduct research across all settings to promote the health and well-being of our veteran patients and students. They are deserving of our efforts.

Brenda Elliott
Katie A. Chargualaf
Barbara Patterson

I

MILITARY AND VETERAN CULTURE 101

THE IMPORTANCE OF VETERANS HEALTH IN NURSING EDUCATION

BRENDA ELLIOTT | KATIE A. CHARGUALAF | BARBARA PATTERSON

Never ... was so much owed by so many to so few.

Winston Churchill

KEY TERMS

military/veteran health issues

all volunteer force

veteran healthcare costs

military caregivers

service-connected disability

joining forces

military/veteran cultural competency

INTRODUCTION

Decades of wars contribute to veterans with a wide range of visible and invisible wounds, temporary and permanent, which can influence their health over a lifetime. The health of veterans is a growing public health concern, yet nursing education is still in the early stages of integrating military/veteran-related content into already content heavy curricula. Nurses at the bedside lack adequate knowledge to care for this population in a culturally sensitive manner. This chapter provides a brief overview of veterans in today's society, the major health issues challenging military service members, veterans and their families, and national initiatives that have been the catalyst for change to meet this population's needs. It also addresses the current status of veteran-related content in nursing education, why it is important, and where we need to go moving forward to ensure nurses are educated to deliver culturally sensitive, patient-centered care to this population.

BACKGROUND

The health of veterans is a growing public health concern, yet nursing education may still be in the early stages of integrating military/veteran-related content into already content heavy curricula. This chapter provides an overview of veterans in today's society, the war eras they fought, the major health issues

The complete reference list for this chapter appears in the digital version of the chapter, accessible at https://connect.springerpub.com/content/book/978-0-8261-3597-1/chapter/ch01

they face, as well as initiatives that have been the catalyst for change to meet this population's needs. To ensure a highly educated nursing workforce capable of meeting the healthcare needs of diverse populations such as military, veterans, and their families, educators must take action and continue to lead change to improve health outcomes for this group within society.

Addressing vulnerabilities of this population across generations, using a holistic and inclusive approach, requires concerted effort and institutional/organizational support. Nurses and healthcare providers need more education, and ideally exposure, to military service members, veterans, and their families to begin developing cultural sensitivity and competency. We know from the growing body of literature that current practicing nurses and healthcare providers generally feel unprepared to care for this population (Bonzanto et al., 2019; Richards et al., 2017; Tanielian et al., 2018; Vest et al., 2019). Thus, the optimal time to gain this knowledge and exposure is during prelicensure education.

According to the National Advisory Council on Nurse Education and Practice (2016), the nursing profession needs to examine the way in which nurses are educated. With an evolving and ever-changing healthcare landscape, a shift from focusing on acute hospital care to population healthcare is needed. One population that needs greater focus are military service members, veterans, and their families (Villa et al., 2002). One barrier to obtaining exposure to this population is access. Therefore, the National Advisory Council on Nurse Education and Practice (2016) recommended that the U.S. Department of Veterans Affairs (VA) also examine ways to reduce the administrative burdens on schools and clinical sites so more opportunities for nursing students can be coordinated. Despite access barriers to VA facilities, opportunities exist to interact with this population with intentional efforts.

VETERANS IN TODAY'S SOCIETY

In American society, we have lived through a number of wars and conflicts over the past century. Millions of men and women have served our country in the Army, Air Force, Marines, Navy, and Coast Guard. Surviving still today, we have war veterans who have lived beyond the age of 100, eight decades since World War II ended. We also have veterans who do not live beyond 20. It seems safe to say that the majority of people in the country are proud of our military service members, veterans, and families as they have made many sacrifices for the privilege of our freedoms. Nevertheless, this pride has varied over the years, depending on political and societal support of certain wars and why we fight them. While not all service members serve or deploy during times of war, training alone puts them at risk for injury, disability, and death. Injuries, visible or invisible, as a result of training or conflict, have an impact on the health and well-being of service members, veterans, and their families. Often this impact can follow them into civilian life and continue over their lifetime, as health needs may not manifest until several decades beyond separation from military service or until research to connect symptoms to military service becomes available (Conard et al., 2015).

For nearly 20 years the United States has been engaged in global military activities, with the most recent war in Afghanistan, also known as Operation Enduring Freedom (OEF), officially ending December 31, 2014 (Defense Casualty Analysis System [DCAS], n.d.). Despite the end of OEF, troops remain present in Afghanistan to take part in a coalition mission to train, assist, and give counsel to Afghan National Defense and Security Forces called Operation Freedom's Sentinel (DCAS, n.d.). U.S. troops conduct operations to counter antiterrorism threats from the remnants of al Qaeda and to date have suffered 69 deaths and 369 wounded (DCAS, 2019). At present, thousands of military service members are deployed globally to provide security and conduct varying missions ("U.S. Military Operations," 2018). An estimated 1.3 million Americans are currently serving in the Armed Services and an additional 800,000 Americans are serving in Reserve and National Guard capacities (Defense Manpower Data Center, 2019). These numbers add to the more than 18 million veterans in the U.S. population in 2017 (VA, 2019a). Alaska, Maine, and Montana have the highest percentage of veterans (VA, 2019a).

The estimated 18 million veterans living today represent service members who served during seven wars or conflicts and peace time. Table 1.1 illustrates the health-related service eras defined by the VA (2019b). In addition to those listed health associated risks, noise exposure and occupational hazards related to the job are a risk regardless of which era a service member or veteran has served. In addition, service members who served during the Cold War Era may have additional health-related issues if they were involved in one of the following projects: Projects 112 or Shipboard Hazard and Defense, The Atsugi Waste Incinerator, The Edgewood/Aberdeen Experiments, Camp Lejeune and Marine Corps Air Station New River, or Fort McClellan (VA, 2019b). Of note is that several wars and eras overlap, meaning that service members serving across multiple eras may have health risks associated with more than one time period. In addition, the number of reported risks has increased over the years and more service-related health concerns arise as research into these health risks continues.

World War II

Based on data from the National Center for Veterans Analysis and Statistics' population projections completed in 2016, an estimated 266,000 WWII (1939–1945) veterans would still be alive by the year 2020 and by 2045 that generation of veterans will be absent (VA, 2019c). Approximately 350 veterans of this era die every day (The National WWII Museum, n.d.). As our oldest living generation, it is important to reflect on the time period in which they served, as it helps to understand how they may now think and behave. For men born in the 1920s, serving in the military during WWII was a normative experience (Pruchno, 2016). These service members emerged from families who suffered hardships during the Great Depression, and they came out of war with many opportunities, including social and economic benefits (Spiro et al., 2016). WWII veterans were welcomed home by a country who was also deeply engaged in the war effort.

Korean War

Approximately 1.1 million Korean War (1950–1953) veterans are alive today, and it is estimated a few hundred could survive to the year 2045 (VA, 2019c). Often coined as the "forgotten war" due to it being sandwiched between a very popular WWII and a very unpopular Vietnam War, veterans of this era served in a war that, to date, still has not been officially resolved (National Veterans Foundation, 2015). Because they fought in the shadow of WWII, less attention was paid to this group of veterans. Yet most were drafted and served their country the same as all other men during the time between WWII and Vietnam. While the Korean War was publicly supported at the outset, its popularity faded with time. As cited by Villa et al. (2002) they are often "lumped" in with WWII veterans when analyzing health and well-being data between and among war eras, making it difficult to pinpoint some outcomes specific to this war era.

Vietnam War

Projections of Vietnam era veterans currently living is just over 6 million, with estimates of half a million still living by the year 2045 (VA, 2019c). The largest living cohort of male veterans served during this era (VA, 2019a). The Vietnam War (1961–1975) was markedly different for the American people as many protested the war and it was the first time in history that the war could be seen from uncensored media clips in any home (Elliott, 2015). It was a long, drawn out war spanning 14 years, more than double the duration of WWII and almost five times as long as the fighting period of the Korean War. The Vietnam War was less "traditional" compared to previous wars, as civilians engaged in guerilla or insurgency type warfare against U.S. troops, making the enemy difficult to identify (Villa et al., 2002). Deployment experiences changed from being gone for potentially several years as seen in previous wars, to returning home more periodically (Way et al., 2019). Advances in evacuating injured service members during combat greatly improved survivor rates, yet many veterans returning home did not

TABLE 1.1 HEALTH-RELATED RISKS BY ERA SERVED

WAR ERA	DATES	ASSOCIATED HEALTH RISKS
World War II	September 1, 1939–September 2, 1945	Ionizing radiation Extreme cold Mustard gas
Korean War	June 25, 1950–July 27, 1953	Extreme cold
Vietnam War	November 1, 1965–April 30, 1975	Diseases related to Agent Orange Diseases related to other herbicides Hepatitis C Liver fluke infection
Cold War Era	1945–1991	Radiation Mustard gas Herbicides (tests and storage)
Gulf War – Operation Desert Shield and Desert Storm	August 2, 1990–present	Extreme heat Toxic embedded fragments Infectious disease Sand, dust, and particulates Depleted uranium Oil well fires Chemical and biological weapons CARC paint Pesticides Vaccinations Pyridostigmine
Iraq War – OIF and OND	March 19, 2003–December 15, 2011	Explosions Extreme heat Toxic embedded fragments Infectious diseases Rabies Sand, dust, and particulates Burn pit smoke Depleted uranium Sulfur fire Chemical warfare agents Chromium Pesticides Side effects of mefloquine
OEF in Afghanistan	October 7, 2001–present	Explosions Extreme heat Extreme cold Toxic embedded fragments Infectious diseases Rabies Sand, dust, and particulates Burn pit smoke Depleted uranium Side effects of mefloquine

CARC, chemical agent resistant coating; OIF, Operation Iraqi Freedom; OND, Operation New Dawn; PB, pyridostigmine.

SOURCE: From U.S. Department of Veterans Affairs. (2018). *Veterans Benefits Administration annual benefits report: Fiscal year 2017.* Retrieved September 27, 2019 from https://www.benefits.va.gov/REPORTS/abr/docs/2017_abr.pdf

receive the same welcome as service members from previous wars. More women and minorities served their country during this war, compared to past wars, making Vietnam veterans all the more diverse (Spiro et al., 2016).

Gulf War

For the purposes of representing an ongoing era in history that continues to today, both Pre-9/11 and Post-9/11 will be included in this section. Post-9/11 includes Operation Iraqi Freedom (OIF), OEF, and Operation New Dawn (OND), which are collectively known as the War on Terror or Global War on Terrorism (GWOT; "A Timeline of the U.S.-Led War on Terror," 2019). According to the VA (2019b), 7.7 million from this era are now veterans. The largest cohort of women veterans served during this era (VA, 2019a). It is expected this group will peak in size around the year 2027 (VA, 2019b). By 2045, there will still be over 7 million veterans from these wars. Even if no additional wars break out in the next 25 years, millions of veterans will continue to need healthcare. The conflicts/wars that occurred during this time period were marked by a different type of battle rhythm, or rather a change in the daily routines and processes often seen during military operations (Spiro et al., 2016). Units and service members experienced multiple deployments, sometimes deploying as individuals and not with the unit in which they were assigned and completed training, with much less time between leaving the war zone and returning home. This complicated the return home for many service members.

All Volunteer Force

The all-volunteer force (AVF) was put into effect during the Vietnam era (Rostker, 2006). Up until that time, the military used a draft to fulfill military needs for most of the 20th century. This practice, generally accepted by American society, began to erode during the 1960s when discussions began to reevaluate military service (Rostker, 2006). Due to the changes brought on by the AVF, the military has become more of a professional military. The composition of the military has also changed. It is more diverse in regard to gender, race, and ethnicity (VA, 2019a), and less diverse in regard to socioeconomic status (Spiro et al., 2016). According to the VA (2019a), by the year 2040 the overall veteran population is expected to drop from 18.6 million to 12.9 million, while the proportion of veterans who are minorities will increase from 23% to 34%. Since the AVF was introduced in 1973, more Reserve and National Guard service members are called upon to augment Active Duty forces, which contributes to even more variation in socioeconomic challenges as these groups are generally older and have more family responsibilities compared to their Active Duty counterparts (Spiro et al., 2016).

According to Lanaras (2016), today's military veterans who served under the AVF may struggle more overall compared to those who served under the draft. Having an AVF is not likely the cause of this shift as challenges with reintegration, loss of camaraderie, or even dealing with physical or mental injuries are not so vastly different among war cohorts. Before the AVF, service members represented people from all backgrounds and from all over the United States (Lanaras, 2016). People in every community across the country knew someone who served. Today, military service members come disproportionately from the South and have close family members who served (Lanaras, 2016). In addition, the closure of military bases over the past two decades has reduced the number of active installations in urban and northeast regions of the United States, shifting more military personnel to rural and southern regions. This results in a large portion of people in the United States not having direct contact with the military or veterans. Lanaras (2016) suggests that veterans who served under the draft were forced to reintegrate, but for today's veterans that process has perhaps changed allowing more of them to be self-isolating, which can lead to greater problems.

Way et al. (2019) postulate that as a result of the switch to an AVF, a higher concentration of service members are entering the military with histories of adverse childhood experiences. This could further explain the variance in today's veterans struggling more after their service ends. Men with a history of service during the AVF era had a higher prevalence of adverse childhood experiences in all 11 categories inventoried, which lends support to the notion that entering military service for men served as an escape from dysfunctional home lives (Blosnich et al., 2014). While women of the same AVF era had higher prevalence in just four of 11 categories inventoried, the researchers postulate their entry into the military is more to improve socioeconomic opportunities. Their reasoning for this is that the military is comprised mostly of men (Blosnich et al., 2014). Of concern is the associated risk of suicide to adverse childhood experiences. Blosnich et al. (2014) reminded us that people who experience adverse childhood experiences can and do go on to live healthy lives, and that those who enlist in the military do it for positive reasons. To avoid unintentionally elevating stigma toward those who have had adverse childhood events, Blosnich et al. (2014) encouraged balanced messaging that demonstrates support. Therefore, it continues to be important when making comparisons of war eras to understand factors that may make veterans quite different with respect to healthcare needs.

HEALTH ISSUES FACING THE MILITARY/VETERAN POPULATION

Military service members are exposed to a variety of hazards, placing them at risk for long-term health problems that range from training injuries to something highly recognizable such as exposure to Agent Orange from the Vietnam era. With the fastest growing cohort of veterans being those who served Post-9/11, more focus will be placed on this sub-group within the larger veteran population. This section includes a discussion of the phenomenon of the healthy solider effect, allostatic load, and a summary of the most common service-related disabilities.

Healthy Soldier Effect

There exists a phenomenon, the healthy soldier effect, which refers to those who served in the military as healthier compared to other populations (McLaughlin et al., 2008). It is proposed that initial screening criteria to determine a person's "fit" for service, physical training, and standards maintained during military service, and access to healthcare while serving may protect the mortality of military service members (McLaughlin et al., 2008). In their systematic review of the literature, the researchers determined military personnel display a healthy soldier effect ranging from 10% to 25%, depending on the cause of death and the period of follow up. Waller and McGuire (2011) proposed that the healthy soldier effect changes over time and may vary depending on the cohorts being compared and by the cause of death. In contrast, Bollinger et al. (2015) conducted a study of OIF/OEF/OND veterans and found this cohort of veterans had either equivalent or higher than expected mortality compared to the general U.S. population. This suggests that the healthy soldier effect may be eroding. Further, a study conducted by Cranston et al. (2017) found that protective health effects of military fitness standards in a group of Air Force personnel are reduced shortly after retirement (6–8 years), with the prevalence rates of metabolic syndrome shifting toward that of the U.S. population in that time frame. Further, Cranston et al. (2017) suggested that healthcare providers educate newly retired veterans of this effect so that preventive measures can be initiated and risks reduced.

Allostatic Load

Allostatic load is a term used to describe the cumulative effects of acute and chronic stress on the body (McEwen et al., 2012). How often a person is exposed to factors that influence allostatic load or the rate at which it accumulates is individual. However, it is postulated that the outcomes resulting from allostatic load can be physiological, psychological, or psychosocial (McEwen et al., 2012). Chronic and repeated stressors, often experienced by military personnel, may be combined by acute stress incidents and, over time, result in a shift from adaptive to maladaptive functioning. This maladaptive functioning can lead to negative health consequences such as cardiovascular, metabolic, immune, and autoimmune disorders. Military deployments are one such stressor that helps support and explain the effect of allostatic load (McEwen et al., 2012).

Through complex processes of homeostasis and allostasis, our bodies adapt to stress or challenges (McEwen et al., 2012). When the body's mediating responses are chronically triggered it can lead to disease, resulting in allostatic load that is manifested by anger, frustration, fatigue, and feeling out of control. Subsequently, this state of allostatic load can lead to disruptions in sleep, anxiety, and other poor coping mechanisms such as drinking, smoking, or overeating (McEwen et al., 2012). This may help explain the increase in sleep issues facing Post-9/11 veterans (Caldwell et al., 2019). While this model is just one of many to help explain the health effects of stress on the body, it is important to recognize the repeated and continuous stress on military service members and their families so that action can be taken to mitigate stress and decrease potential adverse health outcomes.

Service-Connected Disabilities

Military service members participate in physically demanding activities on a routine basis, placing them at risk for a multitude of musculoskeletal injuries. The most prevalent service-connected disabilities include chronic long-term hearing and orthopedic problems (VA, 2018). Table 1.2 displays the most prevalent service-connected disabilities of all compensated recipients. According to a VA annual report, GWOT veterans account for 59% of compensated disabilities (VA, 2018). In addition, 53,770 women and 541,016 men are compensated as 100% disabled.

When specifically examining GWOT veterans, sleep apnea syndromes (obstructive, central, mixed) replace paralysis of the sciatic nerve (Table 1.2), among the top service-connected disabilities (VA, 2018). Caldwell et al. (2019) examined the association of insomnia and sleep apnea with deployment and combat exposure in the entire population of U.S. Army soldiers from 1997 to 2011 and found a major increase in both disorders between 2003 and 2011. Caldwell et al. (2019) found that deployment more than doubled the risk of developing insomnia or obstructive sleep apnea (OSA) compared to non-deployed counterparts. Combat exposure also increased the risk for insomnia (Caldwell et al., 2019). The researchers determined five conditions more than double or triple the risk of insomnia, which were (a) sleep-related movement disorder, (b) posttraumatic stress disorder (PTSD), (c) anxiety,

TABLE 1.2 MOST PREVALENT SERVICE-CONNECTED DISABILITIES OF ALL COMPENSATED RECIPIENTS

DISABILITY	MALE	FEMALE
Tinnitus	1,654,756	92,860
Hearing loss	1,101,363	21,048
PTSD	866,005	81,549
Scars, general	805,971	111,568
Lumbosacral or cervical strain	763,632	144,594
Limitation of flexion, knee	745,186	119,921
Paralysis of the sciatic nerve	609,375	53,226
Limitation of the motion of the ankle	498,027	68,622
Migraine	365,472	121,465
Degenerative arthritis of the spine	409,666	57,000

PTSD, posttraumatic stress disorder.

SOURCE: From U.S. Department of Veterans Affairs. (2018). *Veterans Benefits Administration annual benefits report: Fiscal year 2017.* Retrieved September 27, 2019 from https://www.benefits.va.gov/REPORTS/abr/docs/2017_abr.pdf

TABLE 1.3 HEALTH RANKINGS OF THOSE WHO SERVED COMPARED TO CIVILIANS

CHRONIC CONDITION	SERVED (%)	NOT SERVED (%)	UNHEALTHY BEHAVIORS	SERVED (%)	NOT SERVED (%)
Arthritis	24.7	22.8	Smoking	19.9	16.6
Cancer	10.9	9.8	Smokeless tobacco	8.7	3.5
Cardiovascular disease	9.8	7.2	Excessive drinking	21.4	18.6

SOURCE: Data from United Health Group. (2018). *New data – American's health ranking: Health of those who have served report.* Retrieved September 27, 2019 from https://www.unitedhealthgroup.com/newsroom/posts/2018-11-12-ahr-report-those-who-served.html

(d) adjustment reaction, and (e) acute reaction to stress. The presence of hypertension, gastroesophageal reflux disease, diabetes, PTSD, and overweight/obesity were among the top five conditions that more than doubled the risk of developing OSA. While the researchers attribute some portion of the results related to increased OSA to be related to increased incidence of overweight/obesity in the Army in the past decade, they concluded that more research is necessary to understand the underlying cause. Of concern for nurses is assessing veterans for sleep disturbances, as a number of physical and mental health problems can develop from insufficient sleep.

Brief Comparisons to Civilian Counterparts

Data support that those who have served report high rates of unhealthy behaviors (United Health Group, 2018). Veterans also report better overall health compared to those who never served. Yet, in actuality, veterans face higher rates of some chronic diseases compared to those who have never served (United Health Group, 2018). Table 1.3 illustrates these data. Data suggest veterans also suffer higher rates of depression, anxiety, and mental distress (United Health Group, 2018). In contrast to the negative health effects of service, veterans demonstrate strengths over their civilian counterparts in several measured areas. According to the report, veterans fare better in preventive health measures such as dental visits, flu vaccination, and colorectal cancer screening (United Health Group, 2018). Veterans also had less (8.7%) unmet medical needs due to cost compared to civilians (14.1%).

Aside from chronic disease, one pressing issue that has raised alarm is the rate of suicide plaguing veterans. From 2008 to 2017 the number of veteran suicides exceeded 6,000 per year, averaging about 16 per day (VA, 2019d). An estimated 2.5 suicides per day in 2017 were former Reserve or National Guard members who were never activated. Compared to non-veteran adult women, veteran women had a 2.2 times higher rate of suicide in 2017 (VA, 2019d). The rate of suicide for men was 1.3 times higher in veterans compared to non-veteran adult men in the same year.

DEPARTMENT OF VETERANS AFFAIRS

Military service members, their families, and military retirees and their eligible family members and survivors receive medical care through the Military Health System (MHS), which is the universal health system of the Department of Defense (DoD, n.d.). There are an estimated 600 clinics and over 50 military hospitals, both in the United States and at various overseas locations, which serve this population. In addition, TRICARE™ insurance provides coverage for contracted civilian care when necessary. For service members and their families assigned to areas where no MHS facility is available, there is a higher rate of engagement in civilian healthcare systems.

The VA (2019e) is comprised of three major administrations: (a) Veterans Health Administration (VHA), (b) Veterans Benefits Administration (VBA), and (c) National Cemetery Administration. Across the three administrations, military service members, veterans, and their families may be eligible for a variety of benefits that range from educational assistance, healthcare, or home loan support, to name just a few (VA, 2019f). It is key to understand that not every person who has served in the military is eligible for benefits. Eligibility for each of the benefits varies, is subject to change over time, and can be complex to comprehend even for those who serve. For example, as new research reveals a link between Agent Orange exposure and a specific disease, eligibility for healthcare is also expanded to those affected despite the amount of time that has passed since the Vietnam War. However, not all veterans may be aware of these changes and are therefore not receiving entitled benefits. Due to the complexity of eligibility, healthcare providers are encouraged to visit the VA website (www.va.gov) and contact a representative.

The VHA boosts a wealth of information through their public health sector, which is accessible online (www.publichealth.va.gov). The public, including healthcare providers, can learn a great deal about military and veterans' health ranging from military exposures to chemicals and noise to mental health. The VA develops evidence-based public policy, conducts research, and educates not only those who work within the VA system but also provides resources for healthcare providers who may encounter veterans outside the VA. Within the public health pages one can also find information on current research studies and registries for those who may have been exposed or deployed during a time that has potential risk for long-term effects such as the VA airborne hazards and open burn pit registry (www.publichealth.va.gov/exposures/burnpits/registry.asp).

U.S. Department of Veterans Affairs' Priorities

Based on the 2018–2024 Strategic Plan (VA, 2019g), the priorities of the VA include customer service, implementation of the MISSION Act, improvements in electronic health records, business systems transformation, and suicide prevention. The MISSION Act permits veterans greater access to healthcare in and outside the VA, expands caregiver benefits, and improves the VA's ability to offer the best medical providers to deliver care (VA, 2019h). Of significant importance to nursing is the national crisis to address suicide among military and veteran populations, with potential interaction occurring more frequently in civilian settings. According to Barr et al. (2019), being non-honorably discharged from military service may place veterans at higher risk for poor behavioral and mental health outcomes compared to those honorably discharged. Results of their study showed higher mean scores for non-honorably discharged veterans across all study variables, which included PTSD, depression, alcohol misuse, physical disability, somatic symptoms, and suicide risk (Barr et al., 2019).

The VA has become increasingly interested in the population health indicators that take into account the social determinants of health (SDOH), to assist them in achieving their commitment to both medical and non-medical needs of patients (Duan-Porter et al., 2018; Hatef et al., 2019). The changing demographics of the military include more minorities and women (VA, 2019a), either marginalized or vulnerable populations historically, so this focus is necessary to improve quality healthcare for this population and reduce further health disparities. This notion is further supported in a study examining the impact of SDOH on medical conditions among transgender veterans (Blosnich et al., 2016), another historically marginalized group. The research team found that social determinants of transgender veterans were strongly associated with medical conditions and that documentation of SDOH can help providers identify and address these factors as part of the plan of care (Blosnich et al., 2016).

A mere 6.1 million veterans utilized VA healthcare in 2017 (VA, 2019a). This leaves approximately 60% of today's veterans seeking care in civilian settings, supporting the need for all healthcare providers to have foundational knowledge of veterans' unique needs. Historically, quality and access to VA care has been under close scrutiny. Some veterans may have a positive experience with the VA system, while others may not, leading to distrust of the VA system. Therefore, nurses in all settings should be aware of the "newest VA reform measures and philosophy as it impacts patient care and resources" (Carlson, 2016, p. 7). Whether one practices at the bedside, teaches healthcare providers in the classroom, or has nursing students who are veterans, it is imperative that the momentum continues to self-educate and be able to advocate regardless of the practice setting.

IMPACT OF SERVICE ON HEALTH OVER A LIFETIME

Military service can have both a positive and a negative impact on a person's health. There are a number of factors that influence health, making it complex to generalize. One major factor that contributes to a veterans' health is how they appraise their military service, which can be conceptualized in three ways: overall military experience, wartime experience, and combat experience (Settersten et al., 2012; Spiro et al., 2016). Spiro et al. (2016) proposed an interdisciplinary model that takes into account life span and life course. The five principles outlined in their model are: (a) the effects of military service are lifelong; (b) the effects of service are multi-dimensional, affecting multiple domains of life, including health and well-being; (c) military service leads to both gains and losses; (d) the effects of military service are experienced within a matrix of social relationships that can protect veterans or create risk for them over time; and (e) these effects occur within and are affected by sociohistorical context. Their model (Figure 1.1) takes into consideration pre-military characteristics of a person, entry into the military, military experiences, post-military pathways, and then later-life outcomes. In addition,

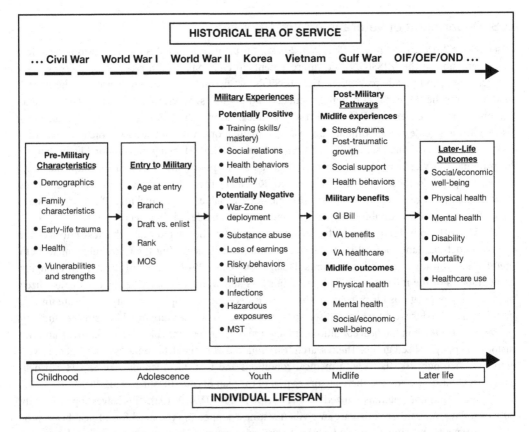

FIGURE 1.1 Long-term outcomes of military service.

MOS, military occupational specialty; MST, military sexual trauma; OEF, Operation Enduring Freedom; OIF, Operation Iraqi Freedom; OND, Operation New Dawn; VA, U.S. Department of Veterans. Affairs.

SOURCE: From Spiro, A., Settersten, R.A., & Aldwin, C.M. (2016). Long-term outcomes of military service in aging and the life course: A positive re-envisioning. *The Gerontologist, 56*(1), 5-13, by permission of Oxford University Press.

physical health, mental health, and socioeconomic domains are suggested to measure outcomes (Spiro et al., 2016). With most military service members entering service between the ages of 18 and 22, early adulthood, their experiences during service occur during a critical point in life (Pruchno, 2016). Spiro et al. (2016) proposed that "rather than asking whether military service has long-term effects, the more appropriate questions are, for whom does military service have long-term positive and/or negative effects, in which domains, and why?" (p. 7).

For the majority of people who enter the military they do so as they enter into young adulthood, defined by Erickson as ages 18 to 35 ("Erikson's Stages of Development," 2019). With parental consent, youth can join the military at age 17 ("Are You Eligible to Join the Military," 2019). During this developmental stage, coined Intimacy and Solidarity versus Isolation, people typically seek companionship, deep intimacy, and satisfying relationships. Some may get married and start families, which are major life changes. If people in this stage do not establish close relationships with a spouse or friends, isolation may occur ("Erikson's Stages of Development," 2019). For those serving in the military, camaraderie has been identified as a common thing people miss when they leave military service (Callahan, 2015). Therefore, it can serve as a protective factor while serving but may be problematic once separated from service. Frequent relocation and deployments during the early years of relationships, marriage, and raising young children, can place significant strain on service members and their families making them vulnerable to emotional and physical health problems. No single factor determines this. However, it can also create strong bonds and resiliency.

Middle-aged adulthood ranges from age 35 to age 55 to 65 ("Erikson's Stages of Development," 2019). Although age limits vary among service branches, a person can also join the military during middle age, with the Air Force allowing people to enter as late as age 39 ("Are You Eligible to Join the Military," 2019). Generativity versus Self-Absorption or Stagnation, the terms used to describe this stage, is a time when people are most focused on a career/work and family. People strive to make a difference in society (generativity), with a common fear of meaninglessness if they do not ("Erikson's Stages of Development," 2019). Major life changes can start to occur during this stage, such as children leaving the home or changing careers. For those who stay in the military until retirement (20 years of active duty), potentially longer if serving the National Guard or Reserves, middle adulthood is the time when they are taking off the uniform and stepping back into civilian life. This transition and reintegration can prove challenging after living and working in the military culture for that length of time.

According to Erikson's developmental stages of life ("Erikson's Stages of Development," 2019), persons in late adulthood (age 55–65 to death) fall into a stage of Integrity versus Despair. As a stage of reflection, individuals may look back on life with a sense of fulfillment and contentment that they lived a life of meaning and their contribution to society was valuable (integrity). On the contrary, individuals may also look back on their life experiences with a sense of failure and struggle, unable to see what purpose their life served (despair). As veterans age and face typical stressors all older adults face such as illness, declining functional ability, and losses, they may simultaneously engage for the first time or reengage with prior military and war time memories in an attempt to find meaning and build coherence (Davison et al., 2016). Davison et al. (2016) call this process later-adulthood trauma reengagement (LATR), postulating that during this dynamic stage of life veterans may be trying to adapt and get "unstuck" from past traumatic experiences so they may find meaning and build coherence with life. Through life review, reminiscing, and facing the issues they are experiencing, veterans may experience delayed-onset posttraumatic growth. The LATR process may help them reconcile past experiences, leading to integrity and not despair, ultimately improving satisfaction with life.

Seligowski et al. (2012) studied the correlates of life satisfaction among aging veterans and found that variables representing personal resources (social support, sense of mastery, and positive appraisal of military experience) appeared to have the strongest relationship to satisfaction with life for older veterans. Both physical and mental health were significantly and positively linked to life satisfaction in their study. Seligowski et al. (2012) suggested that veterans who possessed the belief they have power to influence and effectively manage their own personal domain later in life may be a protective factor against late life distress. Further, Lee et al. (2017) found that veterans of the Korean War experienced traumatic memories and suffering of veteran stereotypes, as well as an increased personal strength and appreciation of life from their service. One participant in their study suggested that even after 60 years, time did little to ease the pain of the traumatic experiences, supporting that older veterans may have unresolved inner conflicts as they age and reach end of life (EOL). Korean War veterans in this study identified membership in veteran associations as a foundational bridge for veterans to support each other (Lee et al., 2017). Active problem solving, planning, and use of non-avoidant coping skills were assessed as strengths in the study group. The researchers stated "nurses and other helping professionals need to be aware of the veteran's strengths and support systems" so they can provide patient-centered care (Lee et al., 2017, p. 235).

Palliative Care and End of Life Considerations

End of life (EOL) can be a difficult time for any human being and their loved ones. Being a veteran and facing EOL may bring with it a number of mental and physical concerns above and beyond what one might anticipate for non-veterans (Elliott, 2017). Progressive illness or a life-limiting prognosis can often magnify psychosocial issues for veterans, compromising their capacity to face the dying process (Antoni et al., 2012). Acknowledging military service is essential and is especially important when caring for a veteran at EOL (Gabriel et al., 2015). Yet, many healthcare providers may not be assessing for veteran status or may lack resources and expertise in addressing issues facing veterans (Antoni et al., 2012). In addition, healthcare providers may feel uncertain what to do with information they obtain (Maiocco et al., 2018), or may not feel comfortable evaluating military-related causes of distress at EOL (Way et al., 2019). Respecting and honoring the veteran and their family for the service and sacrifice to our country can aid in building trust and rapport during this stressful time. Understanding the manner in which a veteran may process guilt from the past, handle symptoms of PTSD that may surface due to the stress of dying, or even differences in the way they cope with pain at the EOL are key pieces to providing veteran-centered care (Elliott, 2017; Way et al., 2019).

Difficulties and symptom burden faced by veterans at EOL can stem from spiritual conflicts or survivor's guilt (Elliott, 2017), as well as adverse childhood experiences, military sexual trauma, PTSD, or moral injury (Way et al., 2019). With a growing number of veterans who have had adverse childhood experiences, "more and more veterans may find their social support to be lacking or find that relationships may be severed as they reach EOL" (Way et al., 2019, p. 712). Therefore, it is critical for nurses and healthcare providers to understand the veteran experience, evaluate their resources and supports, and be cognizant that for those who do have families and caregivers, they may also need support during this challenging time. Although not all veterans want to share their stories, those that do could be carefully guided using gradual reminiscing (Elliott, 2017; Young et al., 2018) or storytelling (Carlson, 2016).

Over the past two decades the VA has made great strides in improving palliative and EOL care for veterans through a variety of initiatives and programs, both internally and externally (Way et al., 2019). One external partnership between the VA and the National Hospice and Palliative Care Organization, which has grown and evolved, is the We Honor Veterans (WHV) program (www.wehonorveterans. org). The WHV program, through education and resources, engages community agencies such as home care and hospice, as well as long-term care and assisted living facilities, to recognize the unique needs of veterans, their families, and caregivers. Expanding from WHV are programs such as the Hospice-Veteran Partnership, the Veteran Community Partnership, the Veteran-to-Veteran Partnership, and the No Veteran Dies Alone program (Way et al., 2019). Collectively, these programs have reached more veterans than could otherwise be reached by VA services alone, especially in rural areas.

SOCIETAL IMPLICATIONS

Over decades of wars, the military has been a main contributor in advancing life-saving measures. With the GWOT, tourniquet use, and better trained medics and soldiers (buddy-care and self-care),

TABLE 1.4 NUMBER OF DISABILITIES PER VETERAN BY WAR ERA

	WW II	KOREAN WAR	VIETNAM ERA	GULF WAR ERA	PEACETIME PERIODS	TOTAL
Disabilities	166,391	286,679	5,345,987	14,889,302	2,528,136	23,216,495
Average no. of disabilities per veteran	2.41	2.45	3.83	6.73	3.34	5.10

SOURCE: From U.S. Department of Veterans Affairs. (2018). *Veterans Benefits Administration annual benefits report: Fiscal year 2017.* Retrieved September 27, 2019 from https://www.benefits.va.gov/REPORTS/abr/docs/2017_abr.pdf

the result has been a higher survival of amputees (Baker, 2014). Changes in fluid resuscitation and blood volume restoration protocols, coupled with the use of mobile forward surgical teams, allowed for quicker stabilization and safe mobilization to higher echelons of care. Critical Care Air Transport Teams enabled the highest acuity of patients to be transported to medical centers for more definitive care. Further, advances in information technology improved how well essential information followed patients from one stage of care to the next so that providers could administer the very best care (Baker, 2014). The result was more wounded service members surviving injuries that would have killed them in prior wars. Cumulatively, Gulf War veterans have approximately 14.8 million service connected disabilities (Table 1.4), with the average number of disabilities per veteran at 6.7 (VA, 2018). Subsequently, the future health, social, and economic impact on healthcare resources will be significant.

Cost of Caring for Veterans

An estimated 61% of GWOT service members are veterans, leaving 39% still in the military (Baker, 2014). Researchers project that in the next 30 to 40 years, the care needs of the most recent war veterans will escalate and have likened it to a tidal wave coming in (Baker, 2014; Geiling et al., 2012). Healthcare for these veterans will shift from the DoD or MHS healthcare system, to the VHA System, and eventually private sectors. The long-term care needs (Geiling et al., 2012), coupled with extensive rehabilitation and restorative care (Baker, 2014), have demanded civilian healthcare providers be prepared to treat this population. Additionally, there is an increased demand placed on caregivers. Geiling et al. (2012) projected that billions of dollars would be not only spent providing this care, but delivering better, more effective care to restore veterans to optimal physical and mental health, and ultimately reducing some of the future financial costs.

Impact on Families and Caregivers

Referring to the collateral damage of war, Baker (2014) stated, "Another huge impact on society for which there is no metric is the tragic effect of this fiasco on veterans' families" (p. 352). Spouses, children, parents, and siblings can be affected by deployments, injury, or death of loved ones; development of mental health issues, change in economic or social status, or substance abuse (Arceneaux et al., 2019). This risk for collateral damage is on top of the stressors a military lifestyle places on service members and families, which requires multiple relocations, changing schools for children, spouses having to find new employment, and changing social supports. This is often all at a distance from immediate family. In addition, children of military caregivers may be at risk to suffer more social isolation, mental health challenges, and poorer quality of life (Elizabeth Dole Foundation, 2018). Parents who are military caregivers may find meeting the needs of their children difficult when balancing caregiving and household tasks.

In a secondary analysis of 2010 National Survey of Veterans data, Schnittker (2019) examined the health spillover effect (the effect of the experience of one person on the health of another) among military spouses. Data revealed that spouses of active duty service members report worse health compared to spouses living with a veteran. Data also supported that the impact of military service experiences on a spouse may extend long-term, beyond the initial transition to civilian life (Schnittker, 2019). The researcher reported that the magnitude of the effects of being married to an active duty service member "are as large as the widowhood effect, which is, in turn, as large as caring for a veteran spouse with a service disability" (Schnittker, 2019, p. 71). Of interest is that lower self-rated health was not explained by active conflict, presence of young children in the home, or high unemployment of spouses, which are typically major stressors for military families. While more research is needed to understand the effects of military service on spouses, this study brings to light the potential impact on the health of close family members.

Based on data from a 2014 Rand report (Ramchand et al., 2014), there are an estimated 5.5 million military caregivers in the United States. Almost 20% are caring for Post-9/11 veterans, who do not resemble military caregivers from previous war eras. According to Tanielian et al. (2013), "the appeal of military service to future generations is based upon our nation's commitment to support our service members, veterans, and military families" (p. 2). Safeguarding that adequate care is available for veterans is a critical piece of this obligation. The burden of this care falls largely on America's military caregivers, many of whom prioritize their veterans' health and well-being over and above their own (Tanielian et al., 2013). Caregivers may experience a great risk of disease or other negative health outcomes such as coronary heart disease, hypertension, compromised immune function, and reduced sleep as a result of the physical strain from being a caregiver (Tanielian et al., 2013).

Military caregivers are typically younger, reside with the individual they are caring for, care for individuals with complex injuries and comorbidities, and navigate changes in eligibility benefits in a complex healthcare system, making them different from civilian caregivers (Tanielian et al., 2013). They experience a great deal of emotional stress associated with caregiving, unduly suffering from mental health problems. Klippel and Sullivan (2018) postulate that caregivers of veterans with PTSD may experience more stressors if behavioral and emotional symptoms are not regulated. Maintaining open and honest communication may be the best way to enhance relationship satisfaction for caregivers at risk of experiencing caregiver burden. This is especially true in the presence of comorbid dementia, which can complicate PTSD symptoms and requires more care (Klippel & Sullivan, 2018). New evidence suggests that veterans who have experienced a traumatic brain injury (TBI) are at increased risk for developing dementia (Peterson et al., 2019). This further complicates the potential long-term care and costs considering that the number of veterans who experienced a TBI during deployment is estimated between 10% and 20 % as reported in several studies conducted since 2008 (Peterson et al., 2019). Compared to previous war eras, those deployed during the Gulf War era are at higher risk for developing chronic traumatic encephalopathy due to repeated blast exposure, which is also of concern for caregivers long-term (Peterson et al., 2019).

In a qualitative study on health-related quality of life in caregivers of individuals with military-related TBI, researchers identified four domains in which caregivers spent the most time discussing their concerns (Carlozzi et al., 2016). Those domains included social health, emotional health, physical/medical health, and cognitive health. Within the social health domain, caregivers voiced difficulties with finances as a result of giving up work, changes in social roles between the person with the TBI and others, including close social systems such as extended family. Caregivers voiced uncertainty with how hard to push the person they cared for who used to be an independent person, switching from spouse to caregiver, reevaluating priorities and future plans, and loss of friends. The emotional domain concerns were caregiver strain/burden, feelings of loss, anger, and anxiety, and depression. In this domain, caregivers shared how military culture influences one to maintain a strong appearance, even when things are not going so well (Carlozzi et al., 2016). Thus, caregivers felt like they were constantly minding their behaviors, and the behaviors of others, as to avoid noticeably upsetting the service member. The last two domains were less commonly spoken about yet are important to consider. Caregivers voiced difficulty keeping up with their own healthcare needs, how the injury negatively affected their sexual health, and how sleep difficulties coupled with caregiving responsibilities left them constantly fatigued. Cognitive concerns related primarily to feelings of not being "sharp" anymore, as if they too had a TBI (by proxy). Overall, military caregivers in this study often experienced caregiver hypervigilance and emotional suppression of anger related to ease of access to the VA or financial services, further differentiating them from their civilian counterparts (Carlozzi et al., 2016).

The Program of Comprehensive Assistance for Family Caregivers (PCAFC) was established in 2011 to support caregivers of Post-9/11 era veterans who required assistance with activities of daily living, or supervision resulting from residual effects of injuries sustained while in the line of duty (Van Houtven et al., 2019). The comprehensive program requires caregivers to complete a training curriculum, including topics such as caregiving skills, caregiver self-care, and managing challenging behaviors. Participants must also meet other eligibility requirements. Van Houtven et al. (2019) examined the early impact of the PCAFC on veteran healthcare utilization and cost and found that enrollment in the program led to increased utilization of VA outpatient care, specialty care, and mental healthcare. Despite not having an impact on reducing acute emergency department usage, the increased short-term utilization of other services could lead to positive long-term health outcomes for vulnerable veteran patients.

NATIONAL INITIATIVES FOCUSED ON EDUCATING NURSES

The efforts of local, state, and federal agencies in response to the needs of veterans, particularly in the past decade with the Post-9/11 era veterans growing in numbers, are vast. Currently, over 7,000 U.S.-based non-profit organizations are helping military service members, veterans, and their families ("Nonprofit Organizations for Veterans," 2019). This section focuses on two key initiatives that were launched as a catalyst to address the healthcare needs of service members, veterans, and their families.

Veterans Affairs Nursing Academy

As a result of the growing numbers of veterans requiring combat-related medical care at the onset of the Iraq and then Afghanistan wars as well as the demand for nurses within the VHA health system, the VA (2017) launched the Veterans Affairs Nursing Academy (VANA). The purpose of the VANA was to expand learning opportunities for nursing students at VA facilities and fund additional faculty at partnership schools so more undergraduate students could be accepted, with the intent of increasing recruitment and retention of VA nurses. The 5-year, $40 million program launched in 2007 and to date there are 18 partnerships between the VA and schools of nursing in the United States. In 2014 the program transitioned to a non-funded program (Carlson, 2016).

There are a few publications describing the implementation of VANA partnerships (Harper et al., 2015) and their effectiveness (Dobalian et al., 2014; Miltner et al., 2015). Perhaps of greater importance and relevance are the lessons learned from the implementation of partnerships and how those lessons can be utilized by anyone working with and caring for military and veteran populations. Within the first 18 months of joining the pilot program, researchers visited each VANA site at least once to gather data on program implementation to determine what elements were critical for partnership effectiveness (Dobalian et al., 2014). The researchers identified both positive and negative indicators of a successful or unsuccessful launch based on the program goals, which were the initial program inputs and implementation activities and outputs for increasing faculty positions, increasing student enrollment, implementing curricular innovations, increasing recruitment and retention, and promoting collaboration. Through the analysis of their data, five themes or key factors, were extracted (Dobalian et al., 2014). The first critical factor in enabling partnerships to succeed was teamwork or collaboration between organizations. A second factor related to blending different cultures and integrating activities across differing organizational practices and constraints. Third, the time required to recruit nurses to take faculty roles, while expanding student enrollment and scheduling clinical and didactic courses, needed to be realistic. The need to plan more strategically was identified as the fourth factor focused on expectations beyond adding faculty and increasing student enrollment. At the time of this research study there was an economic downturn, making the demand for nurses tempered (Dobalian et al., 2014). Therefore, the last factor related to the importance of partnerships being long-term commitments, whereby short-term changes in supply and demand for nurses should not impact the solidity of the relationship.

As nursing education moves forward with curricular changes, considering partnerships that afford student nurses the opportunity for exposure to military service members, veterans, and their families is essential. Harper et al. (2015) reported that through their VA partnership the school of nursing was able to expand its program in a number of ways, enriching student experiences with veteran-specific simulations, an elective course on veteran healthcare, and creation of a veteran-friendly culture. Clinical faculty should require students to inquire about military or veteran status during their initial assessment to maximize their opportunity to engage with this population. Through various publications, nursing programs report on the initial logistical challenges of gaining access to Veterans Affairs Medical Centers (VAMC), but persistence seems to be beneficial. For those who do not have nearby access to these facilities, there are many options to locate and engage veterans outside of the VAMC.

Joining Forces

The *Joining Forces* campaign was spearheaded and launched in 2011 by then first lady Michelle Obama and Dr. Jill Biden (White House Archives, n.d.). The overall purpose of the campaign was to mobilize Americans to support service members, veterans, and their families through employment, education, and wellness. The initiative had six main goals (Box 1.1). On April 11, 2012, the Office of the First Lady

---

BOX 1.1

JOINING FORCES INITIATIVES

Educating America's future nurses to care for our nation's veterans, service members, and their families facing posttraumatic stress disorder, traumatic brain injury, depression, and other clinical issues

Enriching nursing education to ensure that current and future nurses are trained in the unique clinical challenges and best practices associated with caring for military service members, veterans, and their families

Integrating content that addresses the unique health and wellness challenges of our nation's service members, veterans, and their families into nursing curricula

Sharing teaching resources and applying best practices in the care of service members, veterans, and their families

Growing the body of knowledge leading to improvements in healthcare and wellness for our service members, veterans, and their families

Joining with others to further strengthen the supportive community of nurses, institutions, and healthcare providers dedicated to improving the health of service members, veterans, and their families.

SOURCE: From White House Archives. (2012). *America's nurses Join Forces with the first lady and Dr. Biden to support veterans and military families.* Retrieved May 23, 2019 from https://obamawhitehouse.archives.gov/the-press-office/2012/04/11/americas-nurses-join-forces-first-lady-and-dr-biden-support-veterans-and

released a statement that "3 million nurses, through 150 nursing organizations and 500 nursing schools will be educated on PTSD and TBI in the coming years" (White House Archives, 2012, para. 1). In collaboration with the VA and DoD, the American Nurses Association (ANA), American Academy of Nurse Practitioners, American Association of Colleges of Nursing (AACN), and the National League for Nursing (NLN) led the charge to secure commitment from other nursing organizations to educate future and current nurses in military and veteran-specific healthcare issues they might face in their respective practice settings.

In response to the *Joining Forces* initiative, the American Academy of Nursing (AAN) created a Military and Veterans Health Expert Panel in 2011, responsible to develop policy recommendations and facilitate outreach to healthcare providers (AAN, 2015). In 2013, the panel launched their "Have you ever served in the military?"" campaign in 10 states, sparking change in nursing practice to ensure vital military service information was obtained (ANA, n.d.). With quality of care as a driver, this campaign reached all 50 states by April of 2015. The NLN (2019) responded to the call to *Join Forces* by developing resources titled *Advancing Care Excellence for Veterans*. These teaching resources provide faculty with unfolding case studies, simulations, teaching strategies, and other resources to aid in teaching nursing students at all levels of veteran-specific care.

As one of the leading organizations for nursing education, the AACN answered the call for action from the White House and sought the pledge of member schools to join in support of educating students about the military and veteran population. By 2014, just 2 years after the launch of *Joining Forces*, approximately 660 schools pledged support (Elliott & Patterson, 2017). The AACN (2019a) created the *Enhancing Veteran's Care Faculty Tool Kit* as a resource for faculty to implement curricular elements that focus on this population. In addition, the AACN also partnered with the City of Hope to create *End-of-Life Nursing Education Consortium (ELNEC) for Veterans* to enhance palliative and EOL care nationally for this population (AACN, 2019b). A veteran-specific curriculum was created and six nationally held train-the-trainer programs were offered to 745 nurses and interdisciplinary healthcare providers representing over 200 VA facilities and community programs, such as hospice and home care agencies (AACN, 2019b).

Elliott and Patterson (2017) conducted a study to determine how schools of nursing who pledged to support *Joining Forces* incorporated military and veteran health content into their curricula, as well as barriers and facilitators to this process. Within the first 3 years of the pledge, findings suggested variation of implementation with some schools/colleges of nursing exceeding the initiative goals to some still in the process of figuring it out. The majority of respondents felt incorporating this content was important, but lack of time and a content-laden curriculum were identified as common barriers (Elliott & Patterson, 2017). Based on the data, approximately 75% of respondents indicated they had achieved the first goal (Box 1.1). The remaining five goals ranged between 43% and 56% achieved. Nurse educators have an ethical responsibility to teach students culturally sensitive care. Making the pledge was only the first step to change. To date, we are not aware of any further research that examines the long-term impact of the *Joining Forces* pledge. However, it remains the charge for nurse educators to advance curricular changes.

Military/Veteran Friendly

"Military Friendly' is the standard that measures an organization's commitment, effort and success in creating sustainable and meaningful opportunity for the military community" ("What Does Military Friendly Mean," 2019, para. 2). More and more colleges and universities, as well as various organizations, have sought this designation as a way to stand out among the crowd in terms of commitment and excellence to supporting and serving people in the military (active duty, National Guard, Reserve), veterans, and their spouses. Healthcare organizations can also receive this designation. Thus, they are setting a standard of care and improving the outcomes and lives of veterans.

CURRENT STATUS OF NURSING EDUCATION AND PRACTICE

At the time of this writing, it is still unclear exactly what nurses and healthcare providers know about caring for military service members, veterans, and their families. What they need to know is more apparent with a moderate number of publications available in professional journals. Efforts from professional organizations appear steadfast. Many gaps in understanding the difference between education and practice remain. From 2010 until present day the number of publications across disciplines related to the care of military service members, veterans, and their families has escalated. Within nursing publications, authors have focused primarily on what currently practicing nurses need to know in civilian settings or exemplars of curricular changes to enhance nursing education. Table 1.5 illustrates an array of publications, although we acknowledge the list may not be exhaustive and some publications fall into more than one group. The following section summarizes the current status of nursing education and practice literature to date, with a more focused discussion on practice-related research. Section III of this book examines nursing education subject matter in more detail.

Nursing Education

To gauge what students may be exposed to, the authors conducted an informal appraisal of readily available nursing textbooks to evaluate presence of content related to military service members, veterans, and their families. Although it was not an exhaustive or systematic process, we found nursing texts currently in print largely fail to acknowledge the full spectrum of veteran healthcare needs. In fact, a limited number of undergraduate psychiatric nursing textbooks draw attention to veteran care needs and are exclusively linked to PTSD and suicide content. These examples fail to capture the scope and breadth of military and veteran health-related knowledge needed by nurses in practice today and for the future.

A number of authors have evaluated and published competencies for students, nurses, and nurse faculty (Carlson, 2016; McMillan et al., 2017; Moss et al., 2015). Collectively, these publications illustrate the essential knowledge, skills, and attitudes vital to care for or teach military/veteran-centric content. Above all, military culture is the most widely addressed competency when engaging with and caring for this population. Simulation or unfolding case studies are often highlighted as effective teaching strategies. Some schools of nursing have created stand-alone courses focusing on veteran-centered health, while others have illustrated ways in which content can be integrated through various courses or clinical experiences such as Community Health, Mental Health, and Medical-Surgical nursing. Various organizations have collected and packaged toolkits and resources for education and professional development. Yet, educators must know they are available and how to best utilize them. At the advanced practice level, two universities to our knowledge have developed post-bachelors and specialty programs focused on the care of military and veteran populations for nurses and healthcare providers to prepare already-practicing providers.

Nursing Practice

For nurses currently in practice, a number of resources and publications are available. The essential message in these publications is the importance of screening and assessing patients for military or veteran status. Second is knowing what do to with the essential information that is gathered. Research conducted to evaluate non-VA employed or civilian nurses' experiences or comfort level in caring for military and veteran patients and their families is limited. It appears that more is being published regarding the importance of understanding military, veterans, and families' healthcare needs than reports of action taken or interventions trialed in clinical areas to improve care. This may be due to the fact that nurses may be learning what is important, yet translation to practice is its infancy. Table 1.6 highlights currently available empirically based reports.

TABLE 1.5 SELECT NURSING PUBLICATIONS RELATED TO MILITARY AND VETERAN HEALTH (2012–2020)

FOCUS OF PUBLICATION	YEAR	CITATION (AUTHOR)
Nursing care of veterans	2013	Johnson et al.
	2013	Miltner et al.
	2014	Stanton
	2015	Conard et al.
	2015	Counts et al.
	2015	Fullwood
	2015	Elliott
	2016	Conard et al.
	2017	Elliott
	2017	Mohler and Sankey-Deemer
	2017	Waszak and Holmes
	2018	Elliott
	2018	Young et al.
	2019	Elliott
	2019	Conard and Armstrong
Recommendations for educational preparation, including competencies	2013	Allen et al.
	2015	Linn et al.
	2015	Moss et al.
	2015	Olenick et al.
	2016	Carlson
	2016	Cooper et al.
	2017	Champlin et al.
	2017	Elliott and Patterson
	2017	Finnegan et al.
	2017	McMillan et al.
	2020	Finnegan et al.
Exemplars of curricular changes	2015	Keavney
	2015	Jones and Breen
	2015	Morrison-Beedy et al.
	2017	Magpantay-Monroe
	2018	Rossiter et al.
	2018	Crary
Teaching and learning strategies for veteran-related content	2012	Anthony et al.
	2012	Harmer and Huffman
	2013	Beckford and Ellis
	2016	McKenzie et al.
	2017	Champlin and Kunkel
	2017	Kaplan et al.
	2018	Magpantay-Monroe
	2018	Vessey et al.
	2019	Regan et al.
Professional development of nurses or faculty	2016	Merkle et al.
	2017	Erickson-Hurt et al.
	2019	Chargualaf
	2019	Gibbs et al.
	2018	Maiocco et al.
Military cultural competence	2013	Convoy and Westphal
	2014	Koenig et al.
	2015	Westphal and Convoy
	2018	Brommelsiek et al.
	2018	Kautzmann and Lancaster
	2019	Bonzanto et al.
	2019	Vest et al.
Military caregivers	2017	Conard et al.

TABLE 1.6 EMPIRICAL EVIDENCE INFORMING NURSING PRACTICE

AUTHOR	YEAR	TYPE	FOCUS AREA
Bonzanto et al.	2019	Prospective quantitative survey	Examined the capacity of RNs working in non-VA hospitals to deliver culturally competent care to military, veterans, and their families
Elliott	2018	Quantitative descriptive	Assessed home care nurses' knowledge, comfort, and confidence caring for veterans
Elliott	2019	Qualitative descriptive	Examined home care nurses' experiences caring for veterans
Maiocco et al.	2018	Multimethod descriptive	Assessed how nurses are caring for veterans and the challenges they face in delivery of that care
Merkle et al.	2016	Quality improvement	Designed, implemented, and evaluated a screening process to identify veterans in the emergency department
Mohler and Sankey-Deemer	2017	Quantitative descriptive, cross-sectional	Assessed screening practices for military service and PTSD of healthcare providers in a primary care setting
Vest et al.	2019	Qualitative descriptive	Assessed barriers to care and perceptions of what tools are most valuable in developing cultural competency

PTSD, posttraumatic stress disorder; VA, U.S. Department of Veterans Affairs.

Veterans, even those eligible for care at a VA, can and may seek care elsewhere (VA, 2019a). Merkle et al. (2016) designed and implemented a screening process to identify veterans during emergency department visits at a civilian hospital. The authors reported embedding a mandatory screening question "Have you ever served in the military?" in the electronic medical record. The authors noted that screening for TRICARE™ insurance, a practice of some providers, was insufficient and many veterans were either not identified or misidentified (Merkle et al., 2016). Department staff developed a resource guide for veteran patients to be given at encounters in the emergency department. Through their change process and asking about military or veteran status, more veterans were identified and provided a resource guide as part of their discharge instructions. No other outcomes were measured and the authors recommended further required education and training beyond this initial intervention.

Mohler and Sankey-Deemer (2017) conducted a cross-sectional study examining the screening practices of non-VA primary care providers in rural central and western Pennsylvania. Their sample included physicians, physician assistants (PAs), and nurse practitioners (NPs). The researchers aimed to determine first if providers screen for military service and, second, if they then screen for PTSD. Although the sample size was small ($N = 50$), the results do provide a basis for beginning to understand the work that is yet to be done in educating civilian providers. Results indicated 88% of subjects had no education related to the healthcare needs of veterans. Only 8% of providers responded they screen all patients for military service, 40% responded they never screen, leaving the majority (52%) who screen somewhere in between. A mere 10% screened all or most patients for PTSD, after identifying patients as veterans.

According to Maiocco et al. (2018), the state of West Virginia issued a mandate in 2014 of 2 hours of annual education related to mental health issues in veterans. This was a result of the increase in suicides within this population in West Virginia, which was significantly higher than the overall national rate, as well as a high percent of veterans seeking care outside the VA. At the time of the study, West Virginia was the only state requiring this education. Continuing education (CE) was provided between the years of 2015 and 2016 (Maiocco et al., 2018). Upon completion of the CE, the authors conducted a survey using open-ended questions to gain understanding of the impact of CE on nurses. The results of their study revealed that only 16% of nurses consistently asked about military status and of those only 6% document status upon admission (Maiocco et al., 2018). In addition, 85% did not know where to access this information if it were documented, 86% were unaware of hospital resources and services to assist nurses in caring for veterans, and 83% did not know how to refer a patient to the VA. From the open-ended questions, three themes emerged: *uncertainty related to delivery of care, uncertainty related to inexperience talking to veterans, and uncertainty related to potential for violence.*

The researchers reported stopping the study early due to reports of violence from veterans toward nurses found in the survey data (Maiocco et al., 2018). The primary investigator alerted risk management of the unsafe practice environment and steps were taken to ensure documentation of military/veteran status. Based on the results and despite education, "the 'Have you ever served campaign?' has generated mindfulness about military culture, but translation to practice in a non-VA hospital environment is still in its infancy" (Maiocco et al., 2018, p. 5). As of 2019, Connecticut is the only other state mandating similar education, once every 6 years ("Continuing Education Requirements for Nurses by State," 2019).

In a mixed methods study of home care nurses, lack of knowledge of resources available to veterans, war-specific exposures, and veteran-specific health issues were identified practice gaps (Elliott, 2018). Of the 102 subjects in the study, about 50% reported that they screened for military status, and only 18% felt confident in knowing how to make a referral to the VA. This demonstrates that while some nurses are screening for veteran status, they often do not know what to do with the information once obtained. However, home care nurses were able to identify a number of differences in caring for veterans compared to non-veterans (Elliott, 2019). Major themes from the study were: *challenges coordinating care, building rapport takes more time,* and *recognizing the impact of military service on patient's worldview.* This supports that this population does have healthcare needs that are different from other cultures within the United States and that this culture should be included in discussions related to cultural competency. In addition, nurses caring for veterans who utilize both VA and another healthcare system should be alert to medication overlapping (Chui et al., 2018), adherence (Taber et al., 2019), and overall coordination of medication regimens.

Bonzanto et al. (2019) conducted a study to examine the capacity of RNs working in non-VA settings to deliver appropriate culturally competent care to military, veterans, and their families. The researchers used a modified *Ready to Serve* survey (Cronbach's $\alpha = 0.9081$ for the study) to survey nurses within a large multi-hospital system. Factor analysis revealed four factors: (a) knowledge, awareness, and attitudes about military culture; (b) practice behaviors, skills, and comfort; (c) health-related screening behaviors; and (d) beliefs about evidence-based practice. Bonzanto et al. (2019) reported 612 nurses participated out of 6,875 invited (response rate 9%). The overall results of the study revealed few nurses employed at one of the hospitals within the health system possessed the cultural competency to care for military, veterans, and their families. Almost 70% said they never or seldom assess for military or veteran status (Bonzanto et al., 2019). Approximately 80% were unfamiliar with services available to assist with readjustment after military service, or with DoD and VA resources to assist clinicians in caring for those with mental health issues. From a competency perspective, only 25 (4%) of respondents achieved a score of high cultural competence. However, it should be known that 10 of the 25 previously served in the military, 22 of the 25 had family who served, and 10 reported previous experience working in a military or veteran setting (Bonzanto et al., 2019).

Lastly, Vest et al. (2019) conducted a study of non-VA primary care physicians, PAs, and NPs to assess their barriers to providing care to veterans, the training providers perceived as most useful, and the tools and translational processes deemed to be adequate in enhancing cultural competency. Data analysis revealed three themes from the interviews, which were *barriers to caring for patients who are identified as veterans, thoughts on tools that might help better identify and screen veteran patients,* and *thoughts on translating and implementing new care processes for veteran patients into everyday practice.* Barriers included lack of knowledge on the impact military service has on a veteran and how that could change the provision of care, inconsistent knowledge of military culture/population, limited knowledge of resources and support services available in the community, and lack of coordination with the VA healthcare system (Vest et al., 2019). Although only one NP was included in the sample, study results related to challenges coordinating care with the VA were similar to Elliott's (2019) findings of home care nurses.

As the literature continues to expand related to care of the military/veteran population, targeted education of nurses will be needed. A critical first step is determining what health professionals' attitudes and views are in caring for this population. Knopf-Amelung et al. (2018) developed a tool to evaluate health professionals' attitudes toward veterans. Their Health Professionals' Attitude Toward Veterans (HPATV) scale measures three domains: culture, care, and health. The researchers state the tool could be utilized to conduct a needs assessment of health professionals in any setting to identify strengths and weaknesses that can inform professional development activities, or policy and procedure (Knopf-Amelung et al., 2018). Further, the HPATV can be used for program evaluation of veteran-specific education initiatives. Brommelsiek et al. (2018) used the scale to evaluate students' attitudes after completing an interdisciplinary course on military culture and found significant improvement in attitude across all domains of the HPATV. In addition, the researchers found a significant improvement in knowledge pre and post course.

Patient-Centered and Culturally Competent Care

The essentials of nursing practice at all levels mandate cultural competency as part of the nursing curricula (AACN, 2006, 2008, 2011). In making a case for veteran-specific content in nursing education, nurses and nurse educators need to recognize that this is ethically the right thing to do. As societal demographics change, nursing education must also change. To provide perspective to the need for change, consider how much time is spent in current nursing curricula focusing on the care of children newborn to age 5. According to the latest population estimates there are approximately 23 million children from birth to age of 5 in the United States ("POP1 Child Population," n.d.), just three million more than current military and veterans. Yet, curricular changes to include veteran-centered content seem sporadic and appear to remain limited across nursing education (Elliott & Patterson, 2017). In discussions of vulnerable populations, veterans are not always part of the conversation. Yet, many are at risk for homelessness or incarceration as a result of unresolved mental health issues and other complex factors (National Coalition for Homeless Veterans [NCHV], n.d.). According to the NCHV (n.d.), an estimated 40,000 veterans are homeless on any given night. This represents about 11% of the adult homeless population. Demographic and social trends within the United States must be regularly reviewed and considered in curricular changes so nursing students are best prepared for a culturally sensitive practice in today's environment (Elliott & Patterson, 2017).

A small number of studies have examined military, veterans, and family members' perspectives on healthcare. Butler et al. (2015) found that veterans universally wanted care that demonstrated the *importance of respect for personhood,* "the belief that veterans were deserving of care that recognized them as individuals with a unique (military) identity, life history, and experience, and worthy of respect no matter who they were or how successfully they had managed their lives" (p. 119). Veterans described caring behaviors of healthcare providers as communicating effectively, following up to ensure the veteran got what they needed, and using specialized knowledge about unique health issues veterans face (Cohen et al., 2018). Further, results indicated that veterans want providers to explain things to them, so it is clear what they need to do for themselves. Partnering and collaborating on healthcare (Cohen et al., 2018) and being direct in sharing information is important to veterans (Butler et al., 2015). A lack of understanding military culture (Borah & Fina, 2017) or ability to speak military language (Cohen et al., 2018) may cause military service members, veterans, or family members to depart interactions in frustration. While many military service members and veterans may delay seeking healthcare for various reasons, the "need to be listened to and be treated with respect when they seek healthcare" overrides all other actions (Nworah et al., 2018, p. 775).

Worthy of highlighting is that, as a result of injury or exposure to traumatic events during military service, some service members or veterans may present to healthcare providers with symptoms which may be misunderstood or as if the person is behaving in a rude manner. Veterans voiced the importance for healthcare providers to recognize and be sensitive to difficult patients with a military history, and to be able to de-escalate situations because that is "what we need" (Butler et al., 2015, p. 122). Further, providers should be aware of the influence of the military ethos to be strong and stoical, as veterans tend to underreport or complain very little until something is seriously wrong. In a study of homeless male veterans, data supported veterans who utilize emergency departments instead of primary care do so because they have expressed they feel they have *no other option* (Weber et al., 2019). Recognizing that some providers go above and beyond to help and be an advocate, veterans in the study more often shared that not *feeling valued* and *lack of voice* when seeking care made them feel "disposable" (Weber et al., 2019, p. 5). Also important in caring for veterans is not to assume everyone has PTSD (Borah & Fina, 2017).

IMPLICATIONS FOR NURSING EDUCATION AND PRACTICE

Across the literature and related disciplines, there is ample support demanding that civilian providers become more culturally sensitive and competent to provide the best patient-centered care to military and veteran populations, including their families. This same level of competency is necessary of faculty teaching veteran-centered content or teaching students who are veterans (Carlson, 2016). While there may be gaps in essential knowledge for currently practicing nurses and healthcare providers, this trend needs to change. Military service members, veterans, and their families deserve quality care and, with the projections of needing significantly more long-term care for those veterans who have served since the Gulf War era, nurses and nurse educators need to prepare themselves. Preparation begins during prelicensure nursing education.

Carlson (2016) conducted a study of six VANA faculty that produced five thematic concepts and dimensions related to veteran care for faculty competencies and four essential knowledge concepts and dimensions necessary to teach nursing students to provide quality care. Carlson (2016) stressed that cultural competence develops over time and with exposure to the population. A desire to learn and understand more about military service members, veterans, and their families is the first step. To do this, a nurse educator (or any nurse) must understand the importance of always recognizing and acknowledging a veteran and be open to learn about military/veteran culture and their experiences. Appreciating contributions through military service demonstrates sensitivity and can facilitate trust building. Treating them with humanity, respect, and sincerity can also build trust, which is essential to providing care. Being open minded, using open and honest communication, and intentionally listening to veterans' concerns can also demonstrate the care and empathy necessary to build trust (Carlson, 2016). As important is recognizing that military culture is team oriented and the role it plays in engaging and caring for military and veteran patients. Findings from this study can also guide educators outside of academia.

Educators require essential knowledge related to military and veteran populations to teach students and nurses in practice, so quality patient-centered and culturally sensitive care can be achieved. Having a basic understanding of each of the services (Army, Navy, Air Force, Marine Corps, and Coast Guard), rank structures, and historical knowledge of health issues related to war eras is a starting point. Further, unique healthcare needs of this population as a result of their service, impact of service on families, veteran-specific issues across gender and lifespan, and resources available through the VA and other organizations can greatly enhance the nurse-patient relationship when caring for this population. Being able to understand just enough about their experiences can be sufficient for nurses in civilian settings to establish rapport with military and veteran patients. Even inquiring how someone would like to be addressed (first name, last name, or by rank) can demonstrate respect and caring (Butler et al., 2015; Carlson, 2016; Cohen et al., 2018). Creating a respectful environment can increase trust, open up communication, and ideally have a positive effect on follow-up care and health outcomes (Weber et al., 2019).

In order to reduce healthcare risks, contain costs of care, and manage long-term effects of injuries sustained during military service, intentional education is vital. Continuing education (CE) and quality improvement efforts are essential to begin making headway on the health issues facing this population. Chargualaf (2019) argues that "it is not enough to merely acknowledge that veteran care is important" (p. 9). Nurses must seek professional development related to care of this population, and clinical educators and managers must examine processes to improve assessment and identification of military status. This includes developing veteran-centered competencies as part of professional CE for practicing nurses (Chargualaf, 2019).

Student Veterans in Nursing

In light of over two dozen Veteran's Bachelor of Science in Nursing programs that have emerged since 2013, faculty must also recognize veterans as students and how their service experiences can influence the transition to nursing education (Patterson et al., 2019a) and the teaching-learning process (Patterson et al., 2019b; Elliott et al., 2019). Faculty must consider how certain injuries could manifest in the classroom or clinical setting, subsequently determining how they would handle the situation. Applying the same principles of cultural sensitivity and competence of patient-centered care to student-centered teaching is needed. Student veterans bring a wealth of experience to nursing education and maximizing their skills and leadership abilities can add value to the workforce (Patterson et al., 2019a, 2019b). Tapping into these strengths can have a positive impact on student veterans' health and well-being (Elliott et al., 2019).

FUTURE RESEARCH PRIORITIES

For nurse educators both inside and outside of academia, opportunity exists to evaluate nursing and healthcare providers' knowledge, skills, attitudes, comfort, and confidence in caring for military and veteran populations. Development and research on innovative methods in teaching veteran-centered care as well as developing competency are needed. More empirical research is needed on best practices to bridge the gaps between military culture and civilian healthcare settings. Broadly, another look at the impact of *Joining Forces* and what nursing programs are doing to teach future nurses to care for military/veteran populations would help to inform all programs and keep the momentum going.

CONCLUSIONS

Improving veteran healthcare as a national priority, appreciating that nurses can create the greatest impact toward improving veteran health, is the right course of action. While this book is based primarily on research and experiences of U.S. military, veterans, and their families, the content can be transferred to similar populations across the globe. A number of national organizations have put forth efforts to promote the health and well-being of military, veterans, and their families. However, there is more to be accomplished to improve the healthcare for this population. Nurses and nurse educators have the ability and power to increase awareness within the nursing profession, so that veteran-centered care can be achieved.

REFERENCES

The complete reference list for this chapter appears in the digital version of the chapter, accessible at https://connect.springerpub.com/content/book/978-0-8261-3597-1/chapter/ch01

RESOURCES

Educational Resources

AACN – Enhancing Veterans' Care Faculty Tool Kit
www.aacnnursing.org/Teaching-Resources/Tool-Kits/Veterans-Care
NLN – Advancing Care Excellence for Veterans
www.nln.org/professional-development-programs/teaching-resources/veterans-ace-v
RAND – Veterans Health Care
www.rand.org/topics/veterans-health-care.html
WHV – ELNEC – For Veterans Updated Curriculum
www.wehonorveterans.org/elnec-for-veterans-curriculum
WHV – Free Webinars
www.wehonorveterans.org/blog/resource_type/webinar

Military Families

Elizabeth Dole Foundation
www.elizabethdolefoundation.org/
National Military Family Association
www.militaryfamily.org/
RAND – Military Caregivers
www.rand.org/topics/military-caregivers.html

Post-Bachelors Veteran Health Education

Drexel University – Service to Veterans Certificate
www.drexel.edu/cnhp/academics/post-baccalaureate/certificate-pb-veterans-healthcare
University of Colorado – Veteran and Military Health Care Specialty
www.ucdenver.edu/academics/colleges/nursing/programs-admissions/graduate-programs/graduate-specialties/Pages/veteran-military-health-care.aspx

MILITARY CULTURE AND LIFESTYLE

BRENDA ELLIOTT

Valor is stability, not of legs and arms, but of courage and the soul.

Michel de Montaigne

KEY TERMS

military culture	military demographics
military values	military occupational specialties
military training	military structure
military education	military/veteran cultural competence
military stigma	

INTRODUCTION

At present, roughly 2.1 million Americans are serving in the military, including those serving on active duty or in the reserve component (RC; Defense Manpower Data Center [DMDC], 2019). Another 18.6 million veterans are now living as civilians across the United States (U.S. Department of Veterans Affairs [VA], 2019a). Members of the military, and those closely associated with them, belong to an organization that has its own language, customs, and culture. It is an organization of structure, rules, and hierarchy which may be difficult to understand for those who have never served. This culture can have a significant impact on individuals and families who serve alongside them. Healthcare providers often overlook this important factor and how it may influence healthcare. This chapter provides the background and context of military service and culture that can be insightful in understanding the experiences of this population, and are necessary to deliver culturally sensitive care.

BACKGROUND

The first formal branch of the U.S. military, the U.S. Army, was born from the establishment of the Continental Army in 1775 (Greenspan, 2019). Since that time, the U.S. military has sent service members abroad more than 300 times for the purpose of supporting missions that were not peacetime related,

The complete reference list for this chapter appears in the digital version of the chapter, accessible at https://connect.springerpub.com/content/book/978-0-8261-3597-1/chapter/ch02

but has only declared war on five occasions (War of 1812, Mexican-American War, Spanish-American War, World War I, and World War II [WWII]; Greenspan, 2019). The deadliest war in U.S. history was the Civil War and since that time WWII is the next closest war to claim American lives. As of 2019, there remain approximately 266,000 veterans from WWII (VA, 2019a). They represent a small number of the approximate 18 million veterans living today (VA, 2019b). According to the DMDC (DMDC, 2019), an estimated 1.3 million Americans are currently serving on active duty in the Armed Services (Army, Air Force, Marines, Navy, and Coast Guard). An additional 800,000 Americans are serving in Reserve and National Guard capacities (DMDC, 2019).

The purpose of this chapter is to provide readers with an overview of military service, lifestyle, and culture. The rationale for including this content in this book is to offer basic knowledge and understanding of what it is and was like for this population to serve the nation. It is our hope that in gaining this basic information that nurses and other healthcare providers can begin to understand the way in which service members, veterans, and their families think and behave. We also hope that it may enlighten readers in the best ways to establish trust, display empathy, and encourage open communication when it comes to healthcare interactions. This chapter also provides an initial discussion of the various models for assessing or measuring cultural competence.

ORGANIZATIONAL STRUCTURE OF THE U.S. DEPARTMENT OF DEFENSE

The U.S. Department of Defense (DoD) consists of three major uniformed service branches: (a) Army, (b) Navy (including the Marine Corps), and (c) Air Force. The Coast Guard is also a uniformed service that falls under the Department of Homeland Security during peacetime and the Department of the Navy during war time (DoD, n.d.). Within all the service branches, members can serve in an active or reserve status. Additionally, the Army and Air Force have National Guard personnel. The Reserve and National Guard are jointly known as the RC as they only serve intermittently as needed, training one weekend a month and 2 weeks during a fiscal year. Table 2.1 displays the most updated information on the number of personnel in each service branch and respective components. Aside from different components, there are various demographic factors, occupational specialties, rank/grade, gender, and family structures that can influence beliefs, behaviors, and perceptions of service members and their families, and eventually veterans (Hamaoka et al., 2014).

Role of Active and Reserve Components

Personnel who serve in the military on a full-time basis are referred to as active duty. They essentially commit to working 24 hours a day, 7 days a week, and can be called to deploy anywhere around the

TABLE 2.1 NUMBER OF SERVICE MEMBERS ACROSS SERVICE BRANCHES AND COMPONENTS

BRANCH OF SERVICE	ACTIVE DUTY COMPONENT	RESERVE/NATIONAL GUARD COMPONENT
Army	483,153	522,375
Air Force	332,292	176,548
Navy	336,861	59,574
Marine Corps	185,450	38,340
Coast Guard	41,815	6,241
Estimated total	1,379,391	803,078

SOURCE: Defense Manpower Data Center (2019, March). *DoD personnel, workforce reports and publications.* Retrieved May 22, 2019 from https://dcas.dmdc.osd.mil/dcas/pages/report_ofs_type.xhtml

globe on a moment's notice if necessary (National Center for Posttraumatic Stress Disorder [PTSD], 2012). Personnel who serve in the Reserve components (RC) either serve in the Reserves or in the National Guard. The purpose of the Reserves is to provide and maintain service members, or units, who can be called to serve on active duty in times of need, such as war or national emergencies. Historically, Reserve members' primary duty was to fill the gaps in stateside service positions while active duty forces were deployed overseas (National Center for PTSD, 2012). More recently, they have been called to fill the gaps overseas. Those who serve in the Reserves must participate in training (or "drill") one weekend a month and 2 weeks per year to meet duty requirements.

The purpose of the National Guard varies and includes activities such as local emergencies or assistance during times of natural disaster (storms, hurricanes, floods, fires, etc.). The National Guard is state organized and controlled, yet federally funded (National Center for PTSD, 2012). They can become federalized and deployed during times of war and are given veteran status if they serve a minimum of 30 consecutive days in a war zone. While they may see combat overseas, their roles generally encompass activities such as training local peacekeepers or building hospitals/schools (National Center for PTSD, 2012). Like Reserve personnel, they must serve one weekend a month and 2 weeks a year to fulfill their duty.

Rank

The military is a hierarchical organization that uses rank to distinguish its members' place within the organization. Rank is given to individuals the day they enter service, which advances over their career based on criteria such as performance, completion of schooling, or duration of time. Rank is a system used to indicate leadership, expertise, authority, and responsibility within a unit or occupation. Officers and Enlisted personnel are the two distinct groups within the military structure. Some service branches also have warrant officers (WOs). Officers generally enter the military with a bachelor's degree or higher and Enlisted personnel typically join right out of high school (Hamaoka et al., 2014). Officers generally conduct planning and can hold command, directing orders to a unit. They also oversee Enlisted personnel. Enlisted personnel execute plans and training, utilizing non-commissioned officers (NCOs) to lead and supervise. Enlisted personnel become NCOs once they achieve the pay grade of E-5. WOs are specialized experts who progressively attain technical and tactical competence to operate, maintain, administer, and manage equipment, support activities, or technical systems for an entire career ("Everything You Need to Know," 2019).

Pay grades are mostly used as a designation for pay purposes. Pay grades for Officers are O1 to O10 and for Enlisted they are E1 to E9. WOs pay grades are WO1 to WO5. Pay grades and ranks can be viewed in Tables 2.2, 2.3, and 2.4, respectively. Promotion in both the Officer and Enlisted Ranks through the first few pay grades is somewhat automatic assuming the person fulfills their role and responsibilities in an appropriate manner. What is important to note is that while pay grades are the same across service branches, rank may not be. For example, a Captain in the Army is considered an O3 pay grade but in the Navy a Captain is an O6 pay grade. A major difference exists between pay grades O3 and O6.

Pay grade is the most important part of military pay. The second most important part would be an array of allowances that are provided to service members to assist in covering expenses for needs such as housing, food, dislocation, or cost of living for areas that are more expensive to live such as Hawaii ("Military Pay Allowances List," 2019). A list of allowances and pay charts is publically available online at www.federalpay.org/military/army/ranks

Military Occupational Specialties

Military occupational specialty (MOS) is a way to classify career fields or job duties with the military, separate from rank. These classifications include numbers and letters to represent a specialty. For example, in the Army, a medic is a 68W (W stands for "whiskey" in military phonetics) or an Infantryman is an 11B (B stands for "bravo"). There are hundreds of MOSs across the service branches

TABLE 2.2 ENLISTED RANK AND PAY GRADES ACROSS SERVICE BRANCHES

ENLISTED PAYGRADE	ARMY	MARINE CORPS	NAVY	AIR FORCE	COAST GUARD
E1	Private	Private	Seaman recruit	Airman basic	Seaman recruit
E2	Private second class	Private first class	Seaman apprentice	Airman	Seaman apprentice
E3	Private first class	Lance corporal	Seaman	Airman first class	Seaman
E4	Specialist or corporal	Corporal	Petty officer third class	Senior airman	Petty officer third class
E5	Sergeant	Sergeant	Petty officer second class	Staff sergeant	Petty officer second class
E6	Staff sergeant	Staff sergeant	Petty officer first class	Technical sergeant	Petty officer first class
E7	Sergeant first class	Gunnery sergeant	Chief petty officer	Master sergeant	Chief petty officer
E8	Master sergeant/first sergeant	Master sergeant or first sergeant	Senior chief petty officer	Senior master sergeant	Senior chief petty officer
E9	Sergeant major or command sergeant major or sergeant major of the army	Master gunnery sergeant or sergeant major or sergeant major of the marine corps	Master chief petty officer or command master chief petty officer or master chief petty officer of the navy	Chief master sergeant or command chief master sergeant or chief master sergeant of the air force	Master chief petty officer or command master chief petty officer or master chief petty officer of the coast guard

SOURCE: Data from FederalPay.org (2019). *Military pay.* Retrieved December 24, 2019 from https://www.federalpay.org/military/army/ranks

TABLE 2.3 WO RANK AND PAY GRADES ACROSS SERVICE BRANCHES

WO PAYGRADE	ARMY	MARINE CORPS	NAVY	AIR FORCE	COAST GUARD
WO1	WO 1	WO 1	N/A	N/A	N/A
WO2	Chief WO 2	Chief WO 2	Chief WO 2	N/A	Chief WO 2
WO3	Chief WO 3	Chief WO 3	Chief WO 3	N/A	Chief WO 3
WO4	Chief WO 4	Chief WO 4	Chief WO 4	N/A	Chief WO 4
WO5	Chief WO 5	Chief WO 5	Chief WO 5	N/A	N/A

N/A, not applicable; WO, warrant officer.

SOURCE: Data from FederalPay.org (2019). *Military pay.* Retrieved December 24, 2019 from https://www.federalpay.org/military/army/ranks

ranging from administrative roles to pilots to nurses to chaplains. A bachelor's prepared medical-surgical registered nurse in the Army is a 66H (H stands for "hotel") and in the Air Force is a 46N (N stands for "november"). Additional numbers and letters are used to signify specialization. It is common for military service members and veterans to refer to their MOS when asked what they do/did in the military (Hamaoka et al., 2014).

MOS can influence health-related risks for service members. For example, those serving in Infantry units are often at the center of fighting during times of war and are therefore at higher risk for gunshot

TABLE 2.4 OFFICER RANK AND PAY GRADES ACROSS SERVICE BRANCHES

OFFICER PAYGRADE	ARMY	MARINE CORPS	NAVY	AIR FORCE	COAST GUARD
O1	Second lieutenant	Second lieutenant	Ensign	Second lieutenant	Ensign
O2	First lieutenant	First lieutenant	Lieutenant junior grade	First lieutenant	Lieutenant junior grade
O3	Captain	Captain	Lieutenant	Captain	Lieutenant
O4	Major	Major	Lieutenant commander	Major	Lieutenant commander
O5	Lieutenant colonel	Lieutenant colonel	Commander	Lieutenant colonel	Commander
O6	Colonel	Colonel	Captain	Colonel	Captain
O7	Brigadier general	Brigadier general	Rear admiral lower half	Brigadier general	Rear admiral lower half
O8	Major general	Major general	Rear admiral	Major general	Rear admiral
O9	Lieutenant general	Lieutenant general	Vice admiral	Lieutenant general	Vice admiral
O10	General or general of the army	General	Admiral	General or general of the air force	Admiral
O11	N/A	N/A	Fleet admiral	N/A	N/A

N/A, not applicable.

SOURCE: Data from FederalPay.org (2019). *Military pay.* Retrieved December 24, 2019 from https://www.federalpay.org/military/army/ranks

wounds, whereas those who transport equipment may be more at risk for blast injuries from roadside bombs or improvised explosive devices. As the tactics of war change and the "front lines" of battle are not as clear, MOS becomes less of a factor. Nurses or other medical personnel are faced with the stress of caring for the injured, bearing the burden of the outcomes of war and narratives of those they care for. Those who are miles away from the fighting, such as intelligence analysts, have other burdens to bear such as witnessing atrocities from video feeds while monitoring for threats, and the responsibility to safely guide aircraft and drone pilots (McCammon, 2017). As such, inquiring about MOS and what a person did while in the military can not only be a good starting point for engaging in conversation, it can also provide useful information to the potential health risks a person may have faced.

Military Training

Enlisting in the military usually occurs after high school graduation, once a person has talked with a recruiter. To complete the process, recruits must go through a Military Entrance Processing Station, which are located all over the United States (Today's Military, 2019). There are five major steps required to complete military service enlistment (Table 2.5). Full-time enlistment could range from 2 to 6 years, depending on the service branch ("The Benefits of Joining," 2019). Those opting for reserve duty can commit to as little as 1 year. After completion of enlistment, recruits attend basic training, also known as "boot camp." Each service branch has their own basic training course, tailored specifically for that branch of the military. Boot camps range between 7 and 12 weeks in duration, with the Army and the Marine Corps having the longest at 10 and 12 weeks, respectively (Today's Military, 2019).

Basic training, or initial entry training, is a rite of passage for Enlisted service members. It is an intense time of "instruction and indoctrination into military skills, rules, and customs," whereby the

TABLE 2.5 STEPS FOR MILITARY ENLISTMENT ENTRANCE

REQUIREMENTS	DESCRIPTION
Step 1: Take the ASVAB	The ASVAB is a multiple-choice test that helps determine the careers for which a person may be best suited for. Each service branch uses a custom combination of a person's results to yield scores that align with different career fields.
Step 2: Pass the physical examination	Due to physical eligibility requirements everyone must have a regular physical which includes height/weight measurements, hearing/vision screening, urine and blood tests, drug and alcohol test, and muscle group and joint maneuvers. Specialized testing if required may also be done such as pregnancy testing for women or body fat percentage for those who exceed the weight standard.
Step 3: Meet with a Counselor to determine a career	Career selection takes into account ASVAB results, physical exam results, needs of the desired service branch, job availability, as well as recruit preference. At this stage recruits will be given an enlistment agreement to sign and be fingerprinted for security and background clearances.
Step 4: Take the Oath of Enlistment	Recruits must take the oath out loud, vowing to defend the U.S. Constitution and obey the UCMJ. UCMJ is federal law enacted by Congress, which defines the military justice system and lists criminal offenses under military law.
Step 5: After the MEPS	At this point new recruits will do one of two things, either report to Basic Training or opt for the DEP. DEP allows recruits to return home and attend Basic Training sometime within a year (often occurs with those who enroll prior to high school graduation).

ASVAB, Armed Services Vocational Aptitude Battery; DEP, Delay Entry Program; MEPS, Military Entrance Processing Station; UCMJ, Uniform Code of Military Justice.

SOURCE: Data from Today's Military. (2019). *Enlisting in the military.* Retrieved December 26, 2019 from https://www.todaysmilitary.com/how-to-join/enlisting-military

"emphasis is placed on obeying the operational hierarchy, following the direction of superiors, and executing orders efficiently and without question" (Hamaoka et al., 2014, p. 11). Basic training is a time for preparing recruits for the physical, mental, and emotional demands that the military requires of them to be successful in their future roles (Today's Military, 2019). Upon completion of basic training, Enlisted personnel move on to another phase of training called Advanced Individual Training (Army), "A" school (Navy and Coast Guard), MOS school (Marine Corps), or Technical Training (Air Force) depending on the service branch. It is during this time that service members are trained in the knowledge and skills necessary for their MOS (Today's Military, 2019). Once training is complete, service members are typically moved to their first duty station. This move is referred to as a permanent change of station (PCS). For those opting for Reserve duty, they will be assigned a unit near where they live, unless called into active duty ("The Benefits of Joining," 2019).

Officers generally enter the military with a minimum of a 4-year degree and this degree can often influence what career they have in the military. There are several paths to becoming an Officer, which include (a) attend a military college or service academy, (b) enroll in a college or university with a Reserve Officer Training Corps program, (c) attend Officer Candidate School (OCS) after graduating from college, (d) receive a direct commission after earning a professional degree, or (e) advance through the enlisted ranks and complete officer training (Today's Military, 2019). Direct Commission Officers are usually professionals who have already earned a degree but have skills essential to the military such as medical personnel, lawyers, or chaplains. For Enlisted members to compete for OCS slots they must serve at least 4 years, obtain rank of E5 or higher, and have already completed 30 credits of college ("Everything You Need to Know," 2019). Officers entering the military must attend an Officer Basic Course, or initial entry training. These courses varying in length based on MOS.

Service members, whether Enlisted or Officer, can expect to spend much of the first year on active duty attending various schools and training before arriving at their first duty assignment. This of course varies for each MOS and if the service member is selected for additional training such as Airborne School. After this initial time period, most service members generally spend 2 to 3 years at a duty station before getting orders for a PCS. This can vary depending on MOS, promotion leading to a need for a job/responsibility change, or selection for further training/schooling.

Military Education

Professional military education (PME) refers to the continuing education or training needed at different ranks for advancement or perhaps essential for the next role in a particular MOS (Kaurin, 2017). PME varies for Officers and Enlisted personnel, as well as between each branch of the service. However, it often involves leadership and management development to prepare service members for the next level of responsibility they will assume (Kaurin, 2017). Military personnel must also attend/complete education required annually through DoD policy and respective branches (Army, Navy, and Air Force). Examples of annual education may be related to specialized topics such as sexual harassment or suicide prevention.

Demographics

Over the past two decades the U.S. military has become more diverse with the number of women in leadership positions steadily rising (Barroso, 2019). Approximately 15% of active duty military service members in 2015 were women (Parker et al., 2017). The percentage of women varies across branches with the Air Force having the largest percentage at about 19% followed by the Navy (18%), Army (14%), and the Marines (8%; Parker et al., 2017). About 43% of active-duty military in 2017 were from racial and ethnic minority groups (Barroso, 2019). Blacks and Hispanics make up the largest minority groups at about 16% each (Barroso, 2019). Since the end of the military draft in 1973 the average age of both Officers and Enlisted personnel has increased slightly, possibly due to more service members opting to make the military a career.

Demographics within the veteran population have also changed over the past two decades. While the veteran population is projected to decrease between now and 2040, the proportion of minorities among veterans will increase from 23% to an estimated 34% (VA, 2019b). In 2017, minority veterans made up 23% of the total veteran population and 35% of the female veteran population. Minority veterans are younger than White, non-Hispanic veterans and male veterans (median age of 65) are older than female veterans (median age 51). Comparing veterans to non-veterans, the median age of male veterans in 2017 was 65 and for male non-veterans it was 42 (VA, 2019b). For female veterans the median age in 2017 was 51 and for female non-veterans the median age was 47.

The largest living cohort of female veterans served during the Post-9/11 era, which includes Operation Iraqi Freedom (OIF), Operation Enduring Freedom (OEF), and Operation New Dawn. The largest living cohort of male veterans served during the Vietnam Era (VA, 2019b). The states with the highest percentage of resident veterans are Alaska, Maine, and Montana, while the highest percentage of female veterans live in District of Columbia, Virginia, and Alaska (VA, 2019b).

MILITARY LIFESTYLE

Joining the military today is a voluntary act. Individuals decide to join the Armed Forces for various reasons, which may include a desire for specific training, personal or physical challenge, or any number of benefits that come with serving such as healthcare or funding to help attain a college education. Some may choose to join the military based on the perception that it could provide a better future or a way out of undesired/adverse home life or circumstances (Blosnich et al., 2014). But whatever the reason, those entering the military will experience a lifestyle unlike most, especially those serving on active duty (full-time, 24 hours a day, 7 days a week). Entering military service means a person must be willing to give up some freedoms, personal choices, and time as they are entering an organization that demands so much of its people (Segal, 1986).

Members of the military must be willing to obey and carry out lawful orders of their superiors (Coll et al., 2011; Hamaoka et al., 2014). They must also be willing to adhere to a number of enforced standards such as personal appearance, physical fitness, and appropriate conduct both on and off duty. Within the military there is a zero tolerance of drug use. Members of the military, and their families to an extent, must follow specific rules and live wherever the military desires for them to live. While many service members may be afforded the opportunity to rank order selections for future duty assignments, this is not always guaranteed. Therefore, they may end up in locations that they would not otherwise desire to live. At times, service members may be sent to locations where families may not accompany them for up to a year.

Relocation

As mentioned previously, service members can anticipate relocation to a new duty assignment every 2 to 3 years. Each branch of service is slightly different. Members of the military without dependents may be assigned barracks rooms on the military installation if available. Those with families may have the opportunity to live on or off the military installation, depending on location and space availability. If housing on the installation is not available, service members and their families must find and secure housing in the surrounding community. While this is generally not problematic, some locations may have limited availability of housing for rent which may force families to buy homes when they otherwise would not. Regardless of where service members and their families live in relation to the military installation, all service members receive an allowance (basic allowance for housing) to assist in covering housing costs.

With each move, service members and their families must locate new doctors, dentists, and so forth, which can be significant stressors. In most instances, a military health clinic or hospital is available to meet their needs. But this is not always the case and they are sent to civilian providers within the TRICARE™ network for their healthcare needs. While stationed overseas, some may even require the care of providers within the host country medical facilities (Elliott, 2019a). This cross over into the cultural norms of other countries, particularly with health systems that do not operate as they do within the United States, can produce a great deal of stress.

Temporary Duty

Temporary duty (commonly referred to as TDY) is a term used to describe periods of time where a service member may have to leave their duty station to temporarily train or work in another location. TDY can be as short as a few days up to a year. TDY can occur while moving to the next duty assignment, but most commonly service members return to their current assignment. TDY should not be confused with deployment, as these are different assignments with specific mission orders. In addition to being away from the home unit for TDY, service members belonging to certain types of units may experience long periods of time training in the field. These are generally referred to as field exercises. Units, such as Infantry units, must train on rotation to maintain readiness for deployment.

Deployments

Deployments can occur at any time during a person's time in the military, whether serving on active duty, or with the Reserves/National Guard. Service members can be deployed globally in times of conflict/war, peace-keeping missions, natural disasters, or humanitarian efforts. Deployments can

TABLE 2.6 RESOURCES TO SUPPORT FAMILIES DURING DEPLOYMENT

RESOURCE	WEB LINK
National Military Family Association	www.militaryfamily.org/info-resources/deployment/
Operation We Are Here	www.operationwearehere.com/index.html
Military.com	www.military.com/deployment/deployment-guides-and-resources.html
Military One Source	www.militaryonesource.mil/military-life-cycle/deployment
Blue Star Families	bluestarfam.org/for-mil-families/deployments/deployment-resources/

impose a host of challenges for service members and their families (Hamaoka et al., 2014). Changes in family dynamics and roles are particularly stressful and burdensome. Spouses are left to manage the household as a single parent, often living away from other immediate family. It is for this reason many military families will turn to others in their position, building relationships with those who are experiencing similar challenges (Tam-Seto et al., 2018). While many resources are available to spouses (Table 2.6), some will attempt to bear the burden and not ask for help. This can lead to physical and behavioral consequences. Children may be particularly at risk for behavioral challenges depending on age and duration of deployment.

During times of deployment, all the service branches provide some type of deployment assistance (Military.com, 2020). The name or title given to each type of program varies from branch to branch but include services such as family assistance centers, legal assistance, emergency assistance, and individual counseling services. Some military units have family readiness groups (FRGs) in place that can also be a resource for communicating information to spouses about their service members while deployed. For those without FRG support, unit level contacts are usually identified to facilitate any needs the family may have in contacting their service member while deployed. In addition, the American Red Cross works closely with all services in providing and assisting in emergency communications, emergency financial assistance, and various types of referrals for other needs (Military.com, 2020).

HEALTH CONSEQUENCES OF MILITARY SERVICE/DEPLOYMENT

Military service members face a number of occupational hazards by simply volunteering to serve. To maintain basic physical fitness standards, service members must regularly engage in physical exercise, at times carrying heavy loads of equipment for prolonged periods. The physical and mental demands of military training can be rigorous, involving activities such as obstacle courses and field problems in varying terrains/climates. This can lead to a plethora of orthopedic injures such as back, knee, and ankle injuries. Further, weaponry, vehicles, and air craft used during training and deployment exposes service members to extremely loud noise. For some, exposure to noise is almost a daily occurrence. While use of hearing protection has improved in the past few decades due to increases in service-connected disability, tinnitus and hearing loss remain the top two service-connected disabilities reported by the VA (VA, 2018). Because military training is designed to place individuals under stress so they can perform duties under similar circumstances, mental health effects can transpire even without deployment.

Deployment can place additional health risks on individuals. The effects of deployment can be seen in the most recent cohort of veterans, Post-9/11 veterans (Baker, 2014). Blast injuries requiring amputation, embedded fragments of shrapnel, and traumatic brain injury (TBI) are frequent injuries experienced by Post-9/11 veterans. Posttraumatic stress, PTSD, depression, and anxiety are frequently reported behavioral health consequences. Further, rates of suicide and military sexual trauma plague military members and veterans (Olenick et al., 2015). For women or other historically underrepresented groups (specifically LGBT and minorities), receiving appropriate care within the VA has been an uphill battle. But a battle that is beginning to show signs of improving as more focus is placed on these groups of veterans. Lastly, environmental exposures to burn pits, burning oil wells, and sand/dust particles have also been problematic.

Impact of Military Service on Families

Managing relocations but also separations (TDY and training), unpredictable schedules, and spouse employment are among the many stressors military families face. Research supports that deployments and long work hours may results in spouses feeling abandoned or isolated, or second priority as a result of the "mission first" culture of the military (Borah & Fina, 2017). While all service members receive 30 days of paid annual leave per year, some service members have restrictions when their unit takes this leave. This may leave some service members and their families feeling less in control over their lives. Financial costs considered nonessential are not always covered (i.e., pet shipment if moving overseas or a second vehicle; Elliott, 2019a).

As often as service members' move, so must their children change schools or childcare providers. They may also consider house purchases to ensure their children attend higher quality schools, which could later lead to financial strain. Again, this can vary depending on the number of PCSs made over a career. According to the Blue Star Families' annual Military Family Lifestyle Survey (aMFLS) in 2018, relocation stress was top stressor for service member respondents for the first time (Blue Star Families, 2018). Military family participants reported spending more than $1,000 in unreimbursed expenses during their last relocation. Further, 79% of female service members who relocated within a year of taking the survey reported not being able to find reliable childcare.

The aMFLS (2018) respondents of over 10,000 military spouses, full-time service members, veterans and their immediate family members reported time away as the number one top concern for military families. Other top stressors included significant financial insecurity due to the lack of work for spouses of service members and lack of affordable childcare in the relocation areas. The results of the survey regarding the top five issues by each group are available at the following URL: bluestarfam. org/wp-content/uploads/2019/02/2018MFLS-Executive-Summary-DIGITAL-FINAL.pdf. In addition to time away from family, the impact of deployment on children and military pay and benefits were concerns for all three groups.

A study by Borah and Fina (2017) supports that being a military spouse creates barriers for employment and attaining educational goals. Participants in the study reported delaying or not pursuing education because of factors such as not living in one location long enough to complete a course of study, spending more money to repeat courses that would not transfer, or inconsistent in-state tuition policies that created financial hardship for those not granted in-state rates (Borah & Fina, 2017). Further, maintaining professional licensure across states can be expensive and cause delays in finding employment. A number of initiatives have evolved to assist military spouses in finding jobs, or earning a degree, with each relocation. The DoD Spouse Education and Career Opportunities program aims to help military spouses find employment through partnerships such as the Military Spouse Employment Partnership. Many non-profit organizations also exist to assist and support spouses, and veterans, find work. While not an exhaustive list, a few examples of resources are located in Table 2.7.

In regard to receiving healthcare, military spouses and family members generally expect and are accustomed to changes in healthcare providers. Despite relocation every few years and lack of continuity of care, spouses feel a quality healthcare provider and patient relationship, even if new, is a significant factor in their satisfaction of care received (Gleason & Beck, 2017). Dissatisfaction in healthcare often stems from interacting with providers who lack understanding of military culture, life, and families (Borah & Fina, 2017; Tam-Seto et al., 2018). Further, one participant in their study commented that healthcare providers need to know that "everyone doesn't have PTSD; everyone is not a young,

TABLE 2.7 SELECT RESOURCES FOR SPOUSE EMPLOYMENT ASSISTANCE

RESOURCE	WEB LINK
MyCAA	www.military.com/education/money-for-school/military-spouse-career-advancement-accounts-financial-aid.html
U.S. Government	www.usajobs.gov/
Military Officers Association of America	www.moaa.org/content/topic-and-landing-pages/i-am-a-spouse/
Amazon	www.amazon.jobs/en/landing_pages/mil-spouse
DoD SECO	myseco.militaryonesource.mil/portal/
MSEP	www.militaryonesource.mil/education-employment/for-spouses/career-exploration/military-spouses-let-the-military-spouse-employment-partnership-help-you-find-a-job
Hire Heroes USA	www.hireheroesusa.org/

DoD, U.S. Department of Defense; MSEP, Military Spouse Employment Partnership; MyCAA, My Career Advancement Account; SECO, Spouse Education and Career Opportunities.

uneducated spouse" (Borah & Fina, 2017, p. 150). This suggests, and is consistent with findings by Tam-Seto et al. (2018), that even spouses may feel stereotyped when they disclose they are military spouses.

Military spouses can access a number of resources to find information and support during the time their spouse is serving in the Armed Forces (Table 2.8).

Consequences of Deployment on Families

A number of factors may influence the impact that deployment has on service members and their families. These include things such as the number, length, and frequency of deployments, marital status, number and age of children, available spousal supports, ease and frequency of communication during the deployment, and the type of deployment exposures the service member experiences to name a few (Meadows et al., 2016). When service members deploy, power of the household shifts to the spouse, which can be problematic when the service member returns. If shared power is not restored, it can lead to one or both spouses feeling resentment or not needed (Meadows et al., 2016). Injuries such as TBI, PTSD, and some physical injuries can be taxing on families or create family issues, particularly when the service member refuses to seek necessary help (Borah & Fina, 2017).

According to Meadows et al. (2016), the type of trauma (physical – injury to the service member; combat – exchanging fire with the enemy; or psychological – witnessing or vicarious exposure to trauma) experienced during deployment can have different effects on different relationships within a family. Findings from the RAND deployment life study suggest that combat exposure may lead to less psychological aggression between spouses but lead to poorer relationships with teenage children (Meadows et al., 2016), whereas psychological injury can lead to improved relationships with teenage

TABLE 2.8 GENERAL RESOURCES TO SUPPORT MILITARY SPOUSES

RESOURCE	WEB LINK
Military Spouse	www.militaryspouse.com/
Seasoned Spouse	seasonedspouse.com/
Military One Source	www.militaryonesource.mil/family-relationships/spouse/spouse-resources
Military Spouse Advocacy Network	www.militaryspouseadvocacynetwork.org/
Facebook – Search for local groups	www.facebook.com/

children. Overall, the study demonstrated military families are resilient and relationships after the service member returns from deployment generally return to previous levels with a bit of time (Meadows et al., 2016). Preparation for and communication during deployment were considered critical factors for those families who functioned better during deployment. Further, study results suggested a vulnerability for marital strain and psychological problems for service members if they left the military right after returning from deployment (Meadows et al., 2016).

MILITARY CULTURE AND VALUES

Military culture is defined by the values, norms, language, beliefs, behaviors, ideals, and/or traditions that "create a shared value system across organizations and individuals dedicated to defending a nation or national identity" (Convoy & Westphal, 2013, p. 592). It is organized with a chain of command, or social hierarchy, that allows for its members to understand expectations and authority (Hamaoka et al., 2014). It is comprised of "perceptions that govern how members of the armed forces think, communicate, and interact with one another and civilians" (Coll et al., 2011, p. 489). The military, and thus its personnel, generally follow very structured planning to manage risks and reduce any unknowns. This may lend to individuals becoming very structured in planning day to day life. Each branch of the Armed Forces has its own sub-culture, including titles, language, norms, and traditions that makes them distinct from one another (Hamaoka et al., 2014; Table 2.9). Although collectively, they share similar values.

TABLE 2.9 ARMED FORCES' SUBCULTURES

BRANCH	TITLE	JOB	CORE VALUES	MOTTO
Army	Soldier	The largest and oldest service in the U.S. military, the Army provides the ground forces that protect the United States	Loyalty Duty Respect Selfless service Integrity Personal courage	This we will defend – "this" meaning country
Air Force	Airman	The Air Force provides a rapid, flexible, and lethal air and space capability that can deliver forces anywhere in the world within hours	Integrity first Service before self Excellence in all we do	Aim High…Fly-Fight-Win
Navy	Sailor	On, above, and below water, the Navy is America's forward deployed force and is the major deterrent to aggression around the world	Honor Courage Commitment	Non Sibi Sed Patriae – means not self but country
Marine Corps	Marine	As a component of the Department of the Navy, the Marine Corps maintain amphibious and ground units for contingency and combat operations	Honor Courage Commitment	Semper Fidelis (Semper Fi for short) – means always faithful
Coast Guard	Coast Guardsmen or Coastie	The Coast Guard provides law and maritime safety enforcement, marine and environmental protection and military naval support	Honor Respect Devotion to duty	Semper Paratus (Semper Par for short) – means always ready

SOURCE: U.S. Department of Defense. (n.d.). *Our forces.* Retrieved December 21, 2019 from https://www.defense.gov/Our-Story/Our-Forces/

Military culture is influenced by a code of conduct (Exhibit 2.1) and "ethos" that stresses honor, moral and physical courage, self-sacrifice, accountability, discipline, and loyalty (Gettle, 2007; Naval Medical Research Center, n.d.; Speigle, 2013; "The United State Coast Guard Ethos," 2019; "Warrior Ethos," 2011). For example, the warrior ethos of the Army is "I will always place the mission first, I will never accept defeat, I will never quit, and I will never leave a fallen comrade" ("Warrior Ethos," 2011, para. 1). The ethos that defines military culture can have varying influence on service members while in the military, and for some it can become a permanent part of their self-identity (Suzuki & Kawakami, 2016) and worldview (Westphal & Convoy, 2015). Military ethos can be a source of strength in the face of adversity but also a source of vulnerability when beliefs become a barrier to support and hope (Westphal & Convoy, 2015). Further, each branch of the Armed Forces has their own creed that may also influence their self-identity. The creeds for the branches of the Armed Forces are available at the following URL: www.military.com/join-armed-forces/military-creeds.html.

EXHIBIT 2.1

ARMED FORCES CODE OF CONDUCT

1. I am an American, fighting in the forces which guard my country and our way of life. I am prepared to give my life in their defense.

2. I will never surrender of my own free will. If in command, I will never surrender the members of my command while they still have the means to resist.

3. If I am captured, I will continue to resist by all means available. I will make every effort to escape and aid others to escape. I will accept neither parole nor special favors from the enemy.

4. If I become a prisoner of war, I will keep faith with my fellow prisoners. I will give no information or take part in any action which might be harmful to my comrades. If I am senior, I will take command. If not, I will obey the lawful orders of those appointed over me and will back them up in every way.

5. When questioned, should I become a prisoner of war, I am required to give name, rank, social security number, and date of birth. I will evade answering further questions to the utmost of my ability. I will make no oral or written statements disloyal to my country and its allies or harmful to their cause.

6. I will never forget that I am an American, responsible for my actions, and dedicated to the principles which made my country free. I will trust in my God and in the United States of America.

Executive Order (EO) 10631 (1955) as amended by EO 11382 (1967) as amended by EO 12633 (1988)

SOURCE: National Archives. Federal Register. Executive Orders. (2016). *Executive Order 10631—Code of Conduct for members of the Armed Forces of the United States.* Retrieved December 21, 2019 from https://www.archives.gov/federal-register/codification/executive-order/10631.html

Military Mentality – Collectivism Versus Individualism

Individualism can be defined as the "degree to which members of a society define their self-image as an individual or as part of a group … those who define themselves from the social and collective aspects of the self-concept are described with the term collectivist" (LeFebvre & Franke, 2013, p. 133). Individualism and collectivism are worldviews that "make different aspects of the self-concept salient," or more prominent (LeFebvre & Franke, 2013, p. 133). Core elements of each worldview are highlighted in

Exhibit 2.2. In a study of United States and Ghana undergraduate students, LeFebrvre and Franke (2013) examined how cultural norms and values affect decision-making in conflict situations. The results of their study indicated that those who align with an individualist worldview tend to be more rational in decision-making compared to those who align with a collectivist worldview who tended to be more dependent in decision-making. Those from the collectivist mindset were also more likely to prioritize interests of members of the central society identity groups from which they belonged (LeFebvre & Franke, 2013).

EXHIBIT 2.2

CORE ELEMENTS OF INDIVIDUALISM AND COLLECTIVISM

INDIVIDUALISM	COLLECTIVISM
Independence	Duty to in-group
Uniqueness	Maintain harmony

SOURCE: LeFebvre, R., & Franke, V. (2013). Culture matters: Individualism vs. collectivism in conflict decision-making. Societies, 3, 128–146. https://doi.org/0.3390/soc3010128

The military as an organization is generally a collectivist culture that "stresses the necessity of cooperation, communalism, interdependence, and conformity" (Hamaoka et al., 2014, p. 7). This can be seen through the wearing of uniforms and use of a common language that may not be understood by those outside the military. According to Coll et al. (2011), there is little room for individual autonomy in the military and members must learn to act collectively to complete their missions. This collectivism, or forced cohesiveness, can be both positive and negative. Collectivism can positively aid in establishing camaraderie, which can serve as a protective factor during times of conflict/war. It facilitates a units' ability to function effectively (Coll et al., 2011).

Conversely, this collectivism may unintentionally reinforce a military mindset, moving service members further away from a civilian mindset. This can cause issues for service members upon leaving military service as they have been "psychologically distant" from the civilian world (Coll et al., 2011, p. 491). The military as an organization, uses strict drills to teach discipline to its members to ensure that a soldier does not throw down a "weapon in response to his natural instinct of self-preservation" (Pawiński, 2017, p. 5). Drills facilitate desensitization and conditioning for killing, while learned discipline helps facilitate cohesion. Further, discipline is essential to maintain order and control of soldiers, which may also increase obedience and loyalty (Pawiński, 2017). In a study examining the consequences of military cohesion, Pawiński (2017) argues that the loss of autonomy and dehumanization are unintended consequences of this type of training as it is challenging for soldiers when this level of discipline is not needed, such as peacetime.

Stigma

Military service members, veterans, and their families may experience varying types of stigma, both public stigma and/or self-stigma related to various issues that stemmed from military service or culture. Stigma is defined as a mark of shame or discredit, an identifying mark or characteristic as in a sign of disease (Stigma, n.d.). A number of publications discuss the issue of stigma across professional disciplines. A few examples are presented that highlight health-seeking behaviors, as well as barriers to the transition out of the military to higher education and employment.

Within our society, mental health has carried stigma for centuries. It remains a significant barrier in help-seeking behaviors of service members, largely due to their unwillingness to admit existence of a mental health issue (Curry et al., 2014; Harding, 2017; Nworah et al., 2018). This unwillingness may result from the fear of appearing weak or the fear of negative repercussions should the information get back to commanders (Coll et al., 2011). In a study conducted by Ganzini et al. (2013) "veterans concerns [about] admitting their suicidal thoughts originated from experiences of stigmatization and harmful repercussions in the military, where admitting suicidal thought or having mental health problems was perceived as shameful and embarrassing, inconsistent with being a good soldier" (p. 1218).

In an examination of disabilities, stigma, and student veterans in higher education, Flink (2017) highlights that misperceptions about the number of veterans with PTSD or that most veterans have a mental health issue can lead to stigmatization of these invisible disabilities, which may or may not even be present. This stigmatization can be a major stressor for veterans during their transition from the military into higher education, possibly causing social isolation. As cited by Flink (2017), student veterans are twice as likely to have a disability as non-military students. This raises the question about what resources are available on college campuses to support transitioning veterans so they can be successful, as well as initiatives to reduce stigma associated with military service.

As reported by Correll (2019), veterans of military service may be facing stereotyping just from putting military service on their resume and in cover letters, especially for jobs that require social interaction and feelings. A number of veteran organizations took issue to the study conducted by the Duke University Fuqua School of Business (released September 24, 2019), because it promotes the stereotype of "veterans as brooding malcontents" or "the lone wolf idea of what a veteran is" (Correll, 2019, para. 1). However, others feel it gets the biases out in the open in hopes that companies will recognize the labels they give to veterans and change their practices. Further, the military transition program may be able to assist those getting ready to leave military service with more skills and tips to overcome perceptions of those who may consider them less capable of social-emotional interaction. It may be that those who serve in particular MOSs may have more difficulty cultivating these skills while in the service and the military may be able to intervene to prepare them better for life after service.

Transition to Civilian Life

One the biggest challenges military service members face is the transition to civilian life. While research supports that most service members make the transition successfully, it is during this period of time where individuals may be the most vulnerable. While in the military, a person is told what to do, how to behave, what to wear, and where to live (to an extent). Unlike the civilian world, the military is structured in such a way that every person entering can have a 20- to 30-year career, be provided with the education and training needed to achieve this career (or status), and internal supports should they decide to change career paths (Truusa & Castro, 2019). Healthcare, dental care, food and housing allowances, and for some clothing allowances, are all afforded to service members for free. When a person leaves the military it may be difficult to figure out life without structure and discipline, and to deal with the unorganized behaviors of other people (Suzuki & Kawakami, 2016). Further, figuring out the basics of living outside the military may be very difficult for some as they search for new meaning or purpose in life (Atuel & Castro, 2018; Smith & True, 2014; Weiss et al., 2019).

Data from a study conducted by Suzuki and Kawakami (2016) suggest that veterans feel a loss of comradery after leaving the military; a sense that there is no longer a safety net or a common set of values to live by in the civilian world as there was in the military. Further, some struggle to find their place in a society where they do not always feel like they "fit in" (Smith & True, 2014). The transition between cultures can be difficult, but eventually service members find their place in the civilian world. Truusa and Castro (2019) offer unique advice to veterans, which is to "plan every aspect of their transition as if they were moving to another country" because it may be a similar experience to what immigrants face moving to a new country (p. 17). In taking this approach, service members may be better prepared to make the transition.

TABLE 2.10 ESTIMATED NUMBER OF VETERANS BY ERA IN 2016

ERA SERVED	NUMBER OF VETERANS
World War II	299,800
Korean War	1,019,000
Vietnam War	6,058,000
Gulf War – Pre-9/11	2,555,000
Gulf War Post-9/11 (includes OIF/OEF and OND)	3,429,000
Peacetime	4,159,000

OEF, Operation Enduring Freedom; OIF, Operation Iraqi Freedom; OND, Operation New Dawn.

SOURCE: Adapted from U.S. Department of Veterans Affairs. National Center for Veterans Analysis and Statistics. (2019a). *Veteran population. Tables. The nation. Period served. Table 2L: VetPop2016 living veterans by period of service, gender, 2015–2045.* Retrieved May 22, 2019 from https://www.va.gov/vetdata/Veteran_Population.asp

Veterans

Veterans in today's society represent service members who served as far back as WWII. While the number of WWII veterans is diminishing quickly, the number of Gulf War and Post-9/11 veterans, which includes Operation Iraqui Freedom and Operation Enduring Freedom veterans, is rapidly growing (VA, 2019a). Just over 1 million Korean War Era veterans and 6 million Vietnam War Era veterans are comprised in the over 18 million veterans living in the United States (VA, 2019b). Table 2.10 provides a snapshot of the number of veterans in the United States in 2016 by era served. Of note, for those who served in both war and peacetime, they are counted in the war time category. For those who served during more than one era, they too are only counted in the last served era.

Based on a Pew Research Report, the majority of veterans surveyed (68%) say they have felt proud of their military service (Igielnik, 2019). In comparing Pre-9/11 and Post-9/11 veterans, Pre-9/11 (70%) were more likely to say they frequently felt proud of their service compared to Post-9/11 veterans (58%). About eight out of ten veterans said they would advise a young person close to them to join the military, despite experiencing combat or traumatic events during time in the service (Igielnik, 2019). More than twice as many Post-9/11 veterans (47%) reported the transition to civilian life as very or somewhat difficult compared to only 21% of Pre-9/11 veterans. Further, Pre-9/11 veterans felt the transition to the civilian life was easy (78%), creating a large divide among the veteran population (Igielnik, 2019).

VETERAN IDENTITY

Upon leaving military service, individuals may maintain a part of their self-concept or identity that aligns with the values and beliefs of the military. Veteran identity can be influenced by a number of factors such as serving in a politically controversial war/conflict (Vietnam, OEF, or OIF) or during peacetime, participating in combat, or having a negative experience associated with trauma or some type of discrimination (Hack et al., 2017). Person-level traits such as gender, race, ethnicity, sexual orientation, or being born outside the United States may also affect veteran identity. Suzuki and Kawakami (2016) found that veterans reintegrating into civilian life begin to feel cognitive dissonance as they start to recognize that values and behaviors from the military are no longer effective in pursuit of their values in civilian life. Atuel and Castro (2018) postulate that past military experiences function to help people see who they are and who they are not within a civilian society. In some cases, the "warrior" identity can heighten the differences between civilians and veterans, which can slow or prevent full reintegration (Atuel & Castro, 2018). How a veteran views their military service can be important to establishing a trusting patient-provider relationship (Smith & True, 2014).

CULTURAL ASSESSMENT FOR HEALTHCARE PROVIDERS

Across disciplines, a major focus is placed on becoming knowledgeable about military culture. Developing cultural humility, sensitivity, and competence are essential to achieving patient-centered care. A number of research groups are working on the development of scales and models to assist in providing a framework for which to measure knowledge, skills, and attitudes (KSA) or to underpin research studies focusing on the military/veteran population. These are outlined in Table 2.11.

The Military and Veteran Family Cultural Competency Model (Figure 2.1) developed by Tam-Seto et al. (2019) provides a holistic model in which to approach service members, veterans, and their families. The authors offer a number of applications/uses for the model, which include development of education for healthcare providers and educators, curricular development, as well as informing policy related to the provision of care for this population.

Purnell (2014) has developed a model that is broad and pertains to general cultural competence, which can also be utilized as a framework for research and practice with the military/veteran population. With more veterans seeking care outside military health systems and VA facilities, nurses and healthcare providers need to be prepared to care for diverse populations with health issues that may differ from the larger society (Betancourt et al., 2005). Providing culturally competent care links to quality and ultimately patient satisfaction, which has become a major focus in today's healthcare arena. Further, developing cultural competence may reduce healthcare disparities (Betancourt et al., 2005). For nurses, providing culturally congruent care aligns with the American Nurses Association's Scope and Standards of Practice (Marion et al., 2016).

Communication

Being in the military requires learning a new language, such as a phonetic alphabet, acronyms, and lingo/jargon that varies from the everyday linguistic style used in civilian life. This language is in part a necessity to communicate information in a clear and expedient manner. Communication is also hierarchical, or from the top of the chain of command to the bottom (Hamaoka et al., 2014; Howe & Shpeer, 2019),

TABLE 2.11 SCALES AND MODELS FOR RESEARCH WITH MILITARY/VETERAN POPULATIONS

AUTHOR	NAME OF TOOL	DISCIPLINE/ ORIGINATION	DESCRIPTION
Meyer et al. (2015)	AMCC	Psychology/United States	AMCC scale is used to measure KSA related to military cultural competence
Nedegaard and Zwilling (2017)	MCCP Assessment Scale	Social Sciences/ United States	MCCP Assessment Scale measures knowledge/awareness and confidence in skills and abilities related to military culture
Knopf-Amelung et al. (2018)	HPATV Scale	Nursing/United States	HPATV measures attitudes related to military cultural sensitivity and awareness, provision of care to veterans, and veterans' health issues
Weiss et al. (2019)	TCLS	Social Work/United States	TCSL measures how well a service member is transitioning to civilian life
Tam-Seto et al. (2019)	MVF-CCM	Psychology/Canada	MVF-CCM is a framework that can be utilized to guide development of a culturally competent healthcare curricula, continuing education, or clinical practice that focuses on military/veterans and their families

AMCC, Assessment of Military Cultural Competence; HPATV, Health Professionals' Attitudes Toward Veterans; KSA, knowledge, skills, and attitudes; MCCP, Military Culture Certificate Program; MVF-CCM, Military and Veteran Family Cultural Competency Model; TCLS, Transition to Civilian Life Scale.

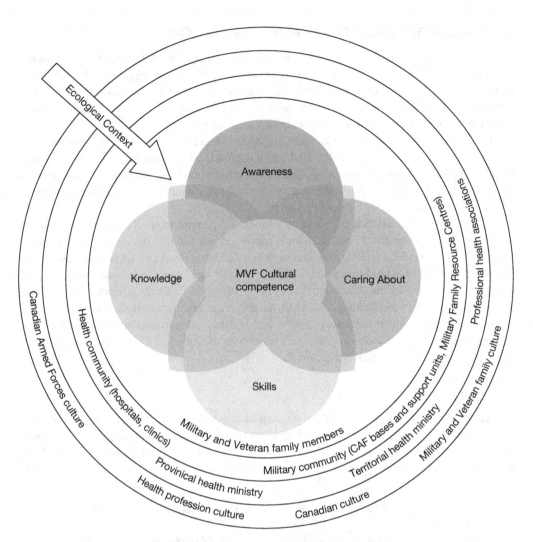

FIGURE 2.1 Military and Veteran Family Cultural Competency Model.

CAF, Canadian Armed Forces; MVF, Military and Veteran Family.

SOURCE: Reproduced from Tam-Seto, L., Krupa, T., Stuart, H., Lingley-Pottie, P., Aiken, A., & Cramm, H. (2019). The validation of the Military and Veteran Family Cultural Competency Model (MVF-CCM). *Military Behavioral Health*, 8, 1–13. https://doi.org/10.1080/21635781.2019.1689875 with permission from Taylor & Francis Group; www.tandfonline.com

with upward communication discouraged. Having an understanding of how communication works within the military can assist others, particularly healthcare providers or educators, in understanding the communication patterns of service members and veterans. This would include both how they prefer to receive communication and how they communicate with others. Examples of how this communication can be understood will be highlighted from two bodies of research, higher education and healthcare.

HIGHER EDUCATION

Chargualaf et al. (2017) conducted a study of 13 military nurse officers (MNOs) transitioning from the military to nurse faculty positions and found that not only did participants discuss significant cultural differences between the military and academia, they also identified communication as a challenge. Through the sub-theme of *recognizing patterns of communication*, participants described how communication and language used in the military differed from an academic setting. While MNOs valued their perceived strength in clear, direct communication, they acknowledged the need to adjust how they communicated to successfully converge into a new workplace (Chargualaf et al., 2017).

In a study by Patterson et al. (2019a), 11 student veterans shared their experiences transitioning from the military to nursing education. Findings from the study support how this group of students transfer core values engrained during military service into their education. Further, *learning how and when to communicate with faculty and healthcare providers* exemplifies that even in this situation, service members must consciously adapt to a new setting. Participants in the study described how to communicate professionally, in a direct manner, and how to use their voice to advocate for patients (Patterson et al., 2019a). This demonstrates that while military service members may enter civilian life with a different style of communication, they can adapt and utilize many patterns learned in the military later in their lives.

Using Communication Accommodation Theory, Howe and Shpeer (2019) investigated the transition experience of 20 veterans to higher education. Represented by three themes, *Culture Clash*, *Perspective Taking*, and *Self-Silencing*, various communication behaviors are seen. These behaviors highlight the communication challenges and ways in which veterans diverge or converge their communication after exiting the military (Howe & Shpeer, 2019). The researchers found that veterans tend to evaluate civilian style of communication through military standards and expectations, which often takes time for them to overcome the frustration they experience during interactions. Through this research, one can glean an appreciation and understanding of how some students are successful in converging into the academic setting and why others opt to "endure" or diverge. The danger in continued self-silencing is that it can lead to diverging communication behaviors, such as verbal conflict (Howe & Shpeer, 2019). Overall, the study findings can assist in understanding a veteran's transition of communication from the military to civilian life and can help inform and explain behaviors faculty may encounter.

HEALTHCARE

Transitioning from the military healthcare system to the VA or other civilian providers may be a deterrent for veterans due to a perception that these facilities lack the same structure and ability to provide effective care (Nworah et al., 2018). Communication plays a big role in the patient–provider relationship and in the case of military service members, veterans, and their families, having knowledge about military culture and lifestyle is necessary. Koenig et al. (2014) suggested that inquiring about what they believe and value from their military service may be useful in establishing rapport, especially if the provider is able to help them apply these beliefs/values positively in civilian life. Veterans appreciate honest, open communication, even if the provider is uncertain of the cause of symptomology. In a study of veterans with medically unexplained symptoms, providers who discussed uncertainty as well as why a more certain explanation for symptoms is not possible (or necessary for treatment), promoted treatment adherence and trust (Phillips et al., 2017). In this study, the researchers found that communication skills were more important to treatment adherence and adherence intention than interpersonal skills (Phillips et al., 2017).

Despite the care setting, the literature supports that veterans give respect and are more likely to adhere to medical instruction if they are treated with respect (Ganzini et al., 2013; Weber et al., 2020). In a study evaluating 34 OEF/OIF veterans' perceptions of the suicide screening and risk assessment process, the researchers found that provider genuineness and empathy, use of understandable and clear language, providing information on the rationale and goals of screening, and attempts to present questions in a personal context (not a medical context) may create more trust and willingness of veterans to disclosing thoughts (Ganzini et al., 2013). Box 2.1 provides a list of recommended empirical studies that further detail ways to improve communication with veteran patients.

BOX 2.1

RECOMMENDED READINGS FOCUSED ON COMMUNICATING WITH VETERANS

Ganzini, L., Denneson, L. M., Press, N., Bair, M. J., Helmer, D. A., Poat, J., & Dobsha, S. K. (2013). Trust is the basis for effective suicide risk screening and assessment in veterans. *Journal of General Internal Medicine, 28*, 1215–1221. https://doi.org/10.1007/s11606-013-2412-6

Howren, M. B., Cozad, A. J., & Kaboli, P. J. (2015). Considering the issue of dual use in Veterans Affairs patients: Implications and opportunities for improved communication and counseling. *Health Communication, 30*, 838–842. https://doi.org/10.1080/10410236.2014.930299

Koenig, C. J., Maguen, S., Monroy, J. D., Mayott, L., & Seal, K. S. (2014). Facilitating culture-centered communication between health care providers and veterans transitioning from military deployment to civilian life. *Patient Education and Counseling, 95*, 414–420. https://doi.org/10.1016/j.pec.2014.03.016

Phillips, L. A., McAndrew, L., Laman-Maharg, B., & Bloeser, K. (2017). Evaluating challenges for improving medically unexplained symptoms in U.S. military veterans via provider communication. *Patient Education and Counseling, 100*, 1580–1587. https://dx.doi.org/10.1016/j.pec.2017.03.011

In talking with service members and veterans a clinician should:

- be emotionally present and attentive (Coll et al., 2011);

- anticipate issues associated with grief and loss, particularly after deployment or right after separation from the service (Coll et al., 2011);

- communicate in a straightforward, clear, understandable, and non-ambiguous manner; be nice and respectful (Ganzini et al., 2013);

- communicate in a direct, clear, necessary, and respectful way (Howe & Shpeer, 2019); and

- use questioning that elicits conservation about challenges, fosters growth, and/or promotes advice giving (Koenig et al., 2014).

Communication is a vital part of providing quality nursing care. It is for that reason the differences between military style communication and what is generally seen outside of the military is highlighted. Koenig et al. (2014) summed it up by suggesting that sometimes providers must change the message veterans hear; that soliciting advice from this population may lead to posttraumatic growth for those who have had negative experiences. It is through these minor alterations in communication that we may be able to connect and engage successfully with service members and veterans.

IMPLICATIONS FOR NURSING EDUCATION AND PRACTICE

Hack et al. (2017) postulated that healthcare providers striving to provide patient-centered, culturally competent care must consider the "many identities consumers can hold, their complexities, and how views of those identities influence their health and experiences in care" (p. 729). In addition, they must recognize the range of experiences during military service among veterans as some may continue to align with the military culture and other may distance themselves more (Coll et al., 2011). Gaining an understanding of how military cultural factors may affect self-stigma and its consequences can arm nurses with essential knowledge to provide culturally sensitive care (Harding, 2017). Applying the Giger and Davidhizar Model of Transcultural Nursing to veteran culture provides an exemplar on how

TABLE 2.12 EDUCATION RESOURCES TO LEARN ABOUT MILITARY CULTURE

RESOURCE	DESCRIPTION AND WEB LINK
Uniformed Services University, Center for Deployment Psychology	Military Culture Course Modules deploymentpsych.org/military-culture-course-modules
U.S. Department of Veterans Affairs	Community Provider Toolkit www.mentalhealth.va.gov/communityproviders/ military_culture.asp
PsychArmor Institute	Online Training for Engaging the Military Community psycharmor.org/military-culture-school/

to change approaches to practice to reduce stigma and develop interventions that take culture into consideration (Harding, 2017).

Based on a systematic review conducted by Beach et al. (2005), evidence supports that cultural competence training improves the Knowledge, skills, and abilities (KSAs) of health professionals. As presented in this chapter, military culture plays a major role in the lives of those who serve and their families. Nurses and healthcare providers are encouraged to seek resources to improve basic knowledge about military culture (Table 2.12). Further, to enhance KSAs, the Military and Veteran Family Cultural Competency Framework (Exhibit 2.3) developed by Tam-Seto et al. (2019) is an excellent resource to inform a military-/veteran-centered practice. Through a family approach, the authors have developed a holistic framework useful in all care settings.

Nursing Practice

Nurses in practice will encounter service members, veterans, and their family members. A major challenge they may face beyond what has been discussed is caring for veterans who receive both VA and non-VA healthcare. Coordination and communication of care in these instances can be very difficult (Elliott, 2019b). In these cases, careful consideration and effort should be taken to reduce duplication in services. Interestingly, in one study of dual healthcare use among veterans (who use both VA and civilian providers), researchers found almost half considered communication between VA and civilian providers their own responsibility (Howren et al., 2015). This indicates that providers should approach veterans about communication preferences as they may facilitate improved care coordination, collaboration, and outcomes for those willing to take ownership of this aspect of care.

Nursing Education

A number of implications exist for nurse educators, both academic and clinically based. First, nurse educators need to examine their own biases that may influence their teaching practice or ability to facilitate learning about this population with students. Second, acquisition of knowledge and skills in the care of military service members, and their families is needed, especially in relation to military culture. Third, faculty need to examine the course(s) they teach and look for ways to integrate content about this population into lectures and classroom activities, followed by specific clinical experiences that will aid in the development of basic competency. Brommelsiek et al. (2018) offer an interprofessional education course and practicum that can serve as an example of not only improving veteran-centered care, but also improving interprofessional practice. Lastly, nurse educators need to evaluate learning to ensure that translation to practice is achieved.

In consideration for student veterans who enter into nursing education, faculty are encouraged to learn about how the military culture can influence this transition and ways in which they can facilitate success (Patterson et al., 2019b). Faculty must also seek ways to improve teaching practices that enhance transfer of learning for this student population (Patterson et al., 2019a). Understanding the impact of invisible wounds, or disabilities, is critical to recognizing student veterans who may be

EXHIBIT 2.3

MILITARY AND VETERAN FAMILY CULTURAL COMPETENCY FRAMEWORK

Awareness
(Internal process; the cognitive acknowledgement of the cultural group)

- Recognizes that military life can affect the health and well-being of military and Veteran families across the life span.
- Reflects on his/her own perceptions, opinions, assumptions, and biases towards the Canadian Armed Forces and military and Veteran families.
- Recognizes that perceptions, opinions, assumptions, and biases towards military and Veteran families may influence the healthcare relationship.
- Engages in ongoing self-reflection, humility, and openness.

Caring about
(Internal process; the emotional acknowledgement of the healthcare realities of the cultural group)

- Is motivated to provide culturally informed health care to military and Veteran families.
- Is motivated to develop cultural knowledge to enhance healthcare for military and Veteran families.
- Is motivated to develop cultural skills to enhance healthcare for military and Veteran families.
- Is sensitive to how military family life events may affect health and health system access.

Knowledge
(Specific health-related knowledge about members of the cultural group)

- Understands that frequent family moves have potential impacts on the health and well-being of military and Veteran family members due to challenges with access and continuity of care
- Understands that familial separation and reintegration due to training and deployment have potential impacts on the health and well-being of military and Veteran family members
- Understands the potential health impacts for military and Veteran families who live everyday with the stress caused by the risk of injury or death of military member.
- Understands that military and Veteran families are at increased risk for certain health conditions and challenges.
- Understands health conditions common among military members and Veterans and how this may impact on the health and well-being of family members.
- Is aware of community resources and supports that supplement and potentially benefit the healthcare of military and Veteran families.

Skills
(Culturally-informed acts used during health care interactions)

- Engages military and Veteran families in an empathetic and non-judgemental manner.
- Engages military and Veteran families in a collaborative, strength-based manner.
- Addresses health concerns as a result of military family life events such as mobility and familial separation.
- Addresses health concerns experienced by military and Veteran family members that emerge as a result of the health and well-being of military/Veteran member.
- Demonstrates flexibility, creativity and support to address health access and system navigation challenges experienced by military and Veteran families.
- Demonstrates awareness, sensitivity, and knowledge of military family life.
- Collaborates with community agencies to support health and well-being of military and Veteran families.
- Demonstrates willingness and openness to learn and further develop skills as a means of enhancing the healthcare experiences of military and Veteran family members.
- Demonstrates professionalism that reflects respect for military culture and unique military family life experiences.
- Evaluates own practice to strive towards equitable access for military and Veteran families.
- Advocates for equitable access to healthcare servies for military and Veteran families.

SOURCE: Reproduced from Tam-Seto, L., Krupa, T., Stuart, H., Lingley-Pottie, P., Aiken, A., & Cramm, H. (2019). The validation of the Military and Veteran Family Cultural Competency Model (MVF-CCM). *Military Behavioral Health*, 8, 1–13. https://doi.org/10.1080/21635781.2019.1689875 with permission from Taylor & Francis Group; www.tandfonline.com

struggling and need additional resources (Flink, 2017). And knowing what resources are available to the student veteran population on campus cannot be understated (Patterson et al., 2019b).

FUTURE RESEARCH PRIORITIES

From a nursing perspective the research priorities seem endless. While empirical studies are starting to emerge and frameworks become available to guide research, much work is yet to be done.

Interventions and teaching strategies aimed at enhancing the cultural competency of nurses and nursing students need to be developed and evaluated so best practices can be established. Research is needed to understand the impact of stigma and disabilities student veterans in nursing education may face. Considering the importance of communication in engaging this population, strategies to improve nurses' communication techniques may be needed. In addition, communication strategies to improve coordination of care between VA and non-VA healthcare settings is vital to ensuring the safe delivery of nursing practice.

CONCLUSION

Military service can have a profound influence on those who serve and their families. This influence can stay with a person for a lifetime. What is important to remember is that the military experience is different for everyone. When entering into the military, individuals are faced with a cultural transition for which they then transition out of years later (Suzuki & Kawakami, 2016). For some, the time in between entering and exiting the military may be short (less than 4 years) and for other it could be 30 years. The experiences each individual has while in the military can shape their future identity and impact health behaviors. Having an understanding of military culture, lifestyle, health concerns for this population, and resources both inside and outside the VA, are paramount to the delivery of patient-centered and culturally sensitive care. As healthcare providers we must avoid making assumptions that all service members, thus veterans, have mental health issues or PTSD. We must advocate for improvements in healthcare delivery within our healthcare facilities. Our nation's military are our nation's veterans and they are deserving of our time and care.

REFERENCES

The complete reference list for this chapter appears in the digital version of the chapter, accessible at https://connect.springerpub.com/content/book/978-0-8261-3597-1/chapter/ch02

UNDERSTANDING THE COMPLEXITIES OF MILITARY TRANSITIONS

Service Member Deployment and Veteran Integration

DONNA M. LAKE | MYRNA L. ARMSTRONG

On the battlefield, the military pledges to leave no soldier behind. As a nation, let it be our pledge that when they return home, we leave no veteran behind.

Dan Lipinski

KEY TERMS

military service member	employment
veteran	education
deployment	caregiving
reintegration	Ecological Model of Veteran Reintegration

INTRODUCTION

Both full-time military service members (MSMs) and part-time Reserve and National Guard component (RC) personnel face multiple transitions related to training, education, deployments, and reintegration to accomplish the Armed Force's missions. This chapter focuses on the latter transitions. Information is provided about the physical, behavioral, and social impacts during the various stages of deployment for the MSM/RC, along with their families/loved ones. With the complex process for veterans to reintegrate into the civilian sector, the Ecological Model of Veteran Reintegration and its four levels of system factors—(a) individual, (b) interpersonal, (c) community organizations, and (d) societal effects—are used to illustrate the interchanging psychosocial and environmental aspects. Specific reintegration challenges of employment, education, and caregiving are also presented. Nurses have a pivotal role in screening psychosocial and physical needs, while promoting healthy coping and parenting, to expand the delivery of family-centered care during these transitions.

The complete reference list for this chapter appears in the digital version of the chapter, accessible at https://connect.springerpub.com/content/book/978-0-8261-3597-1/chapter/ch03

BACKGROUND

Being in the military is tough! Becoming an applicant for any branch of the military presently is difficult with only around 29% able to qualify for the intense readiness criterion (Department of Defense [DoD], 2017). Once accepted, MSMs complete the necessary skills, education, training, and leadership qualifications to face multiple physical and psychosocial transitions throughout their military journey for the fulfillment of their role, whatever the Armed Forces mission. Core values (honor, courage, loyalty, integrity, and commitment) are required, as well as specific standards of conduct such as obedience. Enculturation into the service will also mean there are strong structured criterion expected for both the MSM and their accompanying families/loved ones, regardless of their location, whether within the military unit or the military home (Hall, 2011). When their formative education is completed, MSMs can start meeting the qualifications for promotion to higher rank while they also respond to their ordered missions. These missions might entail encounters with frequent life-changing cross-cultural transitions, moving back and forth from dangerous deployments to subsequent non-deployment circumstances, throughout their career. Later, another major transitional event is the MSM's reintegration into the civilian community, whether it is viewed as returning or re-entering society after they leave the military. Both of these transitions demand equal vigor as they impact MSM, as well as their families and loved ones (Kintzle & Castro, 2018).

Research is providing a better understanding of the complex challenges the MSM and veteran face with these transitional phases (Elnitsky et al., 2017b). This chapter includes a presentation of the dynamism and strength that is needed surrounding both the MSM's deployment, as well as their reintegration into the civilian sector, followed by an emphasis of the pivotal role nursing can have on both of these transitions. Information about the two groups of MSM will be interwoven within this chapter. The first group is employed in the military on a full-time basis with obligations to the service 24 hours a day, 7 days a week; they are always on an Active Duty status. As the military personnel mission can have either a national or international focus, deployments, especially for full-time personnel, can mean there are "frequent separations, regular household relocations, the need to adapt to rigidity, regimentation, and conformity, [concerns of loss at any time, lack of control], and possible detachment from the mainstream of nonmilitary life such as the MSM's family relatives" (Hall, 2011, p. 7). The other group is the part-time MSM of the RC/National Guard component, training on a limited basis (minimum 39 days, most often as one weekend per month plus an additional 2 weeks); when they are deployed they are placed on Active Duty and assume the same responsibilities as the full-time service member (Werber et al., 2013). After the RC deployment is completed, they return to a part time military status until their next deployment. This information on both groups of military personnel should alert the health professional team, particularly nurses who conduct screening and are involved in the care of the MSM, veteran, and/or their family/loved ones, as to what psychosocial and physical needs are present for delivery of family-centered care.

Being a military spouse (93% are women) can be demanding, although they are greatly valued for being the cornerstone of the family unit as the MSM is subject to deployments at any time (Keeling et al., 2019). While there are limited studies on the quality of military life for spouses, Keeling et al. (2019) cited one with a strong associated relationship between the MSM health and the spouse: If one was healthy, the other usually was also, or vice versa. Historically, spouses seeking employment during the MSM military career are often met with disadvantages of frequent relocations, few childcare resources, limited labor markets, and/or employer discrimination. On-line resources have assisted with previous limited education opportunities. More opportunities are slowly being pursued nationally to correct these circumstances (Keeling et al., 2019).

Recognizing that every reader has varying understanding of military terminology, the definition of terms and concepts used in this chapter are further explained:

- **Deployment:** under the direction of their leaders and orders, MSMs complete all role and duty responsibilities to accomplish a specific mission in a prescribed location, including gathering and/or distributing troops, weapons, and various other resources. Types of deployment may be war/conflict environments, peacekeeping, global humanitarian events, and/or natural disasters.

- **Discharge:** every service member (full time or part time) eventually leaves the military. MSM receive a military discharge which, upon receipt, signifies complete severance from all military status gained by an enlistment or commission (Newman, 2010). While most discharges are voluntary, unplanned discharge could be from a "reduction in force, injuries, or other than honorable discharge due to negative physical and behavioral health outcomes ... subsequentially these MSM could feel anger at their forced transition" (Kintzle & Castro, 2018, p. 120). Of the five different types of discharges, the three most common are:

  - **General discharge under honorable conditions:** performance was satisfactory and eligible for most military/veteran benefits except education.

  - **Honorable discharge:** completes duty with admirable personal and professional conduct and is eligible for all military/veteran benefits including education (Newman, 2010).

  - **Medical discharge:** when a service member becomes sick or injured to the point where military duty is no longer possible based on a military medical evaluation. This can occur at any time during their military journey; they are eligible for all military/veteran benefits.

- **MSM:** personnel who serve in the United States Armed Forces to include the full-time and the part time RC.

- **Reintegration:** both a process and outcome of resuming MSM life roles as civilians in the family, community, and society. Full-Time Active Duty personnel begin reintegration when they are discharged and/or retired from the military and become a veteran. Part-time RC personnel encounter reintegration every time they return from deployment, re-entering the community/society as civilians.

- **Separation:** a general term depending on the type of military personnel. For someone in the RC who had been "called-up" or "activated" (placed on Active Duty), they are released from Active Duty ("deactivated") and return to their part-time military status again as a RC member after completing their role and/or mission. For full-time MSM, this term often refers to totally leaving the service either discharged and/or retired following their fulfillment of their enlistment or resigning their commission.

- **Veteran:** former member of the United States Armed Forces. RC do not become a veteran with the potential of receiving any benefits until they have officially served over 30 days of Active Duty. Enlisted RC personnel almost always have more than 30 days of active duty as a result of the time required for Basic Training. RC Officer's Basic Training is typically 2 weeks (Medical, Judge Advocate General, Chaplains). Historically, there could be some RC that did not receive official veteran status.

MILITARY CULTURE

The culture of the military can have a profound effect on those who serve, including their families. To illustrate this, two major areas of military culture that affect deployment and reintegration are first presented to emphasize the impact they will have for the MSM. Inherent in this culture are obedience as a standard of conduct and adherence to mission as the ultimate goal of the military; these commitments "regulate [the MSM and family/loved ones] lives on and off duty on a daily basis ... the MSM must be ready at all times to carry out these prioritizations" (Coll et al., 2011, p. 488). Adherence to direct orders also provides little to no individual autonomy. Instead it includes strong reliance on a trusting dependence on their fellow troops demonstrating the willingness to commit to a larger purpose than self (Coll et al., 2011; Hall, 2011). Missions for RC personnel are not as stringent, as their families remain at their permanent residence, although the MSM can still be sent to national and/or international deployment locations. Additionally, the National Guard MSM are subject to their state Governor's mission demands, with possible deployments for local, regional, or even designated national humanitarian events, and/or natural disaster situations.

Another cultural factor is the distinctive military system of the officer and enlisted personnel roles and rank structure (Hall, 2011). While both systems will often be accomplishing the same mission in the same location, their responsibilities and roles will differ to achieve the task. Usually enlisted MSM operate and maintain technical equipment and sustain support activities while officers plan, organize, and lead troops, along with the provision of professional services (Coll et al., 2011). As the process and outcomes of deployment and reintegration transitions are explained within this chapter, the nurse should be aware that the lifestyles and experiences of the officer and enlisted personnel will vary according to their military expectations and what they encountered during their service time.

DEPLOYMENT

Each service branch, whether full time or RC, have different missions and requirements with varied deployment timeframes, dependent on project needs. To accomplish the various types of assignments (mission and/or roles) the military completes, they commonly use the term "deployment" for the MSM readiness, whether for personal preparation or for their unit. Service branches (Army, Navy, Marines, Air Force, or Coast Guard) provide some type of standard military order process with specific instructions for the location, mission, timeframe (months or 1 year), personal training needs (e.g., chemical warfare training, firearm safety/recertification), family service requirements (e.g., wills, advance directives), and medical preparation (immunization, medical clearance).

Full-time personnel train approximately 240 days per year, whereas RC may or may not work in the same position of their civilian role and training time in their military occupation may average 39 days annually. While healthcare providers usually are working within their chosen role, others (e.g., infantry) may develop skill decay, where aptitude and unused knowledge result in an inability to produce effective responses in the time needed. To combat this problem when deployments are considered for RC units, training time is increased, but this can sometimes lead to cognitive overload, when RC or MSM are provided far more information in a short time exceeding memory capabilities and effective learning (Werber et al., 2013). Another major difference is employment, with full-time personnel consistently paid by the military throughout their service obligation. In contrast, RC personnel often have full-time civilian employment and their employers need to be aware of their employee's military obligations, especially sudden exits for deployments and/or expectations for extra training activities. In addition, trying to interchange military and civilian salary systems to ensure consistent distribution in the appropriate amount during deployment can be arduous (Werber et al., 2013).

During 2001 and then spanning over the next 18 years, more than 2.6 million U.S. MSM were issued military orders to deploy in support of Operation Enduring Freedom (OEF), Operation Iraqi Freedom (OIF), Operation New Dawn (OND), and/or for the reduction ("drawdown") of forces in Iraq and Afghanistan (Statista, 2019). Simultaneously, there were over 37 U.S. special counterterrorism missions carried out under Congressional authorization to prevent further 9/11-type attacks in 14 various hostile isolated countries, such as the Philippines, Yemen, Horn of Africa, Syria, as well as the high seas surrounding Europe and Asia (Congressional Record, 2001; Weed, 2016). At any one time, thousands of American troops can be stationed in non-combat sites globally, such as Japan (>63,000), Germany (>46,000), South Korea (>29,000), Italy (>15,000), and the United Kingdom (>10,000; Statista, 2019).

While all MSM in the Iraq/Afghanistan wars were on Active Duty at the time of deployment and usually served in increments of 12 to 18 months, over 1.37 million MSM were full-time personnel. The Army provided almost 60% of the total deployments since Post-9/11, as well as the Navy (15%), the Air Force (15%), and the Marine Corp (12%; Wenger et al., 2018). In addition, there were over 1.1 million more MSM, who were originally part-time RC that fulfilled their roles and responsibilities as Active Duty personnel during these deployments. This RC cohort tended to be older, married, parents when compared to their full-time military counterparts (Messecar, 2017). Regardless of status during the Iraq/Afghanistan wars many full-time personnel and RC served more than one deployment, in combat situations, with only short periods of time between their deployments (Messecar, 2017). Further, more than 90,000 (6.5%) full-time MSM were married to another active duty member (Danish & Antonides, 2013; DoD, 2012), with the Air Force having the highest number (27,000 Active Duty MSM, 10%). Military policy considers married couples as two separate individuals, notwithstanding living arrangements, which could present separation stressors when children are involved (Mixon, 2013).

Stages of Deployment

The following brief descriptions of deployment phases are presented to illustrate the general activities of the full-time military personnel, as well as any differences the part-time RC may experience during these transitional phases. This further understanding of the military culture and operations will assist with the subsequent physical, mental, and social impacts of deployment transitions for either type of MSM and their families/loved ones (Pincus et al., 2019). One of the most important tools for deployment assistance is providing information through a variety of sources so family members have some idea of what to expect and types of available resources (Pincus et al., 2019). Other family support ideas during deployment include networking opportunities, supporting regular "day out" opportunities for military spouses, establishing communication trees, and discussing the concern of overspending and/or increased alcohol use to overcome stress while the MSM is gone (Pincus et al., 2019). Deployments also affect the MSM's family/loved ones as they go through their own adjustments of intensiveness, anxiety, and separation, with attempts to settle into a new "normal" routine. The spouse/significant other staying behind will now become the sole head of the household, which could be challenging.

The **Pre-Deployment Phase** includes the first notification that a deployment could/will occur. This process could be initiated up to 6 months or less than 48 hours prior to deployment and may include an individual, a small team of troops, or a complete unit. This is a hectic alert time, directed toward completion of intense readiness checklists, concentrated training sessions, financial/family household preparedness, including signing off on death benefit paperwork, and/or possible relocation of family members to another location to stabilize support systems. At this time MSM and families are also busy preparing and lining-up resources, ensuring that all general and detailed plans are in place during the deployment timeframe. What can be problematic during this time is for the MSM and the family/loved ones to focus on all of the details of the dates of departure, the mission, and the specific tasks, as often they are in constant flux; the orders even may be cancelled (Pincus et al., 2019). Rumors run rampant (Pincus et al., 2019). Flexibility and patience during this chaotic period is very difficult for everyone.

The **Deployment Phase** starts when the MSM actually departs from their duty station (local military location). Full-time MSM orders often include a large contingent of troops that are deployed at the same time producing an esprit de corps within the group when they arrive at their newly assigned duty station for the stated mission. Deployment action plans are often designed to be acted upon swiftly and accomplish tasks quickly. Thus, the MSM performing their assigned roles are often lacking in sleep and proper nutrition, are in a constant hyper alert state, and are within unfamiliar circumstances (Werber et al., 2013). Combat experience heightens the situation of being away from your homeland: "spending endless hours in a miserable work environment … punctuated by moments of transcendental terror and unimaginable, horrific destruction of human life and property, [producing] the belief that no one leaves combat without incurring profound physical, psychological and emotional changes" (Coll et al., 2011, p. 491).

During the Iraq/Afghanistan wars, some personnel often found themselves being individually deployed to fulfill an unoccupied position within a team of already deployed MSM. Deploying individually versus within a team may occur with certain military occupations and RC, such as medical personnel and chaplains. For example, security forces deploy together and already have a strong collective alliance as part of a cohesive unit who have trained together as a team. Lack of unit team cohesiveness is problematic, resulting in residual behavioral health issues (Werber et al., 2013).

During this time of deployment, change is inevitable. There can be "major shifts in U.S. foreign policy and the [service branch] roles in extended multinational deployments," creating demands for new skills and longer (and more frequent) commitment requirements (Pincus et al., 2019, p. 2), as well as further impact for the families/loved ones left behind. Everyone, including the MSM, spouse, and children, begins to adjust and grow, whether in dependence or interdependence (Pincus et al., 2019). The military spouse is now "single" and often dealing with children missing the other parent and displaying acting out behaviors or school challenges; as well, they often need respite time without their children for a "day out" (Pincus et al., 2019). Marital/relationship issues that were present pre-deployment are usually not resolved during this time and are often exacerbated. Disrupted family roles, alliances, and routines during the deployment may be difficult to reinstate upon the MSM's return (Brenner & Bahraini, 2019). This can lead to marital dysfunction, parenting changes, and relationship disorders (Allen et al., 2012).

The impact of deployment on military families, specifically the longitudinal data demonstrates an estimate of 300,000 families, including 700,000 children, have been affected by deployments and repeated deployments in support of the Iraqi and Afghanistan wars since 2001 (Agazio et al., 2014). This research team found that families organize themselves for deployment separation in a general process of preparation, survival, and reunion. Additional findings include that the school-age children and adolescents try to demonstrate resiliency overall, which serves as a protective factor, whereas deployments may impact development of younger children and relationship maintenance in the case of an absent parent (Agazio et al., 2014). School-age children may also exhibit behavioral or academic problems in response to the deployment. In their systematic review of nine studies of military children, de Burgh et al. (2011) confirmed that "children of deployed parents are at higher risk than their civilian counterparts, which may reflect the multiple stressors that military children face" (p. 211). The DoD Profile Report (2010) found adolescents may have "more depressive symptoms, decreased academic performance, and peer relationship problems related to parental deployments" compared to adolescents from non-military families (p. 21). Nurses will need to be attentive during pediatric screenings for the effects of military deployment on children, especially preschoolers with higher emotional reactivity, increased temper tantrums, change in eating or sleeping patterns, or increased somatic complaints. This timeframe for many young adults in the military is also stressful, especially those who are away from extended family, as they parent young children, or are simultaneously balancing the demands of working and/or going to school (Elnitsky & Kilmer, 2017). This has affected over 23,000 U.S. military families currently on support programs such as the Supplemental Nutrition Assistance Program benefit (Bushatz, 2018; Jennings & Cai, 2018).

Referrals through service branch specific post-deployment readiness programs can provide resources to assist families during deployment (Messecar, 2017; Werber et al., 2013). They include several military family support agencies/programs such as the DoD military command headquarters, installation, unit, medical center outreach, chaplain support, and/or schools, as well as area communities/schools. RC families may be more reluctant to reach out during deployments as often the distance, time, and complexity of a large bureaucratic military base hinders their exploration for assistance (Messecar, 2017). Instead, often they return to their civilian community agencies, which may or may not be familiar with their issues or be able to help. It is during this time that they may need the nurse's guidance and encouragement in coordination with the social worker assigned to the military health clinic or hospital to come forward with requests for these service referrals.

The **Reconstitution/Demobilization Phase** typically begins with the completion of the specific military order of the deployment/mission or when incoming replacements have arrived. This immediate post-deployment time is usually conducted at a more secure nonthreatening location where the member can remove their deployment body gear (sometimes weighing as much as 40 lbs), including flak jackets, helmets, and attached "loaded" weapons. They can also begin to slowly re-acclimate their circadian rhythm. Specific experiences include debriefings, transitional programs, counseling, quiet rest/sleep areas in clean housing (tent/hard-shell building) with access to warm showers, three freshly cooked nutritional meals, gym facilities, and completion of an anonymous Post-Deployment Health Assessment screening tool to identify physical and/or psychosocial needs requiring rapid intervention (Warner et al., 2011; Werber et al., 2013). This transitional timeframe could vary greatly, from a few days to 2 weeks, and is also dependent on accessible air transportation back to their home units, whether it be in the United States or a residence internationally due to an overseas assignment. While sounding like a restful time, this can still be an anxious occasion for both the MSM and their families/loved ones as they are all eagerly awaiting the reunion. Many emotions are expressed at this time including excitement, fatigue, anxiety, and even frustration that everything is not happening quickly enough (Werber et al., 2013).

The **Post-Deployment Phase** begins upon return to the home duty station and then usually encompasses the next 180 days. Full-time military members, following family/loved one reunification, report back to their military unit used to dealing with deployment and post-deployment activities, moving forward slowly with further responsibilities in their duty station, surrounded by a familiar military environment, including their steady salary. Dependent on the type of unit and service branch (Army, Navy, Marines, Air Force, Coast Guard), there may be very individualized specific post-deployment events held after the return home to help the members/families re-adjust after separation/re-entry (Doherty & Scannell-Desch, 2017).

For the RC and their family members, this is another time when the deployment phase is different. Often, they left for the deployment alone and many were sent home alone during the Iraq/Afghanistan wars, quite unceremoniously, without closure (Messecar, 2017). Then, while it may seem that returning home can be a joyous celebration, RC often feel the pressure to reintegrate back into their "usual" civilian life again quickly, as they no longer have full-time DoD resource support (Messecar, 2017; Werber et al., 2013). This transition can be especially distressful if they are concerned about effective family reintegration, have to again coordinate regular facilitation of civilian paychecks, while trying to adjust smoothly back into the civilian workplace, and/or student academic settings if they are pursuing advanced education (Messecar, 2017). If RC MSM were exposed to combat, they may face more challenges in post-deployment due to any sustained injuries or trauma, which requires RC rebuilding of self, sense of world, and competence in order to reintegrate again into civilian life (Haynie & Shepherd 2011). Concerned about demonstrating weakness or damage to their career trajectory, often RC are hesitant to seek healthcare in a timely manner (Messecar, 2017). While they do receive 5 years of Veterans Health Administration (VHA) benefits, often the distance, time, complexity of a large bureaucratic health system for appointments, and concern of timely treatments, hinder their motivation to seek care (Conard & Armstrong, 2019). Instead, often they will return to their civilian community facility, although the care provider may or may not be familiar with MSM concerns, or the coordination for VHA that might be assistive to the RC. Depending on their enlistment or commission obligations, they may even decide to request a discharge from their part-time RC activities leaving them even more isolated and alienated of further military support (Hall, 2011).

Behavioral Health Screening

Published literature suggests that many OEF/OIF/OND returnees readjust with little difficulty (Institute of Medicine [IOM], 2014). They are provided proactive education about possible behavioral health concerns often during their deployment, especially during demobilization. An integral part of this adjustment is the MSMs' general coping style with life pressures so reviewing the signs and symptoms about behavioral health concerns with them is paramount (Kintzle & Castro, 2018).

Both Danish and Antonides (2013), as well as Dausch and Saliman (2009), estimated that over 50% of the returning MSM population experienced difficulties transitioning back into their family lives and communities post-deployment. In contrast, Sayer et al. (2015) found that 54% of their OEF/OIF/OND veteran participants reported their deployment difficulties were not fully revealed/exposed/uncovered for almost 6 years after returning from their deployments, or sometimes not even until civilian reintegration (IOM, 2014). With Congressional reduction of more in-patient military medical treatment facilities, nurses in civilian health facilities will be seeing an increased number of MSMs after deployment encountering greater struggles upon returning home to their families (McMillan et al., 2017). The stress and increased distress from any of the deployment phases should always be noted for changes in the behavioral health of the MSM.

At higher risk for emotional and physical consequences are those MSMs exposed to combat, killing, seeing someone killed, encountering an injury/disability, and/or other trauma (IOM, 2013, 2014; Messecar, 2017). Behavioral health difficulties, which may or may not be immediately evident, could range from altered sleep-wake cycles, hyperarousal, or hypervigilance, to alcohol misuse, and various levels of depression. With their higher potential risk of posttraumatic stress disorder (PTSD) conditions, MSMs should be encouraged to proactively seek help as soon as possible instead of waiting to try and rebuild themselves, and their sense of world, when they return back to the United States (Haynie & Shepherd, 2011). If unchecked, the MSMs' holistic functional status is disrupted and their issues may build, lead to chronicity, and produce further problems with each future deployment (Baker, 2014; IOM, 2013, 2014). Another outcome is the higher long-term costs, estimated to be in the billions, for veterans; for example, treatment of PTSD ($6 billion), depression ($1.5 billion), and other service-related comorbidities ($3.1 billion; Vyas et al., 2016). Concerns of behavioral health issue observations that may arise during deployments also apply to MSM healthcare providers as they are not immune to these changes (Swearingen et al., 2017).

Wounded Troop Services

During OEF/OEF/OND remarkable recovery efforts using new protective equipment such as body armor and tourniquets, along with effective inter-/intra-service branch relationships, produced unequaled survival of injured MSMs compared to previous war eras. While this feat is outstanding, there is now work to be accomplished for the increasing amount of veterans with multifaceted injuries returning home that will need intensive amounts of care for the rest of their lives (Baker, 2014; Conard et al., 2017). Costs will also be overwhelming for providing medical care and disability services for these returning OEF/OEF/OND veterans; estimates range around $589 billion to $984 billion (Geiling et al., 2012).

When wounded MSMs return with burns, traumatic brain injuries (TBIs), amputations, and other wounds requiring orthopedic needs, the military has specific facilities that can provide exceptional support and care. One such facility is the Center for the Intrepid at Joint Base San Antonio – Fort Sam Houston (Texas). Here, wounded MSMs receive highly technological evidence-based care for rehabilitation and prosthetics; interprofessional personnel are skilled regarding the latest research, education, and training (Spencer, 2017). Sometimes they use extreme sports activities to amplify their rehabilitation. The goal is to maximize the MSMs' potential and return them into being a fully functioning person, whether back into the fighting force, or home.

To date there are also a large amount of civilian organizations that are providing services to wounded warriors and their families (Charity Navigator, 2018). A variety of services can be arranged, from lifting morale to offering financial assistance for food, rent, utilities, and medical expenses. To assist with an evaluation of these helping organizations, Charity Navigator publishes benchmark measures about transparency, progress, and positive results of their assistance. A published *Guide to Intelligent Giving* (Charity Navigator, 2018) identifies several key organizations and ascribes high star ratings to organizations that demonstrate financial responsibility and a commitment to accountability and transparency with best practices regarding wounded warrior services. The most well-known public program, Wounded Warrior Project, has received a three-star rating from Charity Navigator (2018) for their assistance to raise awareness and enlist the public's aid for the needs of severely injured service men and women.

Their top four-star ratings include the Disabled American Veterans (DAV) Charitable Service Trust that supports physical and psychological rehabilitation programs and other direct services to ill, injured, or wounded veterans (Charity Navigator, 2018). DAV Charitable Service Trust also provides food and shelter to homeless or at-risk veterans, accessibility or mobility items for veterans with vision or hearing impairments, and therapeutic activities. Another organization is Homes for Our Troops, a nonprofit agency that builds and donates specially adapted custom homes nationwide for severely injured Post-9/11 veterans that have sustained injuries including multiple limb amputations, partial or full paralysis, and/or severe TBI (Charity Navigator, 2018). The building of these homes is focused on restoring independence for the veteran, and enabling them to focus on their family, recovery, and rebuilding their lives. The Charity Navigator Guide (2018) also gives the Semper Fi Fund a four-star rating. It provides immediate financial assistance and lifetime support to combat wounded, critically ill, and catastrophically injured members of all branches of the U.S. Armed Forces and their families. Since their founding in 2004, they have assisted 22,000 service members with $185 million in grants to ensure they have the resources they need during their recovery and transition back to their communities.

The Army, Navy, Marine, and Air Force also have organizations that provide wounded warrior programs. They include Operation Second Chance, which provides support for men and women MSM (Army and Marines) while they are at Walter Reed National Medical Center (Maryland) to further assist recovery and rehabilitation when they transition either back to duty or back to civilian life. The Air Force Aid Society relieves financial distress of their service branch members and families, as well as worldwide emergency assistance and higher education goals. In partnership with the Wounded Warrior Program, the Navy Safe Harbor Foundation conducts the Caring for Caregivers Program; to date they have assisted over 7,000 Navy and Coast Guard Sailors who were wounded, ill, or injured (Safe Harbor Foundation, 2019).

Transition to Veteran Status

An ongoing U.S. Department of Veterans Affairs (VA, 2018a) Military to Civilian Transitions report states that every year over 200,000 men and women leave the U.S. military service. Of this number only 17% retire and receive full retirement benefits as civilians, whereas the remaining are discharged (U.S. DoD, 2015). Both discharge and/or retirement from their military obligation begins abruptly the day the MSM is released from their service branch. With the variety of discharge conditions, the emotions starting reintegration can be different, whether the veteran is part of a congressional draw down (reduction of force), obtaining a general discharge, retiring after 20 service years or more from full-time military service, or separating due to medical injuries/conditions (Kintzle & Castro, 2018). Each have ramifications for the MSM, including whether they receive DoD/VA benefits, can be employed by a government agency, or even can apply for re-enlistment.

One example of differing policies is when the VA awards veteran status. With full-time military personnel, it is conferred when they are discharged and/or at retirement. RC personnel are required to serve more than 30 days on full-time active duty status before obtaining a veteran designation. For enlisted RC, often their Basic Training requirements fulfills the time for completion. Most RC Officers do have less time for their basic training but depending on their circumstances can apply for extra training experiences. Both RC enlisted and officers are still discharged with specific designations (such as Honorable, Medical, or General) and, depending on the time they have served, could retire from the military with benefits (VA, 2015).

To better understand the veteran transition of reintegration into the civilian society at large, one has to consider the military culture they are leaving, how much the culture lingers with them, and the social and occupational difficulties that may occur when they are re-entering the community. Veteran attitudes, experiences, demographic characteristics, physical and /or psychological injuries, and temporary or permanent disabilities are examples of factors that can affect whether a service member will have an easy or difficult re-entry experience. Morin (2011) provided three examples including:

- those who had emotionally traumatic experiences or suffered service-related injuries were significantly more likely to have reintegration difficulties (56%),

- commissioned officers who have graduated from college are more likely to readjust to their post-military life better than enlisted personnel who are high school graduates, and

- veterans who reported a clear understanding of their missions while serving in the military also seem to experience fewer difficulties transitioning into civilian life than those who did not fully understand their duties or assignments.

REINTEGRATION

The military reintegration revolves around "the dynamic process and outcome of resuming a civilian role … [this experience has been associated with 'joy and a feeling of relief/release' as well as] poor social and family relationships, unemployment, financial strain, homelessness, and poor physical and mental health" (Romaniuk & Kidd, 2018, p. 60). According to Vogt et al. (2020) most veterans in their first year of reintegration "experience high vocational and social well-being," although they are always concerned about any health conditions (p. 1). Multiple losses are also described, including culture, community, identity, and purpose (Romaniuk & Kidd, 2018). Numerous challenges to this military/civilian transition ecosystem can also include the magnitude of returning service members' age, racial and gender diversity, and types/timing of reintegration programs including job placement opportunities, and right skills application for employment (Elnitsky et al., 2017a). To date there is a large amount of "programs, services and supports to assist veterans with the military-civilian transition"; some estimate over 40,000 different kinds of groups (Vogt et al., 2020, p. 2).

Several disciplines, including nursing, have studied the various transitional experiences of veteran reintegration in an attempt to understand and describe the complex process. Examples include Meleis' Transition theory (nursing; Meleis et al., 2000), Schlossberg's 4-S Transition Model (counseling; Anderson et al., 2012), and Military Transition Theory (social work; Kintzle & Castro, 2018). Across theories and models, a challenge exists to capture both the personal and professional identity reformation service members may experience in their transition as they exit the military and re-enter civilian life. This stems from not only leaving a culture, but also the change in roles and responsibilities, adding to its complexity.

The Ecological Model of Veteran Reintegration

To guide our examination of this next military transition, the Ecological Model of Veteran Reintegration (Elnitsky et al., 2017a) is used to project the psychosocial and environmental factors of the complex veteran reintegration process as they begin to function within their new life roles. The ecological systems theory offers a deep-rooted theoretical grounding in an integrated public heath approach and a linkage to psychosocial and environmental factors. This model is based on an extensive public health literature review of 1,764 articles which yielded 186 articles (Elnitsky et al., 2017b). Then Bronfenbrenner's (1979) historical ecological systems theory was selected and incorporated within this theory and followed by 15 years of subsequent research (Elnitsky et al., 2017b).

Various levels of influence during the reintegration process seem to impact this delicate ecological system creating a societal priority (Elnitsky et al., 2017a). The circular Ecological Model of Veteran Reintegration is structured to demonstrate the continuous spherical lifecycle of influential concerns at four system levels, which include (a) individual, (b) interpersonal, (c) community organizations, and (d) societal factors. These four system level factors have been utilized to assess, provide care interventions, and evaluate research outcomes for thousands of veterans in the reintegration process and it can also assist nurses in understanding the key dimensions (Elnitsky et al., 2017b).

The following sections highlight each of the four levels with examples of challenges the veteran and their families may experience. Interventions nurses can apply in their practice with this model are presented later in the chapter.

FIRST LEVEL: INDIVIDUAL FACTORS

As part of the Ecological Model of Veteran Reintegration, the first level, Individual Factors, consists of (a) psychological and physical health, productivity, as well as (b) demographic and cultural characteristics. During their military time many trusted and responded to the military social command structure with resolve, now they describe "it's very hard ... to lose [as when] you put on an uniform ... you had a name badge on and you had rank ... you were identified for so long as being special in my field, and then all of a sudden it's not there anymore ... now to be frighteningly devoid of identity" (Romaniuk & Kidd, 2018, p. 69). These cultural characteristics exemplified their military identity and values when they were within their service branch and often influence the veteran even after leaving, as well as throughout the rest of their lives, whether into their new employment and/or school environment. Their military ethos could be "Army Strong," which signifies "the best of soldiers and/or the solid team," or for the Marines "Semper Fi," meant to build strong cohesiveness, courage, and loyalty, a commitment to mission and military daily life (Danish & Antonides, 2013). Interestingly a RAND Corporation report describes that some of the full-time Army MSM, who had deployed one or two times during the Iraq and Afghanistan Wars and now are reintegrating into the civilian sector, continue to retain their military identity and culture by transferring over and serving in the RC (Wenger et al., 2018).

Unfortunately, this ethos may not promote individual veterans to seek personal attention for their physical and/or behavioral health needs (Romaniuk & Kidd, 2018). Instead, the military culture can be deeply embedded causing the veteran to avoid seeking care due to the social stigma against any behavioral health issues; a phenomenon demonstrated by the veterans' feelings of disgrace on their military reputation, and/or their reluctance to seek help (Danish & Antonides, 2013; Tanielian & Joycox, 2008). These findings became evident in the RAND study results in which 850,000 OIF and OEF service members were eligible for VHA services upon reintegration; however, only 40% sought care or other VA entitlements (Tanielian & Joycox, 2008). In 2018 these figures of VHA use have only increased to 50% to 55% (VA, 2019b). An awareness of this statistic is particularly important for nurses as they plan to deliver veteran-centered care to this population (McMillan et al., 2017).

As part of the Ecological Model, the area of individual factors impacting veterans' reintegration challenges could be demonstrated by the rising rates of suicide and sexual assault (Elnitsky et al., 2017b).

Suicide rates among MSM, as well as veterans, continues to create significant challenges nation-wide. In addition, these rates do not include the 33% of surveyed veterans that have already experienced suicidal thoughts (Castro et al., 2015; VA, 2017, 2018b). Three assessment factors for suicide seem to be predominant, including (a) "thwarted belongingness," producing ideas they do not fit in, (b) "perceived burdensomeness," creating feelings of inconvenience, and (c) "an acquired capability to overcome fears and pains associated with any suicide ideation/attempts" (Saitzyk & Vorm, 2016, p. 343). For the full-time MSM, suicide rates were a record high of 321 who took their lives during 2018, including 57 marines, 68 sailors, 58 airmen, and 138 army soldiers (Pruitt et al., 2019; U.S. DoD, 2019). Numbers for part time RC personnel were almost 200. To improve this situation, the DoD has committed more manpower and resources ($2.7 million) for their military-wide anti-stigma campaign about suicide that has been operational for years (Dingfelder, 2009; Shane & Kime, 2016). Additionally, the DoD, in fervent mandates with all the respective service branches, continues to work diligently to raise awareness, screen more astutely, and train all current and incoming MSMs about preventive suicide measures (U.S. DoD, 2019).

Regarding veterans, an average of 20 die by suicide each day (Shane & Kime, 2016; VA, 2019b). Upon leaving the military, veterans may begin to feel a loss of direction or purpose, a sensation that once was so entrenched during their service experiences. As well, their family/friend relationships may continue to be troubled (Saitzyk & Vorm, 2016). As MSMs they felt a "part of something bigger than themselves … a meaningful contribution to a worthy and noble cause" (Romaniuk & Kidd, 2018, p. 68). Now they "miss the common goals, the way people put aside their own personal agendas … I don't feel the same thing even though I try and pour my heart into things" (Romaniuk & Kidd, 2018, p. 68). As part of preventive services, the VHA Mental Health Services has identified geographical isolation, similar to the first assessment factor described by Saitzyk and Vorm (2016), as a key individual precursor. With this recognition the VHA has begun to target increased social connectives programs such as interactive sports among veteran programs and personalized integrated health training retreats to increase camaraderie among veterans (Kintzle et al., 2018).

Another individual level issue is related to the high rate of sexual assault and/or harassment that could have occurred during deployment, in men (10%) and especially in women (more than 25%; Marino et al., 2019). Sometimes called "non-combat [related] violent assaults," these sexual and/or harassment events were thought to be most prevalent during war-zone circumstances surrounding OEF/OIF/OND (2001–2014). Unfortunately, the statistics continue to rise even in non-deployment locations as evidenced from the 2016 to 2019 DoD SAPRO (Sexual Assault and Prevention Response Office) Report which documents an on-going pervasive and increasing occurrence of sexual violence (U.S. DoD, 2019). Over 20,500 MSMs across the military branches (13,000 women and 7,500 men) were sexually assaulted in 2018.

Sexual assault and/or harassment during deployment has specific impact for reintegration on several levels (Conard & Armstrong, 2018). The International Classification of Disease code, the VHA, and the American Psychological Association all characterize this military sexual assault and/or harassment as "an experience … during one's military service," not a diagnosis, producing a negative psychosocial and economic impact for insurance and treatment benefits (Marino et al., 2019, p. 487). Consequences of underreporting sexual assault and/or harassment, and/or experiencing nonsupport from peers and/or leadership command for it, can produce a long list of symptomologies. These symptoms can include fear, and/or stigma, re-victimization risks, and behavioral health problems, especially PTSD, depression, and anxiety, as well as cardiovascular disease (Conard & Armstrong, 2018).

Further, veteran concerns from past sexual assault and/or harassment during reintegration have produced an increase of women suicide rates of more than 45% between 2001 and 2015 (VA, 2019b). Currently their suicide rates are twice the rate of non-veteran women. Based on the Ecological Model, the individual level can be impacted by "precision targeting" for behavioral healthcare programs. One example of this is the VA-Army Warrior Transition clinic that provides telepsychiatry, and other new telehealth specialty care initiatives, to assist individual veterans access to care, especially in medically underserved areas. Another resource is Moving Forward: Overcoming Life's Challenges, an online course related to stress management, building resilience, and social function among service members and veterans (Tenhula et al., 2014).

SECOND LEVEL: INTERPERSONAL FACTORS

The second level of the Ecological Model of Veteran Reintegration is Interpersonal Factors, associated with the interwoven intimate relationships of the veteran, family, spouses or partners, and children, as well as religion (Elnitsky et al., 2017a, 2017b). This has significant impact for over 3 million dependents, spouses, and children of U.S. service members who served during OEF/OIF/OND (U.S. DoD, 2013). Another group is the younger OEF/OIF/OND combat ground troops (Army, Navy, Marines, or Air Force) with an average age of 18 to 24 years. More than half of these young adults were single, thus within the changing social structure of society, many families were not in traditional married relationships. Instead, the veteran may be living with a "significant other," not a spouse (Hoge et al., 2006; Thomas et al., 2010). This can be noteworthy as only documented spouses are awarded military benefits and services when they are extended. For both of these groups, the interpersonal reintegration factors may be different as they "find civilian employment, a new home and adapt to new roles, reference groups, and cultural norms" (Keeling, 2019, p. 1). An example of frustration includes "Sometimes I get mad at the most slightest of things … because in the military we had a plan and it was all structured … [we] come here and everything's all messed up" (Romaniuk & Kidd, 2018, p. 68). These interpersonal factors are influenced by the strength of the relationship before a deployment, the length of deployment, whether there were military service injuries, the amount of exposure to the horrors of war, and certainly reintegration journey experiences (Walsh et al., 2014).

During reintegration military spouses again bring valuable psychosocial and financial support to the MSM; now more attention is being focused on their role (Keeling et al., 2019). Some of the unique reintegration challenges for them include overseeing, coping, and engaging in an ongoing appraisal of the military transition by finding timely healthcare resources, contributing to the family's goals of acclimation, while often trying to find meaningful employment for themselves (Keeling et al., 2019). Specialized services are now being considered and developed for them. The Department of Labor/Veteran Affairs Transition Assistance Program is including more guidance to spouses, as well as some state agencies such as the Texas Veterans Spouse Network (Keeling et al., 2019). These programs include career counseling and educational, behavioral health and financial supports. With limited information about their effectiveness and/or outcomes of these programs, further interventions and research in this area will be important (Kintzle & Castro, 2018).

Military couples with a MSM diagnosed with behavioral health issues such as depression and PTSD can be impacted greatly as they try to maneuver their relationships in problem-solving, communication, roles, affective involvement, and responsiveness. Perkins et al. (2018) suggests that currently there is an underrecognition of these functional challenges. Freytes et al. (2017) found that as the couples tried to adjust and reestablish their family life during this reintegration transition, four themes became evident including individual changes, coping strategies, changes in the relationship, and adjusting to the new normal. Military service branches, as well as more public/private organizations seeking to help new veterans, are beginning to talk more openly about these transition impacts and mention coping strategies that could change these relationships (Keeling et al., 2019). They include tips to enhance communication during the transition, and discuss times to seek counseling.

Particularly noteworthy, of the 5.5 million caregivers in the nation, over 1.1 million are caring for someone who served in the military Post-9/11 (Ramchand et al., 2014). Their circumstances are different with the potential of creating complex situations as OEF/OIF/OND veterans, caregivers, and injuries are distinctive from other general caregiving situations. Regardless of gender, OEF/OIF/OND veterans are/were in good health and younger before being injured, and will often need 12- to 24-hour care for longer, sometimes over several decades. Over half (58%) of the military caregivers receive some type of monetary compensation for their injury/disease as a result of the veteran's VA disability rating, but often this does not cover all of their medical expenses (Ramchand et al., 2014). These caregivers are also helping the VA avoid potential institutional costs for these veterans with yearly savings estimated to be over $3 billion (Ramchand et al., 2014). Compounded medical problems could include hearing/vision loss, respiratory difficulties, spinal cord injury/paralysis, TBIs, and amputation(s), as well as behavioral health issues. In addition, AARP is supporting veterans and their caregivers. A significant resource is the AARP guidebook and toolkit, *Military Caregiving Guide* (2019), which is available at their website (www.aarp.org/content/dam/aarp/caregiving/2019/05/748002-Caregiving-Guide-Military-Dec-2019-WEB).

The Congressional Caregivers and Veterans Omnibus Health Services mandate of 2010 and 2014 produced the VHA's Program of Comprehensive Assistance for Family Caregivers (VA, 2019c). This program is for veterans who have suffered serious physical or psychological injury through their Post-9/11 active-duty service and require personal care services to complete activities of daily living due to their injuries. When qualified for assistance, the program offers education, financial support (stipend), travel pay, lodging, mental health and counseling services, and up to 30-days per year of caregiver support (respite care; VA, 2019c).

Military caregivers are usually a young spouse (37% are less than 30 years of age), often with dependent-age children, and who still trying to stay employed (63%; Ramchand et al., 2014). Overall three concerns affect this veteran/caregiver situation: the socio-demographic status of the caregiver and recipient, the recipient's disease progression, and perceived caregiver stress (Conard et al., 2017). To assess caregiver stress, the Caregiver Self-Assessment Tool (18 items) highlights an initial identification of their physical and behavioral health concerns (American Medical Association, 2015). In addition, stimulating open discussions, social support networks, and caregiver perspectives are important. "When caregiver concerns are not addressed, it could eventually lead to musculoskeletal difficulties, depression, infectious diseases, cardiovascular risks, including stroke, premature aging, and higher mortality rates" (Conard et al., 2017, p. 368). Several support programs are available including the DoD Office of Warrior Care Policy Military Caregiver Support, The Military and Veteran Caregiver Peer Support Network, and the VA Caregiver Peer Support Mentoring Program. Interestingly, some of those severely injured veterans with PTSD and TBI, who have experienced long-term recovery care with intense family engagement, have experienced better outcomes and improved treatment adherence and functioning after attending these types of programs (Bolkan et al., 2013; Riggs & Riggs, 2011). In turn, better family cohesion has resulted in better recovery times and treatment outcomes (Dausch & Saliman, 2009).

A large part of interpersonal factors is also related to how children cope with post military deployments and reintegration into the community. Influences include their age and development, the behavioral health and coping of the parent that is not deployed, the child/family resiliency, and resources (Trautmann et al., 2015). The relationship of the frequent and longer deployments during their parent's service time can have a cumulative effect on the family and child's behavioral health and coping abilities (Bello-Utu & DeSocio, 2015). In caregiving situations, effects can be seen in the children assuming some veteran care, and/or more accountability for younger siblings, as well as experiencing greater stress and isolation often impacting their education (Conard et al., 2017). Nurses are in optimal roles to assess risks, triage those with higher levels of need, and advocate for enhanced behavioral health services. As noted with the effects on the military spouse and children, the use of the question "Do you have a (spouse or parent) who has ever served in the military?" is also an important inquiry. Mental health nurses and nurse practitioners can provide links to preventive strategies, early intervention programs, and support groups (Bello-Utu & DeSocio, 2015). Among the RC personnel, expanding family and community support can also help to promote healthy coping and parenting among non-deployed partners.

THIRD LEVEL: COMMUNITY SYSTEM FACTORS

The third level of the Ecological Model of Veteran Reintegration is Community System Factors (Elnitsky et al., 2017a, 2017b). This involves a series of adjustments during geographic location changes and their new veteran career development, while building new support and social networks (Castro et al., 2015). This factor also relates to health system access, the availability of benefits and services, job opportunities, training and academic entry, civilian community resources, and legal programs that surround the veteran as they reintegrate. Often veterans feel like they have no one outside their family who has shared or understood some of their MSM responsibilities and experiences. One veteran stated I am "used to a tight knit community but here [in civilian life] it's like you're an island … I miss that camaraderie," while another stated "I feel like I could just not exist and nobody would know, there is just no community … I just [feel] invisible" (Romaniuk & Kidd, 2018). A study of more than 8,500 veterans and their military dependents identified the most significant transition challenges included navigating VHA programs, benefits, and services (60%); finding a job (55%); adjusting to civilian culture (41%); addressing financial challenges (40%); and applying military-learned skills to civilian life (39%; Zoli et al., 2015). Veteran household incomes can sometimes be lower than their civilian counterparts, with 20% to 40% near the U.S. national poverty level (Perkins et al., 2018). To overcome these problems, several national non-profit veteran organizations provide proactive coaching, financial, career development, recruitment, retention, and interface services for veterans during their reintegration process. Yet sometimes one of the leading gaps in veteran and military family services is not a lack of resources or capacity, but a lack of collaboration, coordination, and collective purpose among agencies assisting veterans and their families (Zoli et al., 2015). In addition, there is virtually no evidence demonstrating whether these agencies/organizations are improving the quality of life for veterans (Perkins et al., 2018).

Remembering that veterans may use two or more health systems is particularly important as only 8 million veterans, out of the more than 19 million nationwide, are enrolled with the VHA; 45% of those at the VHA are over age 65 (VA Office of Community Engagement, 2019). Seventy percent of veterans receive additional healthcare from "outside" the VHA (VA Office of Community Engagement, 2019). Health professional teams can best assist the veteran by understanding both the community resources associated with the VHA, as well as the community health facilities close to the veteran and their family. The national initiative, VA Community Partnerships (VCP; 2019), is an example of a VHA health system benefit that ensure all veterans and their caregivers have access to the wide range of choices and services, including a partnership between the VHA offices of Geriatrics and Extended Care and Rural Health and Caregiver Support. Over 50 VHA medical centers have community partnerships with a VCP staff member totally committed to assist with care coordination and available community benefits. Their VCP website maintains an updated list of primary contacts (www.va.gov/HEALTHPARTNERSHIPS/docs/VCPCoordinatorsRoster.pdf).

Families of discharged and retired military members are sometimes also eligible for training and educational benefits. The DoD Military Spouse Career Advancement Accounts can provide up to between $2,000 and $4,000 in aid toward degree programs. The Dependent's Education Assistance from Veteran's Affairs gives 45 months of education benefits for degrees, certificate programs and on-the-job training (Military.com, 2019). Specific state Workforce programs, as well as university/community college educational counselors, also have additional information for reintegration programs in local education centers, as well as knowledge of various benefits for both the veteran and their families (Kintzle & Castro, 2018). These benefits could be different for the veteran and family member depending on their full-time or part time RC status, and eligibility for the GI Bill Program, whether for college degrees, trade, or apprenticeship programs, and/or other professional licensing programs.

For veterans who have lost a sense of mission, identity, and social bonds, some regions provide community resources that have teamed up with private industry and nonprofit organizations connections to assist with health benefit programs, possible medical interventions, transitional planning, and cultivation of community support social networks (Ahern et al., 2015). One community-based non-profit organization is Team Red, White, & Blue (RWB), developed to assist with veteran social connections within communities through consistent physical, social, and service activities. This organization is grounded on a theory-based framework for veteran health called Enrichment Equation and emphasizes three core constructs including health, people, and purpose to harness positive social networks for the improvement of the veteran's reintegration to civilian life (Angel et al., 2018). The membership is inclusive, based on veterans helping veterans. Their purpose is to cultivate local community links and resources for reintegration while continuing to build a leadership-based community of veterans with social activities and community services (Angel et al., 2018). There were 45,000 members in 2014 and in 2017 Team RWB has grown to 217 chapters.

FOURTH LEVEL: SOCIETAL SYSTEM FACTORS

Overall, the value of the nation's veterans is directly proportional to the country's societal provisions for them, thus the fourth level of the Ecological Model of Veteran Reintegration is the social system they will be re-entering (Elnitsky et al., 2017a, 2017b). This level comprises an overarching view of the social, environmental, economic, biological, and gender factors that will impact their reintegration. It will also influence their health outcomes and quality of life, as well as employment and social policies, job placement, and veteran's personal social identity (Elnitsky et al., 2017a). In addition, their relationship to income, occupation, and educational attainment becomes part of the social determinants of health (VA Health Services Research and Development Evidence Review, 2017).

Reintegration of the veteran, regardless of discharge reason, most likely means that they will be seeking further employment. Importantly, their military employment was "a call to service, an identity, a community, and a way of life that produce[d] profound meaning" so they believe it will be essential to find a post-service job that will be the right fit (Kintzle & Castro, 2018, p. 117). They already possess many skills from their military role, achieved progressive ranks, and have extensive leadership skills, (Lake et al., 2018). Their employment will not only be for economics, but it will also be valuable for establishing new community linkages and new civilian identity/purpose (Kintzle & Castro, 2018). Data from Kintzle and Castro's (2018) report document that about 80% had not arranged employment, nor anticipated immediate action for it, mainly because they wanted to take some time off, and believed when they did seek employment, it would not be a problem. About 53% had put aside 3 months of money, and 60% were employed within the first 90 days after their military discharge (Perkins et al., 2018).

From a societal perspective, many veterans have obtained associate, undergraduate, and even graduate degrees during their military service. According to a 2016 survey, published in 2018, approximately 278,000 veterans (17–44 years of age) have entered colleges/universities (Patterson et al., 2019). The challenge is to match the veteran educational/training skill set to the right job in order to provide individual satisfaction, while meeting societal needs (Lake et al., 2018). Depending on their age, they could have gone directly from high school into the military with only their service experience as a reference point (Kintzle & Castro, 2018). Some military jobs can transition easily if there is flexibility within the veteran, employees, and communities. But these positions are often influenced by the economy (job market), availability of transitional assistance/counselors, and training programs to assist the veteran with the right job opportunities/training in their rural or urban hometowns, while physical and behavioral health concerns may impede employment. With unexpected employment difficulties, disappointment and exasperation can occur. Expecting more salary than what they received in the military also may not be realistic. As well, younger veterans often need assistance with resume-writing, interviewing, and networking (Kintzle & Castro, 2018).

Healthcare occupations are a good example of where there may be opportunities among military medics looking for a civilian emergency medical technician job, with a goal of the veteran applying to nursing school and receiving constructive credit for their military service training/role (Perkins et al., 2018; Sikes et al., 2018). With some creative curricula plans, several nursing schools (31) are supporting trajectories for veterans (Patterson et al., 2019). Student veterans discussed two themes about their education reintegration transition. One concern was the great efforts that were needed to overcome their past (structured military environment) and fit into the new academic culture (non-structured). The other theme was the pleasure of transferring some of their skills, while "appreciating the implications and meaning of this education pursuit … where they were again joining something greater than myself … a new purpose to help others" (Patterson et al., 2019, p. 353). Another example is military nurse officers, who have obtained a great deal of clinical experience, perfected their leadership skills, and have already advised/instructed thousands of personnel throughout their career, thus providing reintegration employment possibilities of becoming a faculty within a university or community college (Lake et al., 2018). A 2017 descriptive study investigating this military-to-civilian reintegration transition revealed an "identity reformation" as their individualist perspectives evolved into the academic role (Chargualaf et al., 2017, p. 10). While officers were well-versed about nursing care, they had to shift some of their military culture/values/attributes for the faculty position, especially acknowledging the presence of a "new language and work pace, and a lack of teamwork" (Chargualaf et al., 2017, p. 9). Interestingly they attributed their acquired military leadership skills to successfully overcoming their workplace adjustments.

Social determinants can impact veteran reintegration (Elnitsky et al., 2017b). Veteran underemployment, unemployment, and poverty rates are examples of major concerns that nurses should be aware of as having a critical societal impact affecting veteran health, educational attainment, and/or access to affordable housing (VA Health Services Research and Development Evidence Review, 2017). Some veterans have historically voiced concerns of biases in certain workplaces against hiring veterans; they are employed readily for technology positions but seldom for psychosocial occupations. Correll (2019) reported on a collection of studies that did document employers' belief that veterans are less suited for jobs that involve social-emotional skills (people interaction) than non-veteran counterparts. One solution offered was the emphasis within the veteran's resume to include community service and the ability to work with the public (Correll, 2019).

There are also situational challenges, especially among MSM young infantryman or rifleman leaving the service. They too have a specialized skill set, are highly trained and valued, worked hard to excel at their job but now their military position does not exist in the civilian job market (Kintzle & Castro, 2018). Unfortunately, with no previous employment skills before entering the military, the lower ranking staff (Private/Seaman), as they reintegrate into civilian life, may have to settle for an entry level job, with minimal pay. Or in some cases such as a helicopter mechanic, enter into a new skill training, especially if they transition "back home" to a rural community. During 2016, 453,000 veterans were unemployed, with 40% (approximately 181,200) between the ages of 18 and 44, a time usually considered the adult prime working years (VA, 2017). The remaining 60% (271,800) of unemployed veterans were age 45 or over; 2017 unemployment rates were lower for both veteran men and women, although those with a service-connected disability remained the same (Kintzle & Castro, 2018).

Full- and part-time women MSMs have increased to over 15% and soon the numbers of women veterans will soon comprise 10% of the total veteran population. Women veteran rates of unemployment were 5% in 2015, with poverty rates higher for disabled women (15.3%), when compared to disabled men (9.4%); these rates in 2017 remain similar (Perkins et al., 2018; VA, 2017). Homelessness is also a problem. While information about homeless individuals overall is difficult to capture, 2006 to 2010 data document women veterans becoming the fastest growing segment of the homeless veteran population (Absher, 2018; National Coalition for Homeless Veterans, n.d.). They face barriers of employment, the lack of accessible and affordable childcare, and isolating themselves following their military discharge. Often, they do not know where to obtain assistance, or are too proud to seek critical interventions before becoming homeless.

Experiences with military sexual trauma during a woman's military time can produce nine times the risk of PTSD (National Coalition for Homeless Veterans, n.d.). Safety and security concerns also are present. Multiple VA programs are present to assist the homeless with housing solutions, low-income special programs, and employment (Absher, 2018; VA, 2019a). Supportive Services for Veteran Families programs provide a wide range of assistive services to promote housing stability, as well as helping them to reside in and/or move into permanent housing. Another partner is the U.S. Department of Housing and Urban Development and the VA Supportive Housing Program, both concerned about vulnerable veterans with special services for women veterans with disabilities recently returning from combat zones (VA, 2019a).

Military retirements can also be a challenge for veterans within communities and the society, with age and their embedded military culture as factors affecting a smooth transition into reintegration (Lake et al., 2018). Full-time military retirement is often conferred after providing 20 or more years of service. The veteran, who may have entered around 18 to 22 years of age, could be leaving in their low to mid 40s and can receive retirement pay. With their military retirement occurring at an early age, often the veteran returns to their civilian community and seeks further employment in a second career while in the middle of their work years (Lake et al., 2018). The full-time MSM who is discharged/retired and moves to a second employment career can face a complex process that researchers continue to study (Kintzle & Castro, 2018; Koenig et al., 2014; Taylor et al., 2007).

One finding is that this transition from the military culture to civilian life is a simultaneous mixture of two cultures, sometimes producing an individual "clash of cultures" (Kintzle & Castro, 2018; Lake et al., 2018; Taylor et al., 2007). These veterans speak of "warring identities"; that is, the dissonance experienced between their former MSM self and their view as a veteran in their new civilian life (Kintzle & Castro, 2018, p. 120). Other researchers have described the military-to-civilian life shift resulting in "reverse culture shock," a situation experienced by veterans as difficulty in finding meaning or purpose, as well as disconnection or conflict with people in their communities (Koenig et al., 2014, p. 416). These occurrences have been noted more frequently among the higher ranked enlisted and/or officer veteran with deeply embedded structured cultural values, while their new civilian employment displays "more autonomy and an increased emphasis on personal self-actualization and fulfillment" (Lake et al., 2018, p. 27), or the veteran is upset by the lack of structure in the civilian organizations (Ahern et al., 2015). This can impact their new reintegration employment role and well-being (Kintzle & Castro, 2018; Taylor et al., 2007). Nurses can play an assistive role by encouraging bicultural employment mentorships to help veterans ease into realistic expectations of their new civilian role (Lake et al., 2018).

RC personnel can also retire from their military obligations after 20 or more years of creditable service. Their circumstances are somewhat different in that they are usually older when they entered the part-time military program and often have had previous/present full-time employment in the community throughout their military involvement (Werber et al., 2013). However, the RC could be in the "gray zone" where their retirement military benefit is not dispersed until age 60. While their military pay will most likely be less, the amount is dependent on their monthly training experiences, full-time deployments, rank, and any other services provided for the military. If they retire at the age of 60 they can receive their retirement pay immediately.

Some final thoughts about MSM transitions. Throughout this chapter the strong presence of military identity threads have been noted. During the MSM introductory socialization process of learned customs, habits, practices, norms, and policies was their service/unit bonding especially when deployed, the sense of family and community throughout their various relocations and assignments, as well as the impact of its possible loss during transition out of the military (Kintzle & Castro, 2018). While this identity is very important during the initiation process, this enculturation may stay with the military veteran for their lifetime, affecting portions of their community reintegration, decision-making, and health-seeking behaviors (Lancaster et al., 2018). It could also influence their health outcomes and quality of life, as well as employment and social policies, job placement, and veteran's personal social identity (Elnitsky et al., 2017a), especially as they try to reconcile their military and civilian identities. Currently a Warrior Identity Scale is being validated for "dimensions of demographic and psychosocial variables" to better note the predictive perspectives of military identity on daily functioning; further analysis could provide more awareness of the "development, maintenance, and impact of identifying oneself with military service" (Lancaster et al., 2018, pp. 36/42).

IMPLICATIONS FOR NURSING EDUCATION AND PRACTICE

While deployment processes over the span of 18 years of the OEF/OIF/OND wars have become smoother and more efficient for all MSMs, each deployment transitional period is distinctive and affects the MSM and their family/loved ones differently. Challenges will always be present but proactively helping to stabilize the situation early is important. Thus, when assisting MSM deployment returnees five pivotal factors for nurses are:

- individuals experience their own unique deployment transition following the conflict/mission/war situation and should have individualized healthcare (Conard & Armstrong, 2019);

- awareness of the embedded military culture of disclosure avoidance due to "embarrassment, confidentiality concerns, and fear of adverse career consequence" (Bastian et al., 2015, p. 33);

- knowledge that physical injuries are reported easier than nonvisible behavioral health wounds;

- proactive, frequent nursing use of assessment tools that detect early problems of behavioral health issues are essential during every MSM health encounter, as well as the timeliness for social services, behavioral, and family healthcare referrals/interventions at any time following a deployment (Danish & Antonides, 2013); and

- for a variety of reasons, many of the physical and behavioral health issues that originate during deployment(s), will often not be acknowledged, diagnosed, or treated, during post-deployment.

A snapshot into the military culture and the challenges to and from a deployment and the veteran reintegration into the community are important as nurses become uniquely qualified to assess the veteran's psychosocial, physical, and emotional needs. The nurse caring for this population should be orientated to these resources through their community outreach specialists within the respective health systems. Again, behavioral and sexual assault screening protocols/tools for every veteran, during each health encounter, remains important for it might be the specific nurse's personal relationship that finally opens the door for further response and action for care. The nurse can then connect them to the right care, at the right time by incorporating a strong insightful interprofessional team that leads with advocacy and understanding for the MSM and veterans who have served our nation.

First should be the identification of the MSM (and their family) with the question to everyone who enters the civilian community healthcare system "Have you ever served in the military?" (Conard & Armstrong, 2019). Then, further exploration about where and when they served, their occupation, and their unique experiences can provide an introductory assessment (Conard & Armstrong, 2019). A knowledgeable nursing coordinator of care can assist veterans and their families navigate whatever system of healthcare and community resources they are using, ensuring there is applicable timely access to care to the precise provider and services. Behavioral and physical health issues impede a successful transition and can impact all facets of civilian life, such as obtaining employment, education, housing, counseling, and other necessary care. "Listening" carefully becomes crucial to understanding the veterans' concerns for improving their reintegration into the civilian society. This could be accomplished by meeting family and parenting needs.

Nurses will meet the veteran in many locations such as during home health visits, rehabilitation hospitals, public health clinics, in-patient hospital units, emergency departments, living in city parks, or even at county fair health screening booths. An examination of the four system levels of the Ecological Model of Veteran Reintegration can assist in making a difference for them by understanding the needs of this population. Table 3.1 incorporates the levels and provides specific nurse interventions to work with the key dimensions of reintegration at each of the four system levels. Identifiable actions are important for nurses who are screening and involved in the care of the veteran, and/or their family/loved ones during reintegration, so applicable psychosocial and physical needs for family-centered care can be implemented.

Within nursing education, the more interactive scenarios (and simulations) that can be developed to engage the student with the various facets about MSM deployment situations and veteran reintegration will be helpful, both within didactic and clinical portions of their education. Knowledge of identification, assessment tools, communication skills, and community resources for MSM/veterans remains essential. Nursing faculty could guide students, especially pediatric nurses and nurse practitioners, to design and implement interprofessional healthcare team leadership practica about veteran families transitioning to civilian life. This project could include assistance for family members and children in the form of information, practical skills, support, and parenting programs (Castro et al., 2015).

TABLE 3.1 NURSING SCREENING AND INTERVENTION ACTIONS BASED UPON THE ECOLOGICAL MODEL OF VETERAN REINTEGRATION AND ITS ASSOCIATED FACTOR LEVELS

INTEGRATION INFLUENCES	NURSE SCREENING AND INTERVENTION ACTIONS
Individual level	**Screen** for depression, substance abuse, suicide, less startled response
	Assess for physical improved health, increased ADL with disability
	TBI cognitive improvement, less pain, less hearing loss, improved sleep patterns
	Screen for positive transitions into academic and occupational activities, attending new job/education programs
Interpersonal level	**Assess** relationship with family, spouses/partners, friends
	Screen for social isolation and disruptive behaviors in veterans, families, children, and adolescents
	Identify if attending or need of reintegration programs, support groups, marital counseling, combat support injury group, stress management programs, sexual assault programs
	Observe for stress in single parents, verbalization of socioeconomic stresses, family caregiver fatigue, and relationship difficulties as it relates to depression
Community systems level	**Identify** healthcare access barriers, integrating primary care with specialty care (rural/urban)
	Assist with behavioral healthcare access, scheduling with family work schedules to support the veteran
	Provide community-based job training information or entrepreneurship info, employment opportunity services (VA or non-profit programs)
	Connect to legal, financial, spiritual, social, cultural organizations and support programs/counselors
Societal level	**Be aware of health policies** – Veteran Choice Act and Affordable Care Act and Homeless Vet Programs

ADL, activities of daily living; TBI, traumatic brain injury; VA, U.S. Department of Veterans Affairs.

As noted previously, it will be exciting to see MSM and veteran students in our educational environments, whether in our classrooms and/or on-line to seek entry into civilian nursing careers. They often come with an amazing inventory of battlefield experiences, leadership knowledge, and previous patient encounter situations; their military education, skills, assignments, activation, and deployments are distinctive. Nursing faculty should obtain specialized knowledge of military culture education such as Green Zone Training (Sikes et al., 2018). Then, be involved in applicable, specific preparatory activities for their recruitment, skills assessment, entry, and retention activities to assist their journey for a successful completion of the nursing program. Re-considering traditional approaches to nursing education will be important (Sikes et al., 2018). Their success will be "influenced by a number of factors including military work type, service branch and length, deployment number and length, trauma experienced, type of separation, time since separation, available social support, and/or physical/mental health issues … as well as financial factors" (Patterson et al., 2019, p. 352). Their success is do-able with deliberate planning; with faculty assistance they can become qualified nurses caring for our nation's veterans and civilian clients.

FUTURE RESEARCH

As never before, the 18-year span during OEF/OIF/OND contains a large amount of literature about MSM deployment and veteran reintegration providing rich knowledge about their needs and challenges (Elnisky et al., 2017a). Yet upon review, there are still areas related to transitions that could be researched, such as:

- impact on the new Veterans Choice Act and the Affordable Care Act related policies in facilitating access to healthcare for the veteran;

- nurse's education of veteran's transition experiences from military to civilian life, with the development of culture-centered communication that promotes readjustment to civilian life;

- construct of Transitional Care models during transitions from combat injury, to VA, to civilian care, while identifying key trigger points for success;

- veteran clinical outcomes for civilian community-based care in physical and psychological rehabilitation programs, featuring further collaboration among VA, DoD, and community-based clinicians;

- evidence-based outcomes research and pilot demonstration projects on topics that identify veteran community needs during pre-deployment, deployment, and post-deployment phases, and the appropriate cycle of support through deployments – to reintegration;

- interprofessional collaborative practice team assessments with Advanced Nurse Practitioners on whether subgroups (e.g., race, gender) of veterans are experiencing disparities in particular domains. Also access to services for the Reserve/National Guard;

- the identification of specific skills/behaviors in all levels of nursing students in Ambulatory Care clinics, to facilitate increased MSM and veteran trust and communication about any suicidal ideologies;

- an examination of the effects of longer clinic appointments to facilitate further relationships and trust for veterans with higher risk for behavioral health issues;

- validating evaluation instruments on the veteran's community reintegration process, specifically including content, construct, and predictive values of the instrument;

- "[c]onducting longitudinal research to understand the prevalence and course of the behavioral health of veteran spouses and children as they experience military to civilian transition" (Keeling et al., 2019, p. 12); and

■ "[c]onducting longitudinal research investigating marital/romantic relationships during military to civilian transition aimed at highlighting risk and resilience factors for relationship functioning and adjustment" (Keeling et al., 2019, p. 12).

From an institutional research aspect:

■ review the VA Health Services Research and Development Office identified potential topic needs via their website (www.hsrd.research.va.gov/publications/vets_perspectives/0319Incorporating-Veterans-Perspectives-into-Research.cfm#3), and

■ consider suggested key areas of future research from the Center for Evaluating Patient Centered care, in their 2020 Comprehensive Addiction and Recovery Act Report to Congress, with a major priority area of suicide, and factors that facilitate veterans talking with their providers about suicidal ideation.

Specific areas of women gender studies are needed related to deployment issues including:

■ examining behavioral health screening findings of the Post Deployment Health Assessments on first-time mothers using the DoD survey data from deployment return, and at 3, and 6 months;

■ investigating applicable education and engagement on "prevention, the efficacy of treatment modalities, and long-term consequences of MST" (Marino et al., 2019, p. 489);

■ identifying access to community levels of support for the newly disabled women service members; and

■ validating readiness impact for deploying women MSMs when they are caring for infants, or children, or elderly relatives.

CONCLUSION

This chapter's purpose was to provide a better understanding of the complex transitional phases of deployments and/or the reintegration from the military to civilian life. MSMs, veterans, and their families are known to experience varying degrees of stress-related disorders, disappointments, frustration, and poor services during these transitional changes. Nursing faculty, students, clinical practice nurses, and other interprofessional practice partners can play important roles to assist the MSM, veteran, and their families during these major transitions. While the men and women of our Armed Forces are better trained, educated, and prepared for these transitions, they still face unique challenges in accessing healthcare, attaining education, and establishing careers that necessitate actions to ensure their special needs are met. The screening of the veteran is critical at every healthcare encounter, particularly for women with a history of sexual assault, those men and women who live in isolated rural areas, and those with firearms.

The four levels of the circular Ecological Model of Veteran Reintegration help grasp further opportunities for a better examination of the veteran's involved reintegration process. Descriptions of the complexity and successes of assisting veterans by comprehensively supporting the MSM and veterans to foster a culture of emotional wellness were provided. If there were physical and/or psychological injuries sustained during their military service, they may be heavily impacted, particularly, needing a multifaceted approach during their reintegration process.

REFERENCES

The complete reference list for this chapter appears in the digital version of the chapter, accessible at https://connect.springerpub.com/content/book/978-0-8261-3597-1/chapter/ch03

VETERANS IN THE COMMUNITY

GWENDOLYN M. HAMID | HELENE MORIARTY

There is no greater or higher calling than helping our wounded soldiers heal and transition successfully back to the fighting force or to the community.

Lt. Gen. Patricia D. Horoho

KEY TERMS

Military Health System	community resources for veterans
veterans' health	family members of veterans
veteran homelessness	veteran caregivers
VA resources	MISSION Act
Veteran Service Organizations	

INTRODUCTION

Nurses encounter veterans in numerous healthcare settings in both the Veterans Health Administration and in the private sector. Veterans have many strengths, talents, insights, and resilience related to their service, training, and experience. Yet they may face unique challenges affecting their physical and mental health, many of which are intimately linked to their military service and the transition from military to civilian life. Owing to these complex and unique challenges, it is imperative that nurses be competent to serve and support this population. This chapter includes a discussion of the varying needs of veterans in the community, such as the transition from the Military Health System (MHS) to the VHA, implications of the Maintaining Internal Systems and Strengthening Integrated Outside Networks (MISSION) Act, and issues related to veterans experiencing homelessness. Furthermore, information on services and resources available to veterans and their families to assist veterans as they navigate reintegration to the civilian world are presented.

BACKGROUND

About 20 million veterans are living in the United States; 9.4% of those veterans are females (Bialik, 2016). Veterans live in every state, with the highest numbers of veterans residing in Alaska, Maine,

---

The complete reference list for this chapter appears in the digital version of the chapter, accessible at https://connect.springerpub.com/content/book/978-0-8261-3597-1/chapter/ch04

and Montana; they reside in major cities, suburban settings, and in rural communities. The median age of male veterans is 65 while the median age of female veterans is 51 (The Office of Enterprise Integration & NCVAS, 2017). Gulf War-era veterans make up the highest portion of the current veteran population, followed by Vietnam-era veterans (NCVAS, 2018). Transitioning from military to civilian culture can pose many challenges for veterans and their families. Some of these challenges include securing employment and housing in the civilian sector; transitioning from military healthcare to the U.S. Department of Veterans Affairs (VA) or private sector healthcare; issues around physical and psychological health related to injury or exposure resulting from service; and general reestablishment of life and relationships in the civilian world, commonly referred to as community reintegration. Health-related challenges may include one or more temporary or permanent disabilities, mental health concerns (including substance use disorder [SUD], depression, posttraumatic stress disorder [PTSD], military sexual trauma [MST], and anxiety), and physical concerns (including chronic pain, sequelae of traumatic brain injury [TBI], or other physical injuries; Olenick et al., 2015). Nurses are positioned to provide care for veterans in varied healthcare settings and must ensure competency in caring for this unique population in the communities in which they practice.

To serve as advocates for veteran patients and to ensure competency in caring for veterans, nurses need a general understanding of the process of transition from the MHS to the VA or to the private-sector health system. Further, the provision of culturally competent care for the veteran population is essential not only for nurses within the VHA, but also for those employed in the private sector. Nurses working in the private sector are likely to have increased opportunities to care for veterans as a result of the 2019 MISSION Act. The beginning of this chapter includes a discussion of the structure of the VA system, specifically focusing on the scope of services offered through the VHA, the process of transitioning from MHS to VA care, as well as an overview of the MISSION Act and its implications for the nursing profession.

MILITARY HEALTHCARE TO VETERAN HEALTHCARE

In most cases, active duty service members and retired service members have their healthcare costs covered through TRICARE™ and receive their healthcare through the MHS. The MHS operates under the purview of the Department of Defense (DoD) and is a separate entity from the VA. The MHS is responsible for providing healthcare services to both active duty and Reservists (when activated), for the training of U.S. military healthcare providers, and for providing medical benefits to active duty service members, retirees, and their family members, as well as recent Operation Iraqi Freedom (OIF), Operation Enduring Freedom (OEF), and Operation New Dawn (OND) combat veterans (for up to 5 years after separation from service for service-related issues; Military Health Service, 2019). Upon separation from service, whether voluntarily or under circumstances related to physical or mental health, many but not all veterans are eligible to receive healthcare through the VA (VA, 2019c). For example, veterans must have served a full 24 continuous months or the full length of active duty to which the veteran was called to be eligible. For those veterans leaving service prior to 24 months, or those who did not complete the full period of active duty, the veteran must have been discharged for a service-related condition or a condition exacerbated by service; have been discharged for a hardship or "early-out"; or must have served prior to September 7, 1980 (VA, 2019c).

The VA comprises three separate administrations: VHA, the Veterans Benefits Administration (VBA), and the National Cemetery Administration (NCA; VA, 2019k). The VHA is the administration responsible for the management of health-related benefits. The VBA is responsible for non-health-related benefits, whereas the NCA is responsible for burial and memorial-related benefits. The three administrations are collectively referred to as "the VA."

The VHA is the nation's largest integrated healthcare system. With an annual budget of $68 billion, the VHA provides care to over 9 million veterans (VA, 2019n). The VHA is divided into 18 geographically distinct veterans integrated service networks (VISNs) that strive to provide quality integrated healthcare to veterans. Across the nation, there are 170 VA medical centers and over 1,000 VHA health clinics. Community-based outpatient clinics (CBOCs), community living centers (CLCs), domiciliaries, and Vet Centers all work together within the VHA with the shared mission of honoring veterans by providing exceptional healthcare that improves their health and well-being.

CLCs are the civilian sector equivalent of nursing homes that provide long-term skilled care to eligible veterans. Mandatory eligibility criteria include veterans who require a skilled level of care related to service-connected disability, those with at least a 70% service-connected disability rating, and those with a total disability rating based on unemployability ("VA Community Living Centers," n.d.). Established in the 1860s, VA domiciliaries provided a home for soldiers with disabilities returning from the Civil War. Today, domiciliaries are integrated with Mental Health Residential Rehabilitation Treatment Programs and provide economically disadvantaged veterans with clinical and rehabilitative services for mental and physical health problems (VA, 2019b). Vet Centers are community-based centers that provide readjustment counseling for veterans and their families (VA, 2019l). In addition to the provision of health services in varied settings, the VHA is the nation's largest provider of graduate medical education and is responsible for a plethora of research dedicated to the generation of evidence-based practices that improve health not only for veterans, but for patients in the private sector as well (VA, 2019n).

Broad eligibility criteria for VA care include stipulations related to location and length of service, the presence of a service-connected disability, discharge status, receipt of a Medal of Honor or Purple Heart, eligibility for Medicaid services or a VA pension, and various other circumstances (VA, 2019c). The VA defines priority groups who are given faster access to enroll in VA care dependent upon service history, disability rating, income, Medicaid eligibility, and whether the veteran receives a VA pension (VA, 2019c). VA eligibility enables veterans to receive healthcare through the VA health system. Once enrolled, individual factors (primarily related to income) determine the extent of out-of-pocket costs incurred by the veteran for healthcare services. A detailed description of VA eligibility is beyond the scope of this chapter. However, anyone desiring more information can contact a representative through the VA website (www.va.gov).

For many veterans, the process of enrollment can be daunting; however, there are many resources available to assist veterans in this endeavor. For example, Veteran Service Officers are trained to assist veterans in filing for VA benefits. It is important for veterans and healthcare providers to be aware that eligibility requirements for VA care have expanded or can change over time to include more and more veterans. Older veterans who may not have been eligible for VA care in the past may be eligible to receive VA care under the current guidelines. Hence, veterans should be encouraged to investigate potential eligibility with the assistance of Veteran Service Officers, social workers, and their local VA and veterans' organizations (Erickson-Hurt et al., 2017).

Historically, veterans with other-than-honorable discharges were excluded from accessing VA care. However, veterans are now eligible to apply for discharge upgrades (and thus, receive VA care) if their other-than-honorable discharge was related to any of the following circumstances: PTSD and other mental health problems, TBI, sexual orientation, or MST. In 2018, the DoD and VA announced the launch of an online tool to aid veterans in the process of applying for a discharge upgrade. The tool can be accessed at www.vets.gov/discharge-upgrade-instructions. For military service members, veterans, and their families who are enrolled in VHA services, there are a number of support services that can be utilized beyond the primary, specialty, and inpatient care provided through VA hospitals and clinics. The VA strives to support the health of veterans through a variety of prevention, wellness, and health promotion programs (Box 4.1). With the passage of the MISSION Act, veterans' access to care will expand to an approved network of non-VA medical providers (VA, 2019d).

BOX 4.1

HEALTH PROGRAMS FOR VETERANS THROUGH THE VA

- Blind Rehabilitation
- Caregivers/Caregiving
- Chaplain
- Community Living Centers
- Compensated Work Therapy
- Dental Care Benefits
- Disease Prevention
- Fisher House
- Geriatrics and Extended Care
- Homeless Services
- Mental Health
- MyHealth*e*Vet
- National Center for Post-Traumatic Stress Disorder
- Patient Centered Care
- Prescriptions
- Prosthetics and Sensory Aids
- Readjustment Counseling (VetCenters)
- Rural Health
- Smoking Cessation
- Substance Abuse Programs
- Telehealth
- Veterans Crisis Line
- Weight Management
- Women Veterans Healthcare

VA, U.S. Department of Veterans Affairs.

SOURCE: U.S. Department of Veterans Affairs. (2019o). *Veterans' Health Administration: Health programs for veterans.* Retrieved October 2, 2019 from https://www.va.gov/health/programs/

Despite the vast array of VA services offered at locations throughout the United States, it is estimated that only about 48% of veterans access healthcare through the VA (NCVAS, 2017). A 2015 mixed-methods study of 858 community-dwelling veterans found that over 75% of veterans who did not access VA health benefits cited access to private health insurance as the main reason (Franco et al., 2016). Other commonly cited reasons included uncertainty regarding eligibility, the perception that establishing eligibility or accessing care through the VA would be inconvenient, and previous negative experiences or reports of negative experiences with VA care (Franco et al., 2016).

The Maintaining Internal Systems and Strengthening Integrated Outside Networks Act

The MISSION Act was signed into law in June of 2018. The MISSION Act is intended to improve veterans' access to community care by extending their VA health benefits to the private sector under specific circumstances. Veterans are eligible to access care outside the VA if:

- there is longer than a 20-day wait for an available VA appointment for primary or mental healthcare,
- there is a longer than 28-day wait for a specialty care appointment,
- the veteran must travel longer than 30 minutes for a VA primary or mental healthcare appointment,
- the veteran must travel longer than 60 minutes for a VA specialty care appointment, and
- the veteran and the healthcare provider are in agreement that it is in the veteran's best interest to receive care outside the VA (Kirsh & Davies, 2019).

Although the MISSION Act should provide increased access to care, especially in rural and underserved areas, care within the VA system may be preferable whenever possible. As of 2018, the VA has demonstrated superior quality of care and improved wait times when compared to the private sector, and is often the optimal choice for veterans due to VA healthcare providers' specialized training in veterans' physical and mental health issues (Anhang Price & Farmer, 2018; Kirsh & Davies, 2019; Penn et al., 2019). In addition to improving care access, the MISSION Act will also expand eligibility for individuals to participate in the Program of Comprehensive Assistance for Family Caregivers (PCAFC); facilitate the VA's potential to recruit and retain superior medical staff through grants and scholarships; and enable the VA to strengthen its infrastructure across the United States (VAntage Point: The Official Blog of the U.S. Department of Veterans Affairs, 2019).

Considerations With Dual Care

With the launching of the MISSION Act, there will be challenges around the implementation of expanded access to care for veterans in addition to the need for increased cultural competence for practitioners new to serving the veteran population. For example, veterans are required to receive referrals to private sector providers in order use their VA benefits outside of the VA system. Communication and the sharing of electronic medical records between providers from the VA and the private sector will be necessary to streamline processes and ensure quality and cost-effectiveness of care, and prevent redundancy of tests, procedures, or prescribed therapies including medications. For example, studies have already demonstrated the complexity of care coordination between the VA and the private sector. A study by Elliott (2019) found that nurses cite lack of communication between VA and private sector providers as a major challenge to the provision of care for veterans in community settings. Another study found that dual care users (VA and Medicare Part D) had a two to three times higher risk of high-dose opioid exposure (Gellad et al., 2018) compared to those receiving care solely through the VA. Communication and the streamlining of processes between the VA and the private sector are essential to the successful implementation of the MISSION Act to ensure that veterans receive the full benefit the Act was intended to provide.

The Veterans Health Information Exchange (VHIE; previously known as the Virtual Lifetime Electronic Record [VLER]) is a VA program that enables VA and non-VA providers to share health information through a secure electronic system. The VHIE program utilizes two tools to provide information exchange between private sector and VA providers: the VA exchange (VLER Health Exchange) and VA Direct Messaging program (VLER Direct). The VA exchange allows for electronic information sharing for veterans' lab and diagnostic results, medical history, allergies, vital signs, immunizations, physicals, referrals, medications, progress notes, and discharge summaries. The VA Direct Messaging program allows VA and non-VA providers to communicate in real-time to meet the healthcare needs of veterans receiving dual care. Non-VA providers must enroll in the program to be able to access the VHIE system (VA, 2019p). This may be an administrative challenge for non-VA providers who have to self-initiate and learn the information-sharing process with the VA.

Veterans must be questioned about and should be encouraged by providers to disclose their participation in dual care in and outside the VA system to facilitate information-sharing. Just as in the civilian health system, coordination of care among providers is challenging. Veterans may also face challenges in identifying qualified providers outside the VA system or in securing appointments in a timely fashion. Similar to the VA system, access to private sector mental healthcare can be difficult to obtain. A 2018 study concluded that wait times in the VA system were significantly shorter than those in the private sector (in metropolitan areas) across primary care, cardiology, and dermatology, and that while VA wait times have improved since 2014, private sector wait times have remained static (Penn et al., 2019). In early 2020, the VA Inspector General warned that the MISSION Act is projected to increase the number of veterans seeking care in the private sector from 684,000 to 3.7 million (Benyon, 2020). This enormous growth in non-VA care-seeking is poised to effect the already protracted wait times currently experienced in the private sector. For example, in 2018, data from 206,500 referrals for community care found that veterans had an average wait time of 56 days for private sector health appointments (Benyon, 2020).

VETERAN HOMELESSNESS

Individuals experiencing homelessness are defined by the U.S. Department of Housing and Urban Development (HUD) as "a person who lacks a fixed, regular, and adequate nighttime residence" (HUD, 2018, p. 2). Ending homelessness in the veteran population has been a national priority over the past several decades (Tsai & Roseheck, 2015). It is imperative for nurses to understand the risk factors for housing instability and to be aware of the complex mental and physical health issues faced by veterans experiencing homelessness. Furthermore, nurses who are equipped to deliver culturally competent care to veterans experiencing homelessness are better able to provide effective screening, referrals, and follow up care to this vulnerable population.

In December of 2018, HUD reported that on any given night in January of 2018, there were a total of 552,830 persons experiencing homelessness in America, 38% of whom were classified as living in conditions unfit for human habitation (HUD, 2018). Of the total population of persons experiencing homelessness, just under 9% or 37,878 were veterans (HUD, 2018). HUD segregates individuals experiencing homelessness into "sheltered homeless" and "unsheltered homeless" depending upon whether, at the time of the count (on a single night), an individual was sleeping in a designated temporary shelter or was sleeping on the streets, in parks, or in a vehicle (HUD, 2018). HUD's point-in-time (PIT) counts are intended to provide a snapshot of the population of persons experiencing homelessness, and these counts are submitted to Congress on an annual basis to characterize the scope of homelessness in the United States.

It is important to note, however, that advocacy groups such as the National Law Center on Homelessness and Poverty (NLCHP, 2017) have called on HUD to alter the methodology guiding the PIT counts due to evidence suggesting the current methodology is flawed, resulting in a gross underestimation of the true scope of homelessness in the United States. For example, PIT count methods do not count individuals who are "doubled up" or residing with friends or family on a temporary basis. The count also fails to capture individuals who would be experiencing homelessness were it not for their being hospitalized or incarcerated at the time of the count. Furthermore, "sheltered" or "unsheltered" homeless classifications can be misleading because for those experiencing homelessness, being

TABLE 4.1 VETERANS EXPERIENCING HOMELESSNESS AT A GLANCE

BY GENDER	PERCENTAGE OF VETERANS EXPERIENCING HOMELESSNESS
Male	90.8%
Female	8.5%
Transgender	0.5%
Gender non-conforming	0.2%
By ethnicity	
Hispanic/Latino	10.7% (15% of whom are unsheltered)
By race	
White	57.6%
Black	32.5%
Native American	3.1%
Multiple races	5.2%
By location	
Cities	48%
Suburban	27%
By state	
Highest rates of homelessness among all veterans	Colorado, Oregon, and Hawaii
≥50 unsheltered veterans experiencing homelessness	California, Oregon, Hawaii, Mississippi, and Washington
≤5% unsheltered veterans experiencing homelessness	Wyoming, Nebraska, Rhode Island, New York, Wisconsin, Delaware, and New Hampshire
Highest percent of persons experiencing homelessness who are veterans	Montana: 17% New Mexico: 15% [Note: Montana and New Mexico also have the highest rates of veterans among all adults]
States with high rates of veterans experiencing homelessness disproportionate to their general veteran population	Louisiana, Idaho, and New Hampshire
State with highest rate of veterans among adult population and lowest rate of veterans experiencing homelessness	Alaska
States with increases in homeless veterans since 2009	Oregon, Utah, Vermont, Hawaii, and Alaska

sheltered is a transient state that may change from night to night. As such, the NLCHP recommends that the HUD PIT count data be considered as an underestimation of the true number of individuals (veteran or otherwise) experiencing homelessness in the United States (NLCHP, 2017).

The Face of Veterans Experiencing Homelessness

Veterans are at greater risk for homelessness than their non-veteran counterparts, with an especially increased risk in veterans of the all-volunteer force (Tsai & Rosenheck, 2015). Table 4.1 presents a list of demographic characteristics of veterans experiencing homelessness per the 2018 PIT count (HUD, 2018).

A 2015 systematic review of 31 studies by Tsai and Rosenheck (2015) demonstrated that for veterans, the strongest and most consistent risk factors for homelessness, above and beyond poverty, were SUD and mental illness. More specifically, psychotic disorders such as schizophrenia, along with drug and alcohol abuse disorders, were strongly associated with veteran homelessness across studies. These findings are consistent with risk factors for homelessness in the general population. Despite the higher prevalence of PTSD in the veteran versus the general population, PTSD was not identified as a specific mental health risk factor for homelessness in the review.

Combat exposure was not identified as a risk factor for homelessness among Vietnam-era veterans, whereas OIF/OEF veterans who served in combat theaters had a greater risk for homelessness than OIF/OEF non-theater veterans (Tsai & Rosenheck, 2015). The authors hypothesize that this difference in risk is related to the increased incidence of mental health and substance abuse disorders in combat-exposed versus non-combat-exposed OIF/OEF veterans. Likewise, combat-exposed OIF/OEF veterans have an increased risk of TBI and other neurological injuries that were found to be risk factors for homelessness in several studies (Douyon et al., 1998; Metraux et al., 2013; Tsai & Rosenheck, 2015). Finally, deployed, combat-exposed OIF/OEF veterans may have increased risk for deterioration of social support systems during times of separation from social networks, conferring risk for homelessness as evidenced by numerous studies (Mares & Rosenheck, 2004; Rosenheck & Fontana, 1994; Tsai & Rosenheck, 2015; Wenzel et al., 1993).

Furthermore, Tsai and Rosenheck (2015) revealed that low income and other variables related to low income, including unemployment and military pay grade, along with difficulty with money-managing, were associated with homelessness. Consistent with these findings, research suggests that access to VA service-connected disability payments serves as a protective factor against homelessness (Edens et al., 2011). The authors of the review also identified three additional factors associated with veteran homelessness that require further rigorous research to confirm their roles as risk factors for homelessness in veterans: lack of social support, previous incarceration, and a history of adverse childhood events (Tsai & Rosenheck, 2015).

In a 2016 study of a nationally representative sample of veterans, 8.6% reported homelessness at some point in their adult life, while only 17.6% of this group reported that they utilized VA homeless services (Tsai et al., 2016). Low income, being aged 35 to 44, and having poor mental and physical health were factors associated with lifetime homelessness. Furthermore, veterans who were White and living in rural areas were significantly less likely to have utilized VA homeless services, indicating barriers to service access and use, especially in rural areas (Tsai et al., 2016).

RURAL VETERANS
In 2006, Congress established the VHA Office of Rural Health (ORH) to adress the health concerns and barriers to care faced by nearly 5 million veterans living in rural areas, of which approximately 2.8 million are enrolled in the VA (VA, 2019h). Rural communities tend to have higher poverty rates, more elderly residents, fewer healthcare options or access to preventive care, and less healthcare options compared to more urban areas. While rural populations face unique challenges regardless of veteran status, veterans with extensive healthcare needs may find it much more challenging to acquire the care they need in rural settings. The VA allocates an estimated 32% of its healthcare budget to rural veteran care (VA, 2019p). A higher percentage of veterans living in rural areas (58%) are enrolled in the VA compared to urban areas (37%) with 56% being over 65 years of age. Of all rural veterans, 6% are women, 15% are minorities, 55% have at least one service-connected condition, 27% do not access the Internet at home, and 52% earn less than $35,000 annually (VA, 2019h).

There are about 460,000 OIF/OEF/OND era veterans residing in rural settings (VA, 2019h). In 2017, researchers found that between 2013 and 2016, 15% of veterans who utilized VA homeless services were residing in rural areas (Szymkowiak & Metraux, 2017). Although chronic illness profiles were similar between rural and non-rural veterans experiencing homelessness, rural veterans had significantly higher rates of behavioral health diagnoses than their non-rural counterparts (Szymkowiak & Metraux, 2017). These findings underscore the need to improve access to care for veterans experiencing homelessness in rural settings, especially in terms of behavioral health services.

TABLE 4.2 PROGRAMS OFFERED UNDER ENTERPRISE-WIDE INITIATIVES

CATEGORY	PROGRAM TITLE	PROGRAM DESCRIPTION
Primary Care	Teleprimary Care Hubs	Establishes teleprimary care hubs with branch sites to give veterans access to primary care in areas where providers are not available
	Medical Foster Home	For veterans no longer able to live independently and have no caregivers, this program provides an alternative to a nursing home by providing daily personal assistance
Specialty Care	Rural Veterans Telerehabilitation Initiative	Provides physical, recreational, and occupational rehabilitation service through secure Internet video in veterans' homes
	Teleaudiology	Provides audiology remote fittings and aftercare services, remote diagnostic testing, and automated audiometric testing in a store-and-forward model
Mental Health	Rural Suicide Prevention	Provide veterans comprehensive suicide prevention resources and service through enhanced education, public awareness and community training, crisis support, firearm safety and care management of high risk individuals
	MST Web-Based Therapy	Through the use of telehealth, specialized mental health therapy can be delivered in veterans' home for those who have experienced MST
Workforce Training and Education	Rural Health Training Initiative	Provides clinical training sites in rural areas for health profession students and clinical residents, including nurse practitioners
	VA-ECHO Transgender Program	Provides training to rural providers on providing treatment to transgender veterans through online didactic teaching and case-based consultation
Care Coordination	Rural Health Community Coordinator Health Information Exchange	Provides personnel who facilitate secure and effective data exchange between community providers and the VA
Health IT Modernization	VA Video Connect CVT Patient Table Program	Provides rural veterans with video telehealth tablets to connect them with and transmit data to a remote VA healthcare provider over a secure Internet connection
Research	Rural ChooseVA Access Evaluation	Evaluates VA efforts to improve access to care across the health system
Innovation	VA Farming and Recovery Mental Health Services (VA FARMS)	Provides agricultural vocational training and behavioral healthcare services to veterans from licensed providers at 10 VHA sites of care
Transportation	Veteran Transportation Services	Medical transportation services for veterans, including cost of drives, leased vehicles, and mobility managers

ECHO, Extension for Community Healthcare Outcomes; IT, information technology; MST, military sexual trauma; VA, U.S. Department of Veterans Affairs; VA FARMS, VA Farming and Recovery Mental Health Services; VHA, Veterans Health Administration.

SOURCE: U.S. Department of Veterans Affairs. (2019f). *Office of Rural Health: Enterprise-Wide initiatives.* Retrieved October 2, 2019 from https://www.ruralhealth.va.gov/providers/Enterprise_Wide_Initiatives.asp

The VA has made great strides in developing programs to ensure access to care for veterans in rural settings, and expansion of access for veterans will continue as a result of the MISSION Act (VA, 2019h). Through various programs and initiatives, the ORH is able to reach more veterans where they live. Two types of programs offered are Enterprise-Wide Initiatives (EWI) and Rural Promising Practices (VA, 2019h). EWI range from primary and specialty care to transportation. Table 4.2 is not an exhaustive list, but highlights a few programs offered. Rural Promising Practices are projects that have been identified through Veterans Rural Health Resource Centers (VRHRCs) as proven models that significantly impact care and health outcomes (VA, 2019g). Some programs require mentorship support from the VRHRCs, while others do not. Examples of programs that do not require mentorship support and can be directly implemented are listed in Box 4.2.

BOX 4.2

RURAL PROMISING PRACTICES FOR DIRECT IMPLEMENTATION

- COACH
- Geriatric Waking Clinic: Meeting Rural Veterans Where They Are
- IMPROVE
- Interdisciplinary Clinical Video-Telehealth for Geriatrics and Dementia
- Osteoporosis Risk Assessment Using OST
- Rural OsteoPorosis Evaluation Service
- Telemental Health Clinics for Rural Native American Veterans
- Transforming Advance Care Planning into an Atmosphere of Support and Communication
- VA C-TraC Program

C-TraC, Coordinated Transitional Care; COACH, Caring for Older Adults and Caregivers at Home; IMPROVE, Integrated Management and Polypharmacy Review of Vulnerable Elders; OST, Osteoporosis Self-Assessment Tool; VA, U.S. Department of Veterans Affairs.

SOURCE: U.S. Department of Veterans Affairs. (2019g). *Office of Rural Health: Rural promising practices*. Retrieved October 2, 2019 from https://www.ruralhealth.va.gov/providers/promising_practices.asp

---

When working with veterans who are living in rural and highly rural areas, and may have complex physical and mental health needs, healthcare providers need to be innovative in partnering with community and VA resources. Providers living and practicing in rural areas may benefit from learning about models of care established through the VA as they may also help inform ways in which rural healthcare for all could be improved. For stakeholders who wish to learn more about rural veterans' healthcare needs, one can access the Rural Veterans Health Care Atlas Fiscal Year 2015 at www.ruralhealth.va.gov/aboutus/rvhc_atlas_fy2015.asp

Call to Action

In recent decades, the situation of veteran homelessness has garnered much attention, resulting in increased awareness of the problem, along with funding and the implementation of programs to mitigate and eventually end homelessness in the veteran population. Much research has been devoted to identifying risk factors, increasing screening, and tailoring interventions to end homelessness among those who served. Although these efforts have been successful in lowering the number of veterans experiencing homelessness and unstable housing, much work remains to be done to end veteran homelessness.

In 2010, veterans comprised 16% of the adult homeless population. As of the December 2018 PIT count, veterans make up 8.6% of all homeless persons in the United States, representing a 49% decrease in veteran homelessness (HUD, 2018). Comparatively, the population of non-veteran homeless persons has seen only a 13.2% decrease since that time, due in part to displacement related to natural disasters such as hurricanes and wildfires (HUD, 2018). More recently, between 2017 and 2018 alone, veteran homelessness decreased by 5%, while the number of homeless female veterans decreased by 10% (HUD, 2018). Efforts by the Department of Veterans Affairs National Center on Homelessness Among Veterans (the Center) and collaborative programs between federal agencies and the private sector have been instrumental in decreasing veteran homelessness over the past decade.

The Center, founded in 1987, has been responsible for developing pilot programs aimed at providing community outreach services for veterans who are homeless. Since then, the Center has grown to become the largest provider of integrated homeless services in the nation. Working in conjunction with the VHA's Homeless Programs Office, professional organizations, and community partners, and in collaboration with academic medical centers at the University of Pennsylvania, Massachusetts, and South Florida, the Center is on a mission to serve veterans experiencing homelessness. The Center's primary goal is to promote the development of policy, clinical research, and education to facilitate homeless services that enable veterans to live independently in their communities (VA, 2019e).

Another major contribution to reducing veteran homelessness was a federal initiative introduced in 2010 by President Barrack Obama. *Opening Doors: Federal Strategic Plan to Prevent and End Homelessness* was focused on the reduction of homelessness in the general U.S. population, with a specific goal to end homelessness in veterans by 2015. The initiative called on federal, state, and local leaders, in collaboration with advocacy groups, service providers, as well as faith-based and philanthropic organizations, to work together to develop programs to end veteran homelessness. The program focused on five key evidence-based focus areas specific to veterans: (a) provision of affordable housing, (b) provision of permanent supportive housing, (c) increasing meaningful, sustainable employment, (d) reducing financial vulnerability, and (e) transforming homeless services to crisis response services. The alignment of resources between the VA, HUD, the Department of Health and Human Services, and Department of Labor has facilitated great progress in decreasing veteran homelessness since 2010 (United States Interagency Council on Homelessness, 2010).

One example of how resource alignment among agencies has facilitated a decrease in the number of veterans experiencing homelessness is the HUD-VA Supportive Housing (VASH) Program (2019). The HUD-VASH program was implemented as part of the *Opening Doors* initiative and has been successful in decreasing veteran homelessness through the provision of HUD housing vouchers in combination with VA supportive services to provide housing for veterans and their families. Among VA homeless programs, the HUD-VASH program supports the largest number of veterans, with over 78,000 veterans in housing using HUD-VASH vouchers as of the end of 2018 (HUD/VASH, 2019).

In addition, the Supportive Services for Veteran Families (SSVF) program was created in 2012 to help prevent homelessness in veterans and families experiencing housing instability who were at increased risk for homelessness. The SSVF has been instrumental in preventing homelessness through its funding for community-based organizations focused on rapid re-housing of veterans, case management services, employment support, assistance with community reintegration, mental health services, and moral injury repair initiatives (Volunteers of America, 2019). Finally, while numerous VA and community-based programs have been successful in significantly decreasing veteran homelessness over the past decade, much work remains to effectively manage the high rates of mental health and substance abuse disorders, along with social isolation factors known to pose significant risks for homelessness in the veteran population (Tsai & Rosenheck, 2015).

Housing Instability as a Social Determinant of Health

Housing instability is a social determinant of health that is associated with poor health status secondary to exposure, acute and chronic disease, and multiple comorbidities (Weber et al., 2017). As with civilians, veterans experiencing homelessness are likely to suffer from one or more chronic illnesses such as diabetes, hypertension, cardiac disease, chronic lung disease, and cancer (Goldstein et al., 2010). Additionally, comorbid substance use and psychiatric disorders including schizophrenia, bipolar disorder, depression, and PTSD are common in the homeless veteran population (Goldstein et al., 2010). Veterans who are homeless also have an increased risk of suicide. Homeless veterans have a suicide rate of 81 per 100,000, compared to the suicide rate of 35 per 100,000 for veterans overall, and 26 per 100,000 for civilian adults (VA National Center for Homelessness Among Veterans, 2018).

In a 2018 qualitative study of 32 homeless veterans, the investigators identified four chronic illness management subtypes among the study participants. Veterans were either not actively engaged in healthcare, attempting active engagement in care, actively engaged in care, or participating in sustained activity in care (Weber et al., 2018). Consideration of the necessary resources, teaching needs, and support systems of veterans in each of these subgroups is paramount and challenging for healthcare providers and social workers in both the VA and the private sector, whether in acute care, emergency settings, or in primary care or mental health clinics. Veterans not actively engaged in care who present to emergency departments for their care should be connected to needed resources to begin engaging in healthcare.

Promoting engagement in disengaged veterans experiencing homelessness is likely to require an interprofessional team approach that may entail multiple encounters. Care for veterans in this group is likely to require trust-building over time and special attention to teaching, along with referrals to social workers and case managers who can connect veterans with needed services. For those attempting engagement, it is necessary to assess barriers to engagement and to work with providers across specialties to provide resources that address barriers and can facilitate active involvement in health promotion such as regular primary care visits. Those actively engaged in care or participating in sustained involvement in care should be treated with respect and praised for their effort to take control of their health and wellness, while continuing to assess any new or developing barriers to continuing engagement.

Table 4.3 provides a short list of resources for veterans experiencing homelessness. Nurses are encouraged to become aware of homeless services specific to the geographic region in which they practice in order to facilitate referrals and advocate for veterans.

TABLE 4.3 RESOURCES FOR HOMELESS VETERANS

PROGRAM NAME	PROGRAM WEBSITE
HUD-VASH	https://www.va.gov/homeless/hud-vash.asp
HVRP	https://www.dol.gov/agencies/vets/programs/hvrp
SSVF	https://www.voa.org/supportive-services-for-veteran-families
National Coalition for Homeless Veterans	http://nchv.org/index.php/help/help/locate_organization/
The Salvation Army	https://www.salvationarmyusa.org/usn/provide-shelter/
National Alliance to End Homelessness	https://endhomelessness.org/homelessness-in-america/who-experiences-homelessness/veterans/

HUD-VASH, U.S. Department of Housing and Urban Development-VA Supportive Housing; HVRP, Homeless Veterans Reintegration Program; SSVF, Supportive Services for Veteran Families.

COMMUNITY SUPPORT SERVICES FOR VETERANS

Numerous support services and programs within the VA system, federal government, and the community are available to veterans and their families as potential resources that address many different areas of need. Nevertheless, a challenge exists in connecting veterans and their family members to these resources. Education of nurses and other health professionals around the range of available resources and how to refer veterans and family members are critical. To this end, the following section provides detailed information on select resources that pertain to veteran and caregiver support services. The subsequent section offers brief descriptions of other resources with contact information and online links to obtain more detailed information.

Veterans Service Organizations/Advocacy/Resources

Veterans Service Organizations (VSOs) are community-based organizations that serve as important resources in the lives of many veterans and their families and enhance quality of life for both groups (Harada & Pourat, 2004). The VA has published a directory of hundreds of VSOs available for public access online at www.va.gov/vso/VSO-Directory.pdf. Of note, inclusion of an organization in the VA VSO Directory does not constitute an endorsement of the organization by the VA or the U.S. Government. However, some VSOs are "chartered," signifying that "they are federally chartered and/or recognized or approved by the VA Secretary for purposes of preparation, presentation, and prosecution of claims under laws administered by the Department of Veterans Affairs" (VA, 2019m, para. 2).

VSOs offer veterans varied services, such as assistance with VA disability benefits claims and navigating the VA health system, education, job training and fairs, resume writing, financial grants, opportunities to participate in community service projects and social activities, and more. The opportunity to interact with fellow veterans in social and community activities through VSOs can be very helpful and meaningful to many veterans. Some VSOs provide services that are instrumental in supporting family members of active military and veterans. VSOs have also been very active and influential at the national level in lobbying Congress around areas related to veterans, proposing legislation, and offering testimony for this legislation (Harada & Pourat, 2004; VA, 2019m).

Five VSOs—the American Legion, Veterans of Foreign Wars (VFW), Vietnam Veterans of America (VVA), Team Red, White, and Blue, and Wounded Warriors Project—are described in the following in more detail because they are based throughout the United States and serve many veterans and family members. This is followed by a description of the VA Comprehensive Caregiver Support Program and the VA Caregiver Resource Directory. Other services and programs offered by VSOs, VA, and other community groups are presented in the Tables 4.4, 4.5, and 4.6.

AMERICAN LEGION

The American Legion, chartered by Congress in 1919 as a patriotic veterans' organization, focuses on service to veterans, service members, and communities. As the nation's largest VSO, it has over 2.4 million members at over 14,000 posts. Although it was initially launched as a veterans' advocacy group, it grew into having a major social and community role. Posts throughout the country are committed to community service, particularly for families of active military and veterans. Most posts have monthly meetings to carry out its business, implement activities, and offer venues for socialization (American Legion, 2019; Whittle et al., 2010).

The American Legion provides a broad array of programs within local communities and at the national level, where they lobby on behalf of our nation's veterans. Their programs include assistance with VA benefits claims and VA education benefits, employment assistance, and medical coverage for certain wounded, injured, or ill veterans through the Heroes to Hometowns program and Operations Comfort Warriors program. The Legion also raises millions in donations to help veterans and their families in times of need and to fund college scholarships (American Legion, 2019)

Some VSOs such as the American Legion and VFW have participated in health-related initiatives for their members. For example, the Posts Working for Veterans Health (POWER) intervention was evaluated with 219 veterans with hypertension recruited from 58 VSOs throughout southeastern Wisconsin. This peer-led intervention was designed to improve self-care behaviors that promote better blood pressure control. One to three members of each post were trained to be peer leaders who then trained other veterans to serve as leaders for the peer-led intervention arm (Mosack et al., 2012). POWER was part of a community and academic collaboration that involved a college of medicine and two VSOs. This study serves as an excellent example of a research partnership between investigators and VSOs for health promotion among veterans.

VETERANS OF FOREIGN WARS

The VFW organization was established in 1899, when veterans of the Spanish-American War and the Philippine Insurrection started local organizations to attain medical care and other services. These local groups subsequently came together to form the larger organization. Comprised of veterans and military service members from active duty, National Guard, and Reserve forces, the VFW currently has over 2 million members. Its mission is "to foster camaraderie among U.S. veterans of overseas conflicts. To serve our veterans, the military and our communities. To advocate on behalf of all veterans" (VFW, 2019, para. 1). The VFW aids veterans in the processes for VA benefits claims, separation benefits, education benefits, grants veterans' scholarships and financial aid, and offers services to support families and communities. Furthermore, the VFW has been a strong advocate at the national level that supported the establishment of the VA, the cemetery system, compensation for Vietnam veterans with toxic exposures, passage of the GI bill for educational benefits for veterans, and more recent initiatives to improve services for female veterans (VFW, 2019).

VIETNAM VETERANS OF AMERICA

The VVA, represented by 600 local chapters in 43 states, offers fellowship with other veterans, claims assistance, financial assistance, volunteer opportunities, and community service. It offers one-on-one counseling for benefits and claims through a Veteran Service Officer. At the national level, it works to promote legislation pertaining to key veteran issues, such as toxic exposures and VA improvements. Its goals are to address broad issues pertinent to Vietnam veterans and to create a positive public perception of them. VVA advocates for veterans on many key issues such as access to quality healthcare, full accounting of prisoners of war and those missing in action, identifying disability and illnesses related to military service, and supporting the next generation of war veterans (VVA, 2019).

TEAM RED, WHITE, AND BLUE

Team Red, White, and Blue is a community-based, nonprofit organization founded in 2010 to assist veterans facing reintegration challenges to reestablish relationships and social connectedness in their communities. When compared with earlier war cohorts, the 2.7 million service members who served in OEF/OIF/OND had longer and more frequent deployments that made it more difficult for some to return to and reintegrate with their families and communities after deployments (Geiling et al., 2012; Institute of Medicine, 2013; Johnson et al., 2013). Reintegration refers to the process through which the veteran resumes family, community, and employment roles (Berglass & Harrell, 2012). The mission of Team Red, White, and Blue is to build social connections and "to enrich the lives of American's veterans by connecting them to their community through physical and social activity" (Angel et al., 2018, p. 555). The organization uses a strength-based approach guided by positive psychology that emphasizes positive attributes of persons and the strengths that enable them to recover from life stressors. This underlying theoretical framework emphasizes finding meaning and belonging through relationships. The organization defines health "as creating frequent opportunities for team members to connect through fitness, sports, and recreation to improve physical, mental, and emotional well-being" (Angel et al., 2018, p. 556).

In September 2019, Team Red, White, and Blue launched a mobile phone application (or "app") that provides veteran members with access to thousands of physical, social, and service-oriented events hosted by volunteer leaders and members in communities throughout the United States. The app enables members to connect with others who are attending activities, to track past and future activities, and to receive notifications of events of interest (Personal communication with Caroline Angel, December 16, 2019; Team Red, White, and Blue, 2019). With over 217 chapters in the United States as of June 2017, and over 123,000 members consisting of veterans, active duty, and civilians, the organization is starting to gather evidence to assess its outcomes. The inclusion of civilians in Team Red, White, and Blue is purposeful to further expand the veterans' social network beyond an all veterans' group. This also enables civilian members to develop a deeper appreciation and knowledge of the military experience and culture, which enhances community support for veterans (Angel et al., 2018).

Wounded Warriors Project

The Wounded Warrior Project (WWP), a nonprofit organization, was founded in 2002 to provide support for and raise public awareness of service members injured during service on or after September 11, 2001. Serving 113,000 registered warriors, the organization has created and implemented many types of programs, as well as provided grants to other community partners to expand services to warriors and their families. WWP conducts numerous programs that aim to nurture the mind and body, as well as promote economic well-being. Programs address many diverse areas and strive to connect veterans and their families to resources, such as legal services, marriage and family counseling, acquiring a service dog, and medical services. WWP also assists veterans and families to manage VA or DoD benefits claims, apply for emergency financial assistance, and work with resources for job placement, resume writing, and interview skills. Activities are designed to help veterans and family members to connect with other warriors, family members, caregivers, and the local community. The WWP offers an array of mental health services to help warriors with combat stress, PTSD, and TBI, along with their families. The WWP Resource Center offers information to warriors and their family caregivers on the best available programs and services to meet their needs (WWP, 2019).

The Independence Program, offered by the WWP, is designed to assist warriors suffering from moderate-to-severe brain injury, spinal cord injury, or other neurological conditions to progress toward more independent living. To reach this goal, services consist of social and recreational activities, wellness programs, volunteer work, education, and programs on other life skills. The organization hosts peer-led support groups and events throughout the United States, recognizing the profound impact of peer support from fellow warriors who understand one another's experiences. Since 2012, WWP has granted $88 million to 165 military and veteran-connected organizations that offer support services to injured veterans and their family members (Krull & Haugseth, 2012; WWP, 2019).

Other Programs for Caregivers and Veterans

In addition to the five VSOs previously described, there are a multitude of other VA, federal, state, and community-based organizations that serve as resources to caregivers and veterans.

VA GENERAL CAREGIVER SUPPORT FOR CAREGIVERS OF ALL VETERANS

Results from a RAND national survey indicate there are 5.5 million family caregivers of veterans in the United States, with 1.1 million of those supporting a Post-9/11 veteran (Ramchand & Tanielian, 2014). In May 2011, the most sweeping support for U.S. family caregivers of veterans came with the Caregivers and Veterans Omnibus Health Services Act, P.L. 111–163. This Act provided a General Caregiver Support Program for caregivers of all veterans who need it. This program offers monthly telephone educational support with tips on self-care, free online educational workshops, peer support mentoring, and a caregiver support phone helpline (VA, 2019j).

The Caregivers and Veterans Omnibus Act also funded the PCAFC (Van Houtven & Smith, 2017). This program offers expanded assistance to a more specific population as described in the following.

PROGRAM OF COMPREHENSIVE ASSISTANCE FOR FAMILY CAREGIVERS

The PCAFC is a clinical program in which services are given directly to family caregivers of eligible veterans, defined as veterans who incurred or aggravated a serious injury during military service on or after September 11, 2001. The program provides caregivers with required caregiver training, education about VA resources, a monthly stipend ranging from $600 to $2300 per month, healthcare for caregivers without it, mental health services, and respite care (Malec et al., 2017; Shepherd-Banigan et al., 2018; Van Houtven et al., 2019). Findings from a recent evaluation of the program revealed that veterans of caregivers in the PCAFC had significantly greater use of outpatient services, including primary, mental health, and specialty care, and therefore appeared to have greater access and engagement in VA care (Van Houtven et al., 2019).

The 2018 VA MISSION Act states that expansion of the PCAFC will start when the VA has fully implemented a required information technology system to support this expanded access. Once the information technology system is implemented, the PCAFC will also be open to family caregivers of eligible veterans who experienced or aggravated a serious injury in the line of duty on or before May 7, 1975. In the final phase of the expansion, about 2 years later, the PCAFC will serve family caregivers of eligible veterans who developed or worsened a serious injury in the line of duty between May 7, 1975 and September 10, 2001 (VA, 2019i). Of note, many programs are now available to support caregivers of enrolled veterans of all eras. For more information, family members and veterans may call the Caregiver Support Line toll free at 1-855-260-3274 and refer to the 2019 Caregiver Resource Directory.

THE CAREGIVER RESOURCE DIRECTORY WITH RESOURCES FOR CAREGIVERS AND VETERANS

The 2019 Caregiver Resource Directory (DoD, 2019) includes the most commonly referenced resources, organizations, and programs that offer support to the caregivers of wounded, ill, or injured service members and veterans, but many resources can also be accessed directly by veterans. The goal of the directory is to connect communities with caregivers and to increase public awareness and support for caregivers. All the resources and programs in the Caregiver Resource Directory "have been reviewed and vetted in accordance with the National Resource Directory's participation policy, which can be found at www.nrd.gov." (DoD, 2019, p. 2). The plan is to update the directory on a regular basis, and it is available at warriorcare.dodlive.mil/caregiver-resources.

The directory was developed to assist caregivers in four ways: (a) to find and connect with the specific assistance they need, (b) to become more educated about their ill or injured service member's condition, (c) to connect caregivers with other communities of caregivers and caregiver supporters, and (d) to assist caregivers to take care of themselves (DoD, 2019). The 101-page directory is an excellent and comprehensive reference that describes resources for caregivers and veterans on a wide range of topics: helplines for information and assistance, advocacy and benefits, employment, caregiver support, military caregiver lifestyle, children's needs, education and training, financial support, healthcare needs, special equipment, legal assistance, online social networking, peer support, pet assistance, rest and relaxation, smartphone apps, sports and recreation, suicide prevention, and women veterans. The following tables provide some examples of supports described in the Directory in three areas: Telephone Helplines for Information and Assistance for Caregivers and Veterans (Table 4.4); Benefits and Advocacy Information and Services (Table 4.5); and Support Services for Caregivers' Knowledge,

TABLE 4.4 TELEPHONE HELPLINES FOR INFORMATION AND ASSISTANCE FOR CAREGIVERS AND VETERANS

VA Caregiver Support Line	A live operator is available to answer questions related to supporting caregivers. 855-260-3274 More information is also online at www.caregiver.va.gov
VA Coaching Into Care	Provides confidential coaching to help caregivers and others talk with their veteran about their concerns and opportunities for treatment. 888-823-7458
DoD Centers of Excellence	Offers access to resource consultants with expertise in mental health and traumatic brain injury. 866-966-1020 More information is online at resources@dcoeoutreach.org
VA Veteran Crisis Line	Provides assistance and crisis intervention to veterans and family members in crisis and at risk of hurting themselves or others. 800-273-8255
National Suicide Prevention Lifeline	Assists distressed veterans; connects them to a trained counselor at a local crisis center. 800-273-TALK (for veterans, press 1)
VA Operation Enduring Freedom/Operation Iraqi Freedom/Operation New Dawn Care Management Program	Assists service members, veterans, and caregivers to navigate VA programs during their transition from deployment to home. 877-222-8387
VA Veterans Benefits Administration	Provides information for veteran healthcare, benefits, and other services. 800-827-1000
VA PTSD Treatment Help	Provides assistance with PTSD and domestic violence and grief, confidential assessment. 877-259-5637
VA Vet Center Combat Call Center	Offers a confidential call center where combat veterans and their family members can talk with a staff of peers.
VA Women Veterans Call Center	Offers a call center where female veterans can seek support and services. 855-VA-WOMEN

DoD, Department of Defense; PTSD, posttraumatic stress disorder; VA, U.S. Department of Veterans Affairs.

TABLE 4.5 BENEFITS AND ADVOCACY INFORMATION AND SERVICES

Disabled American Veterans (Veteran Service Organization)	Provides assistance in filing for VA disability compensation and benefits. www.dav.org
DoD in Transition Mental Health Coaching and Support	Assists service members receiving mental health treatment to transition between healthcare systems and providers. https://www.pdhealth.mil/resources/intransition
Paralyzed Veterans of America (Veteran Service Organization)	Helps veterans with spinal cord injuries and other conditions with VA benefits, entitlements, and other benefits. www.pva.org

DoD, Department of Defense; VA, U.S. Department of Veterans Affairs.

TABLE 4.6 SUPPORT SERVICES FOR CAREGIVERS' KNOWLEDGE, SKILLS, AND WELL-BEING

VA Building Better Caregivers Workshops	Offers 6-week interactive group sessions (2 hours per week). https://www.caregiver.va.gov/docs/BBCworkshop.pdf
Coaching Into Care	Offers support and problem-solving to family and friends around encouraging and connecting veterans to VA care programs or other programs. www.mirecc.va.gov/coaching
Easter Seals Caregiving Training Program	Offers training to caregivers on home safety, self-care, caregiver skills, managing difficult behaviors, and support services. www.easterseals.com
Elizabeth Dole Foundation	Aims to empower, support, and honor our nation's 5.5 million military caregivers. Programs provide military and veteran caregivers the support they need at local, state, and national levels. https://www.elizabethdolefoundation.org/about-the-foundation/
Family Caregiver Alliance National Center on Caregiving	Provides educational resources, fact sheets, telephone conferences, discussion groups related to caregiving. www.caregiver.org/caregiver/jsp/home.jsp
VA SAFE	Offers 18-session family education modules for those caring for veterans with PTSD and other mental illness. www.ouhsc.edu/safeprogram
VA Caregiver Support	Provides tools for family caregivers, videos of caregivers and veterans. Gives info on closest VA caregiver support coordinator. www.caregiver.va.gov
Veterans Restorative Project	Offers deep relaxation and meditation to active duty military, veterans, and families, in addition to classes, retreats, and workshops. https://veteransrestorativeproject.org

PTSD, posttraumatic stress disorder; SAFE, Support and Family Education; VA, U.S. Department of Veterans Affairs.

Skills, and Well-Being (Table 4.6). These tables are meant to be illustrative, not exhaustive, given that over 600 resources are described in the Directory.

Veterans are residing in all areas of the United States, and they face unique challenges that may affect their mental and physical health and well-being. Whether related to transition from military to civilian life in general, to managing specific healthcare issues, housing, or care-access transitions, veterans and their families often require the assistance of healthcare team members across specialties to address these complex needs. Furthermore, veterans represent a population of men and women with unique skillsets, experiences, and leadership abilities. As a discipline that focuses on holistic patient-centered care, nurses across healthcare settings play a crucial role in the provision of care and education for veterans. Nurses should act as veteran advocates during times of transition and beyond. The remainder of this chapter focuses on the role of the nursing profession in providing care to veterans and their families in the community.

IMPLICATIONS FOR NURSING EDUCATION AND PRACTICE

Given that nurses interact with veterans in many community settings, they should screen all patients for veteran status by asking "Have you ever served in the military?" (American Academy of Nursing, n.d.; Collins et al., 2013). After this screening, nurses should inquire whether the veteran is enrolled in the VA health system. Nurses serve in a pivotal role to encourage veterans to seek guidance to determine VA eligibility, correct any misperceptions about eligibility, and connect veterans to social workers or VSOs who can aid them in the enrollment process. Basic knowledge of military culture and how to establish rapport when working with veterans is central to providing competent care. Basic understanding of the VA structure, eligibility requirements, and enrollment process, and the ability to connect veterans to needed resources can aid in establishing rapport with veterans that can improve their healthcare access and overall well-being.

With the potential for increasingly greater numbers of veterans who seek care in the private sector secondary to the MISSION Act, nurses are called upon to recognize veterans as belonging to a unique cultural entity and to recognize their many strengths and contributions, as well as the potential for complex mental, physical, and emotional conditions resulting from their military service. It is imperative that healthcare providers assess veterans for their reliance on dual healthcare services, and provide them with education on the importance of disclosing the use of dual health services to all providers to enhance communication among providers, prevent redundancies, and control healthcare costs.

Nurses in Practice

Persons struggling with homelessness face numerous multifaceted barriers to healthcare, such as financial barriers and stigma, while simultaneously facing health risks from exposure and poor living conditions. A 2015 study of 185 veterans who were homeless found that stigma was a factor that significantly contributed to veterans' delays in seeking care for needed primary healthcare services. Perceived stigma, specifically around embarrassment about being homeless and around substance abuse, significantly contributed to veterans' attitudes around healthcare (O'Toole et al., 2015). Veterans who are homeless represent an especially vulnerable population who require specialized, culturally sensitive and competent care from healthcare providers. Nurses work on the frontline of healthcare, are trained to provide whole-person care, and are often the first healthcare providers to interact with patients. Furthermore, nurses practice in multiple and varied settings whether in the VA or the private sector, in acute care settings, emergency departments, primary care offices, mental health clinics, and nursing homes that provide care to veterans experiencing homelessness (Weber et al., 2017). Given these unique roles, nurses are called upon to develop competencies to care for homeless veterans and to ensure correct and adequate screening, interventions, and follow-up care to this unique population are provided.

In a 2017 literature review of 21 studies, researchers identified four areas of focus to inform practice for nurses caring for veterans experiencing homelessness: chronic disease care, emergency care, barriers to care, and models for improving care (Weber et al., 2017). Just as in the civilian population, nurses play an important role in helping veterans to understand and effectively manage chronic disease on both a physical and psychological level. Nurses must provide veterans with appropriate teaching on the management of chronic diseases and common comorbid medical conditions, including information related to medication teaching, scheduling, side effects, and monitoring; self-care practices; when to notify a healthcare provider, and interactions among comorbid conditions. Furthermore, nurses are called upon to educate veterans on the association between substance abuse disorders and chronic medical conditions (Weber et al., 2017).

To provide veteran-centered care, it is imperative for nurses, whether at the bedside or in advanced practice roles, to be aware of the chronic conditions that veterans may experience related to their military service. Conditions such as TBI, PTSD, and depression have received much attention as the "signature" or "invisible" wounds of the wars in Iraq and Afghanistan (Tanielian & Jaycox, 2008). However, relationships between military exposures and the development of chronic health conditions are continuing to unfold over time. Furthermore, service-related exposures in veterans from previous war eras continue to affect the health of aging veterans.

For example, correlations have been found between exposures encountered during deployment to Iraq or Afghanistan and the development of chronic health problems such as asthma and chronic obstructive pulmonary disease, likely resulting from exposure to burn pits and other chemical exposures (Pugh et al., 2016; Szema et al., 2010). Additionally, much research has focused on symptom clusters referred to as "Gulf War Illness," including chronic respiratory, gastrointestinal, and dermatological problems, pain, fatigue, and cognitive dysfunction, believed to be the result of exposure secondary to military operations in the Persian Gulf (Kerr, 2015; Mawson & Croft, 2019). These examples represent just a few of the chronic health issues found to be related to military service. Nurses providing care to veterans experiencing homelessness should be aware of these associations in order to provide veteran-centered care and provide appropriate teaching to veterans in whatever health setting they may be encountered.

Nurses working in emergency department settings in the VA or the private sector should be aware of the high utilization of emergency services by veterans experiencing homelessness and the importance of comprehensive discharge planning to prevent return visits and encourage follow-up in primary care settings. Discharge planning should include education on specialized homeless services for veterans and referrals that may require collaboration with social services providers within and outside the VA. In a qualitative study of homeless male veterans' experiences of emergency department care, veterans reported feeling undervalued by healthcare providers and perceived a lack of empathy in the care they received from providers (Weber et al., 2019). Nurses practicing in emergency departments play a crucial role in providing compassionate care that is free from bias and in creating an environment of respect for persons of all cultures, backgrounds, and living conditions.

Increased understanding of the role of the social determinants of health on patient outcomes has led many healthcare systems to implement screening tools that address the social determinants including homelessness and housing instability. Integration of social determinants data into the electronic medical record enables providers to screen, triage, refer, and share data to improve outcomes for vulnerable populations (Gottlieb et al., 2015). Within the VHA, routine screening for housing instability was implemented in 2012 in the form of the Homelessness Screening Clinical Reminder (HSCR) embedded in the electronic health record to identify at-risk veterans. Veterans who are experiencing or are at-risk for homelessness can then be referred for additional services (Montgomery et al., 2013). The HSCR consists of two questions:

1.   In the past 2 months, have you been living in stable housing that you own, rent, or stay in as part of a household? (negative responses indicate housing instability)

2.   Are you worried or concerned that in the next 2 months you may not have a stable housing that you own, rent, or stay in as part of a household? (positive responses indicate risk)

Establishing rapport prior to screening for housing instability is key whether in the VA or private sector, and screening should occur across encounters and settings to ensure adequate care and referrals for services. Research has demonstrated that behavioral health and social service providers are responsible for a higher proportion of positive HSCR screens within the VHA, which researchers speculate may be explained by VA providers in these disciplines being more attuned to the struggles faced by veterans, their intimate knowledge of available housing services, and the level of trust they provide for veterans to feel comfortable to disclose housing concerns (Cusack et al., 2019). Hence, it is necessary for nurses in all settings to provide safe spaces for veterans to disclose their concerns, to be aware of the housing services available to veterans, and to work in collaboration with social services and other disciplines to ensure referral for needed services. These skills are especially important for nurses working in urban areas and those working in counties known to have a large population of homeless veterans.

Nursing Education

The provision of patient-centered care is essential to build trust and improve outcomes for patients in all healthcare settings. Veterans represent a vulnerable population with unique healthcare needs, complex mental and physical concerns, and barriers to care. Nurse educators in healthcare and academic settings have a responsibility to provide students with a solid foundation to ensure the provision of veteran-centered care and family-centered care for their family members. Now more than ever, it is imperative that nurse educators incorporate veteran-centered care competencies into nursing curricula and training modules for nurses. Many universities now have Joining Forces Committees and centers to support students who are active service members or veterans, and their families. Nursing students and faculty could be invaluable resources to assist these groups to implement their mission.

Although basic medical-surgical nursing courses are a good place to embed veteran-centered information, community or public health courses also present a unique opportunity to teach nursing students about the physical and psychosocial needs of veterans. Students should be encouraged to assess how veteran status has affected the veteran's health outcomes, to implement interventions to help veterans manage physical, mental, and psychosocial issues, and provide teaching on local resources to support the veterans they serve. Students should also have the opportunity to interact with veterans in simulated and real-world clinical settings such as the local VA hospital or outpatient health centers that provide care to veterans. Partnerships between schools of nursing and VA Medical Centers can prove invaluable in fostering nursing competence around veterans' health issues and can encourage students and nurses seeking to enhance their competency to serve as veteran advocates through community outreach and research partnerships. Further, utilization of CBOCs, CLC, or Vet Centers may be viable options to promote educational opportunities for nursing students to work with the veteran population.

One strategy that can foster relationships between the VA and schools of nursing is the recruitment of faculty that hold dual appointments between the VA and local colleges of nursing. These appointments can enhance not only the undergraduate curriculum but can also encourage graduate students to pursue advanced practice nursing careers working with veterans and inspire doctoral students to engage in research around veterans' issues. Strategies to incorporate veteran-centered content into nursing curricula include hiring veterans into faculty positions at colleges of nursing or inviting veterans or speakers from the VA to present veteran-centered content in either undergraduate or graduate-level courses (Olenick et al., 2015). Increased knowledge of and exposure to the unique issues faced by veterans and their families can inspire students at all levels to serve as veteran and family advocates at the community, state, and federal levels and to engage in research around veterans' and families' issues.

Furthermore, the value of interprofessional collaboration cannot be overlooked and should be emphasized throughout the nursing curriculum and in healthcare settings. Emphasis on interprofessional collaboration and the provision of exemplars for this will foster relationships between disciplines and lead to increased quality of care for veterans. For example, fostering interprofessional collaboration between nurses and social workers or case managers can help nurses connect veterans to local resources and programs that have the potential to improve their health and well-being. Education of nursing students on the importance of interprofessional collaboration promotes the team approach necessary to manage the complex mental, physical, and social needs of veterans and their families. Engaging in interprofessional education between students of nursing and social work may help to facilitate such collaboration.

Nurses and nursing students should also be encouraged to consider the potential to serve veterans in the role of an advanced practice nurse or in the field of nursing research. The University of Colorado Denver School of Nursing offers a graduate certificate in Military and Veterans Health Care, as well as Doctor of Nursing Practice and PhD degrees in nursing and Military and Veterans Healthcare. For more information on these programs visit www1.ucdenver.edu/online/online-programs/online-masters/master-of-science-in-veteran-and-military-health-care. There are also numerous opportunities for nurse scientists to pursue research opportunities within the VA or through academic partnerships that can serve to improve care for veterans and their families, building the science around the specialty of military and veterans' health nursing.

FUTURE RESEARCH PRIORITIES

Nurses are called upon to extend the knowledge base around evidence-based practice through participation in and the development of research related to the populations they serve. Research opportunities for nursing students and faculty, along with other nurse and interprofessional scientists, could be cultivated through partnerships with VA medical centers, CLCs, CBOCs, VSOs, and other community resources described in this chapter. Developing research partnerships with these organizations requires time to navigate systems and the commitment to work together to build trust. This includes an appreciation for the many strengths of veterans and their families along with the struggles that some may experience.

Within the VA health system, there is an increased appreciation for community-based participatory research approaches with veterans and their family members to elicit their voices and enhance understanding of their experiences and needs. For example, in recent studies using photovoice elicitation, some veterans and family members are part of the research team and are involved in the planning, implementation, and dissemination of the research (e.g., Mitchell et al., 2016; Rodriguez et al., 2019; True et al., 2015; True et al., 2019).

Research priorities related to care for community-dwelling veterans encompass many areas, such as

- the impact of increased screening for homelessness among newly returning veterans when completed by nurses and other health professionals;

- the efficacy of varied community programs in reaching homeless veterans and connecting them to services;

- additional rigorous studies on risk factors for homelessness in the veteran population, such as lack of social support, previous incarceration, and a history of adverse childhood events;

- the impact of early education of nursing students around veterans' health issues on their cultural competence in working with veterans and their families;

- the outcomes of programs that educate nursing students, nurses, and other health professionals to screen all patients by asking, "Have you ever served in the military?";

- the impact of providing nursing students with at least one clinical experience working in a VA hospital; and

- the experience of nursing students and nurses who are partnering with VSOs and other community organizations to provide health promotion and disease prevention initiatives.

CONCLUSION

Nurses are responsible for the care of veterans and their families in numerous and varied community healthcare settings—from the VA to private sector hospitals, to outpatient medical and mental health clinics, to CLCs, nursing homes, homeless shelters, and urgent care centers. Schools of nursing and healthcare systems striving for excellence in patient-centered care must provide education to their students and staff on the unique constellation of mental, physical, and psychosocial issues faced by veterans and their families, and how social factors and unique military experiences may present specific challenges to veterans' well-being. It is paramount that nurses be educated to screen for veteran status and housing instability, to work collaboratively with other disciplines to connect veterans and their families to local, state, and national resources, and to develop cultural humility around this vulnerable population whom they have the honor and privilege to serve.

REFERENCES

The complete reference list for this chapter appears in the digital version of the chapter, accessible at https://connect.springerpub.com/content/book/978-0-8261-3597-1/chapter/ch04

II

VETERAN-SPECIFIC HEALTHCARE ISSUES

OCCUPATIONAL AND ENVIRONMENTAL EXPOSURES IN VETERANS

CARMA ERICKSON-HURT | JULIE L. DECKER

Let us strive on to finish the work we are in, to bind up the nation's wounds, to care for him who shall have borne the battle and for his widow, and his orphan, to do all which may achieve and cherish a just and lasting peace among ourselves and with all nations.

Abraham Lincoln

KEY TERMS

noise exposure	Vietnam
radiation exposure	Korea
Agent Orange	Gulf War
hepatitis	burn pits
liver flukes	toxic embedded fragments
environmental exposure	depleted uranium
occupational hazards	chemical warfare agents
service-connected	oil well fires
veterans	

INTRODUCTION

Military service is often associated with combat-related injuries (i.e., gunshot wounds); however, individuals serving in the military are often subjected to non-combat-related hazards. This chapter highlights the common occupational and environmental exposures attributed to military service. Occupational exposures tend to occur within the workplace where the individual may be exposed to chemical substances or equipment safety-related concerns. Examples of occupational exposures covered in the chapter include noise, faulty equipment, exposure to chemical solvents, burn pits, and radiation. Environmental exposures occur in the surroundings in which humans inhabit, particularly

The complete reference list for this chapter appears in the digital version of the chapter, accessible at https://connect.springerpub.com/content/book/978-0-8261-3597-1/chapter/ch05

TABLE 5.1 OCCUPATIONAL AND ENVIRONMENTAL EXPOSURES BY WAR ERA

EXPOSURE	KOREAN WAR	VIETNAM WAR	COLD WAR ERA	GULF WAR	IRAQ WAR OIF, OND	OEF/ AFGHANISTAN
Occupational hazards	■	■	■	■	■	■
Cold injuries						■
Noise	■		■	■	■	■
Agent Orange or other herbicides		■				
Hepatitis C		■				
Liver fluke infection		■				
Ionizing radiation			■			
Project 112/ Project SHAD			■			
Mustard gas			■			
Atsugi waste incinerator			■			
Herbicide tests and storage			■			
Edgewood/ Aberdeen experiments			■			
Camp Lejeune water supplies			■			
Fort McClellan				■		
Vaccinations exposures				■		
Oil well fires				■		
Chemical and biological weapons				■		
Depleted uranium				■	■	■
CARC paint				■		
Pyridostigmine bromide				■		
Pesticides				■		
Sand, dust, and particulates				■	■	■
Toxic embedded fragments				■	■	■
Infectious disease				■	■	■
Heat injuries				■	■	■
Traumatic brain injury					■	■
Mefloquine					■	■
Sulfur fire					■	■

TABLE 5.1 (continued)

EXPOSURE	KOREAN WAR	VIETNAM WAR	COLD WAR ERA	GULF WAR	IRAQ WAR OIF, OND	OEF/ AFGHANISTAN
Burn pits						
Rabies						
Chemical warfare agents						
Chromium						

CARC, chemical agent resistant coating; OIF, Operation Iraqi Freedom; OND, Operation New Dawn; SHAD, Shipboard Hazard and Defense

SOURCE: Adapted from the U.S. Department of Veterans Affairs, 2019 (a, d–z).

water, soil, and air. Environmental exposures presented within the chapter include extreme temperatures, pesticide/herbicide use, contaminated water supplies, and poor air quality.

BACKGROUND

Veterans seek healthcare in civilian, military, and U.S. Department of Veterans Affairs (VA) health facilities. Being positioned at the center of patient care, it is imperative for nurses to have a basic understanding of the potential exposures and conditions incurred by veterans, active duty personnel, and their families. Many healthcare providers are now aware of the health problems associated with Agent Orange exposure in Vietnam veterans, but for those who served in the Gulf War, Iraq and Afghanistan, the research is still developing. Therefore, in many cases there are insufficient data to identify long-term health effects of hazardous exposures. Obtaining an accurate medical and deployment history is essential in providing accurate diagnosis and appropriate treatment (Olenick et al., 2015).

Exposure risks can vary significantly as deployment experiences are unique to each military service, mission, length, and frequency of deployment, as well as numerous other factors. In addition to deployment in areas of conflict, veterans may have been at risk for hazardous exposure in their everyday work environment, humanitarian and disaster assistance, peacekeeping missions, and other significant events throughout the world. Veterans have their own unique stories in terms of their service; taking the time to conduct a thorough interview to compile a military history, while paying attention to types of duty and location of duty, can provide information regarding potential exposures. This chapter is not inclusive of all the environmental and occupational exposures faced by veterans but addresses the exposures noted as posing significant health risks by the VA (Table 5.1).

OCCUPATIONAL HAZARDS

Occupational hazards of serving in the military are numerous and can vary from injuries sustained on active duty to exposure to substances that may have long-term effects. Injuries will not be discussed in this chapter as injuries are very specific to the individual and incident. Noise, radiation, and asbestos exposure are usually monitored during military service and may qualify veterans for disability compensation from the VA.

Noise Exposure

While each era of military service has unique health concerns, noise exposure tends to be common among all veterans and active duty personnel due to the nature of warfare as well as occupational duties while a member of the U.S. Armed Services. Sources of detrimental noise arise from a variety of

TABLE 5.2 COMMON SOURCES OF MILITARY EXPOSURE TO SOUND

SOURCE	DECIBEL LEVEL
Aviation	
Jet taking off from approximately 25 m/82 ft	150
Aircraft carrier	140
Military jet aircraft take-off from aircraft carrier with afterburner at 15.24 m/50 ft	130
UH-60 Blackhawk helicopter flying at 100 knots/115 mph	108
Jet flyover at 304 m/1,000 ft	103
Munition	
9 mm pistol and M16 Rifle firing	156
M26 Grenade exploding at 30 m/100 ft	157
0.50 Caliber machine gun firing	161
60 mm M720 mortar at 1 m/approximately 3 ft	180
M198 (M203) Z8S 155 mm Howitzer	181
Transportation Sources	
M88A1E1 Recovery vehicle traveling at 15 mph	105
HMMWV Traveling at 50 mph	88
PLS Truck traveling at 55 mph	87
Heavy Equipment/Machinery	
Riveting machine	110
Welder/torch at 50 ft	74
Jackhammer	89
Dump truck	76
Concrete saw	90
Pneumatic tools	90

HMMWV, high mobility multipurpose wheeled vehicle; PLS, palletized load system.

SOURCE: Adapted from Purdue University. (2000). *Noise sources and their effects.* https://www.chem.purdue.edu/chemsafety/Training/PPETrain/dblevels.htm; U.S. Army Public Health Command. (2014). *Readiness though hearing loss prevention-Technical Guide 250.* https://phc.amedd.army.mil/PHC Resource Library/TG250.pdf; U.S. Department of Transportation. (2017). *Noise.* https://www.fhwa.dot.gov/environment/noise/construction_noise/handbook/handbook09.cfm

sources and may occur in varying settings. As a result of this type of exposure, individuals may develop hearing loss, tinnitus, or both (Humes et al., 2006).

Sources of noise may vary among branches of military service according to activity and specialty area of training. The obvious sources of excessive noise may include weaponry, jet engines, vehicles, watercraft, and communication systems, as well as in industrial-type settings (Humes et al., 2006). Service members may be exposed to harmful levels of noise during training exercises, day-to-day military operations, and active combat. Individuals often encounter high levels of noise during their day-to-day activities associated with a specialty area; for example, maintenance of vehicles and aircraft, military construction, and demolition. According to the Hearing Health Foundation, in 2017, 1.16 million veterans were awarded disability compensation for hearing loss related to military service (Hearing Health Foundation, 2019).

Current guidelines for safety, as documented by The National Institute on Deafness and Other Communication Disorders (NIDCD, 2019), suggest that sounds at or below 70 A-weighted decibels (dBA), even after long exposure, are not likely to cause hearing damage. However, long and repeated exposure to sound at or above 86 dBA is likely to negatively impact hearing quality in an individual (NIDCD, 2019). Table 5.2 offers examples of sources of sound exposures experienced by military personnel.

Recognizing the damage to hearing that military service may cause, the U.S. Department of Defense (DoD) has instituted methods to decrease the potential adverse effects of sound. In the military setting, noise exposure may be decreased through isolation (increasing distance from the source of the sound as well as physical barriers), the dampening of the vibrations, insulation as well as proper maintenance of equipment (Humes et al., 2006). As an additional method of reducing the adverse effects of noise, the DoD is mandating the use of individual hearing protection devices in the forms of foam ear plugs, triple-flange earplugs, combat arms earplugs, and noise muffs (DoD, 2019). While these methods are effective in decreasing exposure to sound, compliance with use and ensuring proper fit of the devices are essential to maintaining overall auditory health.

Exposure to loud noises, regardless of the venue, can lead to a negative outcome with regard to hearing quality for individuals. For current members of the military, hearing acuteness and quality are essential from a tactical and survival point of view. For veterans, the loss of hearing may cause a decreased quality of life as well as safety concerns. Proper use of hearing protective devices, even years following exposure, may assist in decreasing hearing damage.

Veterans with hearing loss often have difficulty hearing and understanding speech when they are in situations with background noises. Because most social settings and activities involve multiple people and conversations, this creates background noise which can make it difficult for the veteran to hear, answer questions, and participate in conversations. Veterans may avoid situations that make them feel overwhelmed, leading to social isolation at home and reduced productivity at work (Bressler et al., 2017).

While veterans may be the primary focus of hearing concerns, the family and support system may also be negatively impacted by this health issue. Verbal communication is the most frequent manner by which humans interact with each other. Additionally, effective communication is vital to a harmonious relationship among families and support systems. Unfortunately, when hearing is impaired in one or more members of the family, frustration and impatience may surface leading to anger, disappointment, or even isolation for the family member. Negative feelings may surface among the family/support system because they may feel that communication with their veteran family member(s) is reduced to a "shouting match." The continual frustration with communication may impact the family and support system strength leading to an overall negative environment and lack of support for all parties.

Radiation Exposure

Many individuals attribute radiation exposure to the use of the atomic bombs on the Japanese cities of Hiroshima and Nagasaki in August 1945. While the use of these bombs did expose many individuals, military and civilian, to high levels of radiation, service members may also have received exposures in many forms other than the use of the atom bombs.

Radiation, as defined by U.S. Department of Health and Human Services, Radiation Emergency Medical Management (2019), is a type of energy, in the form of waves, rays, or particles, that is in motion. Two basic types of radiation exist: non-ionizing and ionizing. Whether radiation is non-ionizing or ionizing influences the health risks. Non-iodizing radiation is low-energy radiation that includes radiation from sources such as sunlight, microwaves, radio frequencies, radar, and sonar. While not as dangerous as ionizing radiation, non-ionizing radiation can cause health effects.

Ionizing radiation is the high-energy radiation that attributes to most of the concerns about radiation exposure during military service. Ionizing radiation is basically defined as any form of radiation that can shift electrons from atoms (ionization) which can pose health risks by damaging tissue and DNA in genes (Environmental Protection Agency, 2019). The health concern with this form of radiation is the potential damage to the DNA in the cells of exposed individuals.

During military service, individuals may be exposed to both forms of radiation, ionizing and non-ionizing. The sources of exposure are often found in industry, healthcare settings, nuclear power plants, and research centers. Military members may also receive exposure during operations from sources such as x-rays, nuclear weapons handling/detonation, dirty bombs, radioactive material along with calibration and measurement sources (Blake & Komp, 2014; VA, 2019k). Following specific investigations, the VA (2015) has listed specific circumstances and locations where military members may have been exposed to radiation:

- **Radiological cleanup of Enewetak Atoll:** the U.S. conducted 43 nuclear tests on Enewetak Proving Ground at Enewetak Atoll from 1948 to 1958. Radiation at the test site was cleaned up from May 1977 to May 1980.

- **U.S. Air Force plutonium clean-up mission, Palomares, Spain:** a nuclear weapons mishap occurred on January 17, 1966 when a U.S. Air Force (USAF) B-52 bomber and KC-135 tanker aircraft collided. The result of the mishap led to the release of four nuclear weapons; two weapons were damaged and upon ground impact, released plutonium. While no detonation of the weapons occurred, nearly 1,600 military and civilian personnel were potentially exposed to airborne dust and debris that was contaminated with plutonium.

- **Fukushima nuclear accident:** service members may have been exposed to low doses of radiation in Japan from March 12 to May 11, 2011, following a nuclear accident on March 11, 2011.

- **Radiation-risk activity (includes "Atomic Veterans"):** those with documentation of participation in nuclear weapons testing and the American occupation and cleanup following the bombing of Hiroshima and Nagasaki.

- **military occupational exposure:** various military occupations, such as nuclear weapons technicians and dental technicians including routine, usually safe exposures, to radiation.

- **Depleted uranium (DU):** during an explosion, pieces of DU used in tank armor and some bullets can scatter and embed in muscle and soft tissue.

- **long-range navigation (LORAN) radiation:** U.S. Coast Guard veterans who worked at LORAN stations from 1942 to 2010 may have been exposed to x-ray radiation from high voltage vacuum tubes.

- **McMurdo Station, Antarctica, nuclear power plant:** the U.S. Navy operated a small nuclear plant at the McMurdo Station, Antarctica (1964–1973). The nuclear plant was decommissioned after a leak was discovered.

- **Nasopharyngeal (nose and throat) radium irradiation treatments:** certain pilots, submariners, divers, and others were given this treatment during service in 1940 to the mid-1960s to prevent ear damage from pressure changes.

- **Radiation therapy:** ionizing radiation can be used to treat disease, most commonly cancer.

- **Prisoners of war in Japan**

- **Service during the Korean War:** radiation exposure occurred in several ways for Korean War veterans. Some common sources were an involvement in nuclear weapons testing and proximity to areas where radioactive bombs were dropped.

- **Service in the Gulf Wars as well as deployment locations in Bosnia and Afghanistan:** during these periods, DU may have been ingested or inhaled. DU is a byproduct of the uranium enrichment process used by the U.S. military in projectiles and tank armor during the Gulf War in 1990. It is most hazardous when internalized through shrapnel, contaminated wounds, or inhalation (American Academy of Nursing, 2014; VA, 2016a; VA, 2019k).

The U.S. Veterans Administration currently recognizes a number of diseases related to exposure to ionizing radiation, especially among those individuals classified as Atomic Veterans, groups of

U.S. military personal who participated in one or more above-ground nuclear tests during their military service between 1945 and 1962 or were part of the U.S. military occupation forces in and around Hiroshima or Nagasaki, Japan, before 1946 (VA, 2015). The following types of cancer have been closely linked with radiation, regardless of the circumstance and location of the exposure (Box 5.1).

BOX 5.1

IONIZING RADIATION DISEASES

Diseases related to ionizing radiation during military service

- Cancers of the bile ducts, bone, brain, breast, colon, esophagus, gallbladder, liver (primary site, but not if cirrhosis or hepatitis B are indicated), lung (including bronchiolo-alveolar cancer), pancreas, pharynx, ovary, salivary gland, small intestine, stomach, thyroid, urinary tract (kidney/renal, pelvis, urinary bladder, and urethra)
- Leukemia (except chronic lymphocytic leukemia)
- Lymphomas (except Hodgkin disease)
- Multiple myeloma

Diseases which are possibly caused by exposure to ionizing radiation during service

- All cancers
- Non-malignant thyroid nodular disease
- Parathyroid adenoma
- Posterior subcapsular cataracts
- Tumors of the brain and central nervous system

SOURCE: Adapted from the U.S. Department of Veterans Affairs. (2019k). *Facts about radiation.* https://www.publichealth.va.gov/exposures/radiation/basics.asp

---

While radiation exposure is commonly linked with cancer, it merits mentioning that other disease processes are also part of the concern. Non-malignant thyroid nodular disease, parathyroid adenoma, posterior subcapsular cataracts, and tumors of the brain and central nervous system are also linked with radiation exposure (VA, 2019k).

Asbestos

Exposure to asbestos can be a serious health risk if asbestos-containing material is disturbed in such a way that the particles and fibers become airborne. Symptoms of asbestos-related diseases, such as shortness of breath, coughing, and chest pain, often do not appear until 20 to 50 years after the exposure (VA, 2019a). Veterans who served in any of the following occupations may have been exposed to asbestos: mining, milling, shipyard work, insulation work, demolition of old buildings, carpentry and construction, manufacturing and installation of products such as flooring and roofing. Veterans who served in Iraq and other countries in that region could have been exposed to asbestos when older buildings were damaged and the contaminants were released into the air. Exposure to asbestos can cause permanent lung disease (Box 5.2).

BOX 5.2

LUNG DISEASE ASSOCIATED WITH ASBESTOS EXPOSURE

Asbestosis

- Scarring of lung tissue which causes breathing problems
- Usually occurs in workers exposed to asbestos in workplaces before the federal government began regulating asbestos use in the 1970s

Pleural plaques

- Scarring in the inner surface of the ribcage and area surrounding the lungs which can cause breathing problems
- Usually not as serious as asbestosis

Cancer

- Exposure to asbestos can cause lung cancer and mesothelioma
- Mesothelioma is a cancer of the pleural membrane (lining of the lung)
- Mesothelioma may also affect the peritoneum (lining of the abdomen)
- Mesothelioma is rare and is usually caused by asbestos exposure

SOURCE: Adapted from the U.S. Department of Veterans Affairs. (2019a). *Asbestos.* https://www.publichealth.va.gov/exposures/asbestos/index.asp.

Families and caregivers of veterans with mesothelioma can find resources and support through the VA. If the veteran develops mesothelioma as a result of exposure during their service they may be eligible for healthcare and compensation.

Unknown Exposure: Amyotrophic Lateral Sclerosis

Amyotrophic lateral sclerosis (ALS) is a progressive neurodegenerative disease that affects nerve cells in the brain and the spinal cord, causing the brain to lose the ability to initiate and control muscle movement resulting in patients becoming totally paralyzed in the later stages of the disease (ALS Association, 2019). Military veterans, regardless of the branch of service, the era in which they served, and whether they served during a time of peace or a time of war, are at a greater risk of dying from ALS than if they had not served in the military and they are twice as likely to develop ALS than the general population (ALS Association, 2019).

The connection between ALS and military service was first identified in Gulf War veterans and numerous subsequent studies have validated a connection between military service and ALS. Specific exposures have not been identified as definitely causing ALS and the etiology remains unknown. A study of over 600 veterans with ALS found a positive trend toward ALS and the total time of all deployments (Beard et al., 2016). This same study found ALS was more common after specific exposures including pesticides, chemicals and radiation in World War II, Korea, Vietnam, and Gulf War veterans (Beard et al., 2016). Despite numerous studies identifying correlations, the VA has not identified specific exposure criteria and presumes ALS diagnosed in all veterans who had 90 days or more continuous active military service is related to their service, and therefore they are eligible for care and disability through the VA.

All healthcare providers should immediately ask patients diagnosed with ALS if they are a veteran. Qualifying veterans with ALS are entitled to receive VA disability compensation, which is a monthly compensation. The VA offers healthcare, prescriptions, medical supplies, prosthetic items, and home improvement and structural alteration grants to pay the cost to make the home more accessible (ALS Association, 2019). In addition to benefits for the veteran, spouses and children may receive dependency and indemnity compensation, which is a monthly payment to eligible survivors and an allowance to pay for care providers.

ENVIRONMENTAL EXPOSURES COMMON TO ERA OF MILITARY SERVICE

Wounds and death are commonly associated with ammunition and explosives used during combat; however, environmental exposures may also adversely impact the short- and long-term health of veterans and, possibly, their offspring. The health of military personnel and their families may be at risk due to exposures from chemical, environmental, or physical sources. While each era of military service is described by signature wounds, the different eras also possess common environmental exposures.

Korea

The Korean War, often referred to as "The Forgotten War," began in June of 1950 as troops loyal to North Korean People's Army, with the assistance of the Chinese Communists, crossed the 38th parallel, a border marking the line between North and South Korea, into United Nations (UN) forces as well as those from South Korea. United States military presence numbered nearly 1.8 million (VA, n.d.).

The years of the war in Korea produced much loss of life and injury. Total deaths (battle related, deaths occurring other than in battle, and other deaths in service) numbered just over 54,000 and non-mortal wounds slightly exceeding 103,000 (VA, n.d.). An armistice was signed by both sides on July 27, 1953 ending 3 years of bloodshed.

Aside from the combat-related dangers, military members who served in Korea often endured extremes of temperature, especially troublesome were the cold winters. Due to the extremely cold conditions, individuals commonly suffered frost bite, immersion foot, and hypothermia (VA, 2019h). The extent and degree of cold-related injuries were dependent upon many factors: temperature, wind chill factor, moisture, degree of physical activity, length of exposure, and access to and use of protective clothing (VA, 2019h). While the summer months exposed the individuals to heat, humidity, and harsh rain, the extreme cold, fierce winds, long periods of exposure to the elements, periods of inactivity, and poor shelter define the experiences of those who fought during the winters in the Korean War.

A pivotal battle took place early in the conflict that caused significant exposure-related concerns. The occurrences of frostbite and immersion foot posed a major issue for U.S. military personnel throughout the war, especially during the Battle for the Chosin Reservoir. The Chosin Reservoir, a man-made lake located in the northeast area of the Korean peninsula, held strategic significance for South Korean, United States, and UN forces. During the months of October through December of 1950, the opposing forces fought for control of the 78-mile stretch of road that connected Hungnam and Chosin Reservoir. The road served as the only route of retreat for the South Koreans and their support forces.

Those who served in this area experienced the challenges of maneuvering through very rough terrain that required military personnel to participate in steep vertical climbs with deep drops. Adding to the adversity, roads were in poor condition. In mid-November of 1950, a sustained cold front from Siberia reached the Chosin Reservoir plummeting temperatures to an estimated −36 °F to −50 °F with a wind chill factor of −100 °F (Appleman, 1990; VA, 2019q). Not only did the extreme temperatures place individuals at risk for frostbite but it also negatively impacted the care of the wounded. Icy roads prevented the evacuation of the injured to aid stations delaying medical attention, thereby placing the individual at risk for serious health-related complications such as frostbite or gangrene (Appleman, 1990).

In addition to frostbite and gangrene, immersion foot also developed in some individuals. Immersion foot, commonly referred to as *trench foot*, is a painful disorder of the foot when damage occurs to the skin, nerves, and muscle resulting from prolonged exposure to cold and dampness. Regardless of the era of military service, this type of injury is common among service members whose feet are exposed to wet and cold for prolonged periods of time. Initial symptoms of immersion foot may include reddening of the skin, numbness, leg cramps, tingling sensation/pain, blisters/ulcerations, bleeding under the skin, and the darkening of the foot to shades of dark purple, blue, or gray that strongly suggest that gangrene may be occurring (Occupational Safety Heath Administration, 2018).

Injuries due to cold exposure/cold related injuries during the Korean War were significant. The VA (2019h) estimates that 16% of the Army non-battle-related injuries required hospital admission and over 5,000 U.S. casualties related to cold injuries required evacuation from Korea during the winter of 1950-1951. Complicating matters, the extreme cold prohibited medical care to be given to those in need (VA, 2019h).

Long-term complications of extreme cold exposure include peripheral neuropathy, melanoma in frostbite scars, arthritis in the area of involvement, chronic tinea pedis, fallen arches, stiffness occurring in the metatarsals, nocturnal pain, and cold sensitizations (VA, 2019h). These conditions may be exacerbated due to aging process whereas overall circulation becomes compromised as well as the acquisition of such disease conditions as peripheral vascular disease, arteriosclerosis/atherosclerosis, venous stasis, and diabetes mellitus.

Vietnam

During the early months of the Korean War, the United Sates became involved in another quest to halt the spread of Communism into Vietnam. The United States sent advisors to support France in their effort to combat the Viet Minh forces. By early March 1965, the first U.S. combat ground troops arrived in Vietnam joining 23,000 American military advisors currently in Vietnam. The Vietnam War (1964–1975) saw the utilization of conventional tactics and weaponry as well as other methods. While the risk of injury and death due to combat was ever present, individuals also suffered injuries related to environmental exposures.

Vietnam is a country with a tropical climate consisting of monsoonal weather patterns, high heat, and humidity. For these reasons, individuals stationed in the jungles faced the challenge of staying dry for long periods of time. The ability to properly bathe was scant. As a result of the environmental conditions and infrequent opportunities to perform hygiene, many service members in the jungles suffered from bacterial and fungal infections of the skin and their feet often developed into immersion foot. Also presenting among the troops was several cases of malaria, diarrhea, and cholera (VA, 2019q).

DEFOLIANT/HERBICIDAL AGENTS

During the Vietnam War, several defoliant/herbicidal agents were used by the U.S. military. The purpose of their use was to reduce the density of the jungles of Vietnam thereby decreasing the number of strategic hiding places for the enemy as well as depleting enemy food sources. The herbicides were known by the color painted around the 55-gallon container in which they were shipped and stored; examples included Agent Purple, Agent White, Agent Blue, and the most often used, Agent Orange. Estimations suggest that nearly 17 to 19 million gallons of herbicides were sprayed over nearly 6 million acres in Vietnam (VA, 2008). While the numbers illustrate the geographical coverage of use, estimates suggest that 3 million veterans were exposed to Agent Orange (Vietnam Veterans of America [VVA], 2017).

Agent Orange was sprayed over the jungles, near landing zones, along rivers, and any other area deemed necessary. The compound was sprayed by fixed-wing airplanes and helicopters, trucks as well as backpack devices. Estimates suggest that between 1962 and 1971, 11 million gallons of Agent Orange were sprayed in Vietnam, primarily during "Operation Ranch Hand" (VVA, 2017). Exposure to the chemical agents is not limited to direct contact in the jungles of Vietnam. Other sources of exposure are residue on airplanes, ships off the shore of Vietnam, service in the demilitarized zone in Korea during 1968 to 1971, military bases in Thailand, and herbicidal testing and storage facilities (VA, 2017b).

While Agent Orange exposure is commonly associated with service in Vietnam, approximately 1,500 to 2,100 U.S. Air Force personnel who maintained and traveled in the C-123 may have been exposed (Institute of Medicine [IOM], 2015) as the aircraft was used to transport and spray Agent Orange during Operation Ranch Hand. In the years following the end of the Vietnam War, these planes were used to train and transport members of the military in addition to being used as medical and cargo transport. Samples obtained from 1979 to 2009 confirm the presence of Agent Orange residue in the air and on the surface of some of the planes (IOM, 2015). The Health and Medical Division of the National Academies of Sciences, Engineering, and Medicine (NASEM), formerly known as the IOM, reports that reservists who served as flight crews, ground maintenance crews, and aero-medical crews likely would have received some degree of exposure to Agent Orange (VA, 2017d). Individuals who may qualify for benefits related to Agent Orange exposure are:

- active duty personnel who served in a regular USAF unit location where a contaminated C-123 was assigned who had regular contact with the aircraft through flight, ground, or medical duties between 1969 and 1986, and who developed an Agent Orange related disability; and

- reservists who were assigned to flight, ground, or medical crew duties at the following locations between 1969 and 1986, and who developed an Agent Orange related disability:

  - Lockbourne/Rickenbacker Air Force Base (Ohio; 906th and 907th Tactical Air Groups or 355th and 356th Tactical Airlift Squadron);

  - Westover Air Force Base in Massachusetts (731st Tactical Air Squadron and 74th Aeromedical Evacuation Squadron); and

  - Pittsburgh, Pennsylvania, International Airport (758th Airlift Squadron; VA, 2017a).

For perspective, Agent Orange is a mixture of several toxic substances including 2,4-D and 2,4,5,-T (VVA, 2017). During the manufacturing process of 2,4,5,-T a contaminant, known as 2,3,7,8-tetrachlorodibenzo-paradioxin results. The resultant compound is commonly known as dioxin. The potency of the dioxin compound is serious and severe. Dioxins are described as persistent organic pollutants due to the extended length of time it takes to breakdown once in the environment (U.S. Environmental Protection Agency, 2019). The current scientific evidence suggests that dioxin is a potent carcinogen as well as appearing to possess concerning non-cancer health and environmental hazard effects that include reproductive, developmental, and immunological defects (Birth Defects Research for Children, Inc., 2019). Dioxin appears to act like a persistent synthetic hormone interfering with important physiological signaling systems that have the capability to adversely affect cell development and function.

In the years following the end of the war, many returning veterans began to develop a sundry of symptoms and serious health concerns; these include chloracne, skin lesions, liver damage, decreased libido, photosensitivity, changes in skin pigmentation, numbness of extremities, joint pain, cancers, and birth defects in their children (VVA, 2017). Mounting health concerns prompted several agencies to launch investigations to explore whether Agent Orange was related to the acquisition of the illnesses.

Research conducted by IOM, National Academy of Sciences, VA, and the Centers for Disease Control and Prevention (CDC) over multiple years yielded conflicting and inconclusive results (Beaulieu & Fessele, 2002). However, continued investigations have offered enough evidence of health conditions associated with Agent Orange exposure to merit recognition of the compound as possessing health-related complications. Because of the recognition of the potential adverse effects of Agent Orange, compensation benefits may be awarded to those who qualify. The VA considers veterans who served anywhere in Vietnam between January 9, 1962 and May 7, 1975 as presumed to have been exposed to herbicides. These veterans do not need to show that they were exposed to Agent Orange or other herbicides in order to be eligible for disability compensation for diseases related to Agent Orange exposure.

Current illnesses/diseases recognized by the Veterans Administration as connected to Agent Orange include the following (Box 5.3).

BOX 5.3

AGENT ORANGE CONNECTED ILLNESSES/DISEASES

- Acute peripheral neuropathy
- Adult onset type II diabetes mellitus
- AL amyloidosis
- Chloracne
- Parkinson's disease
- Peripheral neuropathy
- Porphyria cutanea tarda
- Spina bifida
- Sub-acute peripheral neuropathy

SOURCE: Adapted from Vietnam Veterans of America. (2017). *The VVA self help guide to service-connected disability compensations for exposure to Agent Orange for veterans and their families.* Author.

During the investigatory phase, incidents of cancer among Korean and Vietnam veterans merited examination into possible connections to Agent Orange exposure. Over time, studies were conducted and yielded large bodies of evidence that suggested a plausible link between exposure and cancer diagnosis. While investigations on potential health connections continue, current empirical data point to Agent Orange exposure as being connected to cancers, specifically soft tissue carcinoma, non-Hodgkin and Hodgkin lymphoma, chronic lymphocytic leukemia including hairy cell leukemia as well as other chronic B-cell leukemias, and monoclonal gammopathy of undetermined significance, a precursor to multiple myeloma (American Cancer Society, 2019). Additionally, limited evidence also suggests cancer of the respiratory system, particularly the lungs, bronchus, trachea, and larynx; prostate and bladder cancer; and lymphoma as being linked to Agent Orange exposure (American Cancer Society, 2019).

Upon returning home from Vietnam, some couples had trouble conceiving and maintaining a pregnancy to full term. Many returning veterans attributed these issues to Agent Orange exposure. There has been a great deal of discussion and concern on this subject among Vietnam veterans. Various studies were conducted from governmental and private agencies. Following years of research, current results from the NASEM (2018b) reported that there is inadequate/insufficient evidence to support the claim of an association between Agent Orange exposure and changes in semen quality. Additionally, studies independent of the work of the NASEM (2018b) have not established a definitive link between infertility and Agent Orange Exposure. While many studies explore the effects of Agent Orange on males, the effects of Agent Orange on females merits mentioning.

During the Vietnam War, more than 7,500 women served and of this number nearly 6,000 were nurses and medical specialists (The Women's Memorial, 2017). While females, particularly nurses, were not officially recognized as serving in direct combat, they may have been exposed to Agent Orange through the spraying of the compound around the perimeter of the bases as well as the chemical residue remaining on the injured who were transported directly from the combat area. Unfortunately, studies of the relationship of chemical agents and fertility were, and continue to be, less common (NASEM, 2018b).

The NASEM (2018b) reviewed various studies exploring the effects of Agent Orange on female reproductive health. Interpretations suggested that there is insufficient/inadequate evidence to determine an association of Agent Orange exposure to endometriosis, hormonal levels, and diseases associated with pregnancy disturbances, spontaneous abortions, stillbirths, neonatal deaths, infant death, low birth weights of babies, and birth defects (NASEM, 2018b). Additionally, the same source (NASEM, 2018b) reports insufficient/inadequate evidence to link Agent Orange exposure to birth defects. Despite the research reports, the VA recognizes spina bifida as being associated with the exposure of herbicides, including Agent Orange (VA, 2019b).

Additionally, birth defects occurring in children of women who served in Vietnam, are recognized but not related to herbicide exposure (VA, 2019c). Current recognized birth defects included the conditions listed in Box 5.4.

BOX 5.4

RECOGNIZED BIRTH DEFECTS ASSOCIATED WITH FEMALE MILITARY SERVICE IN VIETNAM

- Achondroplasia
- Cleft lip and palate
- Congenital heart disease
- Congenital talipes equinovarus (clubfoot)
- Esophageal and intestinal atresia
- Hallermann–Streiff syndrome
- Hip dysplasia
- Hirschsprung's disease (congenital megacolon)
- Aqueduct stenosis leading to hydrocephalus
- Hypospadias
- Imperforate anus
- Neural tube defects
- Poland syndrome
- Pyloric stenosis
- Syndactyly (fused digits)
- Tracheoesophageal fistula
- Undescended testicle
- Williams syndrome

SOURCE: U.S. Department of Veterans Affairs. (2019c). *Birth defects in children of women Vietnam veterans.* https://www.publichealth.va.gov/exposures/agentorange/birth-defects/children-women-vietnam-vets.asp

Vietnam veterans continue to have concerns about the effects of Agent Orange on the health of their children and grandchildren. The most recent Agent Orange update from NASEM (2018b) reported that, despite new information, insufficient/inadequate evidence exists to determine an association of Agent Orange exposure and health-related effects occurring in children and grandchildren of Vietnam veterans; however, organizations continue to claim a link.

The VVA, a non-profit organization committed to serving the needs of all veterans, has compiled many accounts suggesting potential links of health issues in the children and grandchildren of Vietnam veterans. VVA is encouraging Vietnam veterans to file a claim with the VA for their children and grandchildren who may have Agent Orange-related health issues or birth defects as well as registering with the Birth Defect Research for Children (BDRC; VVA, n.d.). Research conducted by the BDRC (2019) report illustrates the differences in structural and functional birth defects in children of Vietnam veterans compared to children of nonveterans. The VA advocates for further investigations by the Health and Medicine Division of NASEM. In addition to encouraging registering with the BDRC, the VVA has created an Agent Orange/Dioxin Children's Registry to gather and document information regarding post-exposure generational health issues.

In the years following the Vietnam War, veterans and their families filed a class action suit against the major manufacturers of the herbicides for injuries allegedly experienced from exposure to the products during service in Vietnam. The suit was settled out of court in 1984 for a reported $180 million dollars. As part of the settlement, a Payment Program and Class Assistance Program were established. The Payment Program provided monetary compensation to 100% disabled veterans as well as to the survivors of deceased veterans whereas the Class Assistance Program supported funding for social services organizations and networks for the purpose of establishing and maintaining programs to benefit those affected by the herbicides. The Payment Program was operational from 1988 to 1994 during which time the Settlement Fund distributed $197 million in cash payments to those who qualified (VA, 2018a).

LIVER FLUKES

For U.S. forces in Vietnam assigned to remote outposts and firebases, the source of food came in the form of a pre-prepared meal commonly referred to as meal, combat, individual (Figure 5.1), otherwise known as Combat Rations or "C" Rations. In the 1980s the name changed to Meal, Ready-to-Eat. Additional sources of food for service members in remote settings were plants and wildlife. Due to availability of fresh water sources, fish was often consumed. The health concern was that the fish may have been consumed raw, undercooked, or in fermented forms; possibly causing a liver fluke infection and cholangiocarcinoma (Cholangiocarcinoma Foundation, 2019; VA, 2018b).

Liver flukes are part of the environment in many geographic areas around the world. *Clonorchis sinensis* and *Opisthorchis viverrini* are the two main public health concerns in Southeast Asia and East Asia due to being closely associated with clonorchiasis and opisthorchiasis, two common forms of liver infections (Psevdos et al., 2018; Zheng et al., 2017). Concern occurs if flukes, especially *C. sinensis* and *O. viverrini*, were ingested due to their ability to proliferate and reside in the biliary duct of their human host for some 25 years. During that time, infections may occur resulting in scarring and irritation of the bile duct, perhaps leading to cholangiocarcinoma in some individuals, especially those in their 60s.

While liver fluke infection is a potential cause of cholangiocarcinoma, hepatitis B and C present additional risk factors. Primary sclerosing cholangitis, chronic ulcerative colitis, Caroli disease, bile duct cysts, cirrhosis of the liver, diabetes, obesity, alcohol use, smoking, and a genetic link may also predispose a person to cholangiocarcinoma (Psevdos et al., 2018; VA, 2018b). By the time the Vietnam veteran presents to the healthcare provider/facility, the fluke is likely dead, however, symptoms of cholangiocarcinoma may present as jaundice, abdominal pain, dark urine, clay colored stools, fever, itchy skin, nausea and vomiting, and unexplained weight loss (VA, 2018b).

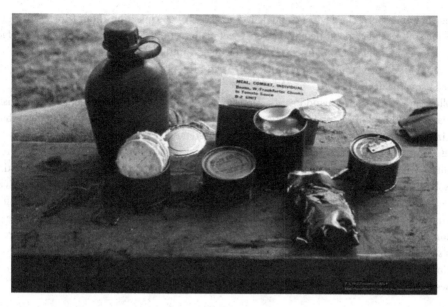

FIGURE 5.1 Meal, combat, individual served in Vietnam.

SOURCE: Image shared with permission from Paul Mashburn Photography.

According to Boyle (2018), experts from the National Institute of Allergy and Infectious Diseases, Johns Hopkins Bloomberg School of Public Health, the Uniformed Services University of the Health Sciences and the VA questioned the research results of Psevdos et al. (2018). While information on the connection of liver flukes and cholangiocarcinoma remains uncertain, veterans who served are encouraged to be alert and informed in the disease process and manifestations.

HEPATITIS C

Hepatitis C is a major public health concern. The CDC (2018) estimate that some 2.4 million Americans are living with hepatitis C; the highest incidence are those born between 1945 and 1965. The hepatitis C virus is described as the most common blood-borne pathogen in the United States as well one of the leading sources of morbidity and mortality (Kim, 2016). Of greatest concern is that up to 50% of those with hepatitis C virus may not realize they are infected (CDC, 2018).

Veterans are at a high risk for hepatitis C, especially those who served during the Vietnam and post-Vietnam eras. Recognizing the significant health concerns of hepatitis C infections, the VA veterans established the VA National Hepatitis C program, now the National Viral Hepatitis Program (VA, 2016b). Following investigations, reports suggested that veterans are at an increased risk of hepatitis C infections (Boscarino et al., 2014; VA, 2016b; VVA, 2019).

Sources for hepatitis C exposures during military service may occur when caring for a wounded/injured comrade in the field/hospital who is bleeding or by receiving blood transfusions, receiving medication from reused vials, or unsanitary dental procedures. Non-battle related exposure sources may include unsterile tattoo equipment, or the sharing of razors or toothbrushes with an infected individual. The use of contaminated needles to inject illicit drugs is another potential source of hepatitis C.

Mandatory vaccinations may serve as yet another source for hepatitis C infections as members of the military received a battery of service vaccinations. The mode of delivery for the numerous inoculations was through a needleless system, "jet guns." The principle behind the "jet gun" was to force the vaccine under the skin by high pressure blasts. At the time, the military embraced this method due to its efficiency and safety. The devices could deliver in excess of 600 injections/hour (Boyle, 2016). Upon reviewing empirical data published by the Ped-O-Jet manufacturer, Scientific Equipment Manufacturing Corporation urged the DoD to cease using the device until information confirmed that there was no risk for blood-borne transmission (Boyle, 2016). In response to the recommendation, the military stopped using the device in 1997.

Following years of concern and investigations into a possible connection of "jet gun" administered vaccinations and hepatitis C, the VA National Hepatitis C Program Office issued a statement that the organization recognized the interest of veterans and veterans' organizations; however, no cases had been documented but it is reasonable to consider a connection may exist (Boyle, 2016). A 2005 review of military immunizations practice reports that the "jet gun" device used unsterile nozzles and fluid pathway to inject consecutive patients and may have allowed for blood-borne pathogens in civilians (Boyle, 2016). As late as 2018, the VA (2018c) continued with their position that discovery of a link to the acquisition of hepatitis C being transmitted by a jet injector had not been discovered but the organization does consider this connection a possibility. Current guidelines from the VA (2018c) recommend screening for hepatitis C for individuals born between 1945 and 1965, regardless of risk factors. Additionally, screening should be performed on those who present with one or more risk factors (Box 5.5) or a desire to be screened.

BOX 5.5

RISK FACTORS FOR HEPATITIS C SCREENING

- Used a needle to inject drugs; even if only once and a long time has passed
- Had a blood transfusion or organ transplant prior to 1992
- Received long-term hemodialysis
- Contact with hepatitis C-infected blood on non-intact skin to mucous membranes
- Snorted drugs and shared equipment
- History of alcohol abuse
- Current/former sex partner with hepatitis C
- HIV infections
- A healthcare worker who has a blood exposure to mucous membranes or non-intact skin or a needlestick
- Born to a mother with hepatitis C at the time of birth
- Served during the Vietnam War era
- Tattoos or body piercings
- Diagnosed with liver disease or told that liver function test was abnormal
- History of hemophilia
- 10 or greater sex partners over life span
- Other instances of potential blood-to-blood exposure during military service or at another time

SOURCE: Adapted from U.S. Department of Veterans Affairs. (2018b). *Bile duct cancer and liver fluke infection – what you need to know.* https://www.publichealth.va.gov/docs/agentorange/reviews/ao-newsletter-2018.pdf

Cold War Era

The Cold War era lasted from shortly after the end of World War II in 1945 to the breakup of the Soviet Union in 1991. The Cold War consisted of a political rivalry between democracy and communism, mostly between the United States and the Soviet Union. This period of time was unique as the "Cold War" was also a war of ideas and threats, as both the Soviet Union and the United States were in a military race to develop the best weapons and defense systems, while facing the constant threat of nuclear war. Several incidents occurred during this period of time in Asia, Africa, and Central America as the United States fought communism by supporting anti-communist groups in countries such as El Salvador, Nicaragua, and Afghanistan. The Cuban missile crisis of 1962 was the closest the United States came to nuclear war. Because of the fears of nuclear attacks, the United States performed numerous nuclear weapons testing experiments and as a result of this testing the main health risks associated with Cold War era service are related to nuclear exposure. Veterans from this era are often referred to as "Atomic Veterans."

Following are the VA categories of potential exposures in Cold War era veterans.

IONIZING RADIATION

Veterans may have participated in "radiation-risk activity"; therefore, the VA has recognized that specific diseases are related to ionizing radiation exposure during military service (Table 5.3).

The VA may consider the possibility that other diseases not listed in Table 5.3 were caused by radiation. Eligibility for disability compensation or survivor's benefits depends on how much radiation the veteran received and other factors, such as the period of time between exposure to radiation and the development of the disease (VA, 2019o). The VA decides these claims on a case-by-case basis.

PROJECT 112/PROJECT SHIPBOARD HAZARD AND DEFENSE

Project 112/Project Shipboard Hazard and Defense (SHAD), was a series of tests conducted by the DoD from 1962 to 1973 to determine the potential risks to U.S. warships and troops from chemical and biological warfare agents. The tests were classified information for years and many of the military involved were unaware of the nature of the tests being conducted at the time. In the 1990s, some of the approximately 6,000 Navy and Marine Corps veterans who participated in the tests, began to raise concerns about exposures. In 2007, the first study of this group of veterans found no evidence of long-term

TABLE 5.3 ILLNESSES RELATED TO GULF WAR SERVICE

ILLNESS	CRITERIA
ME/CFS	Long-term and severe fatigue that is not relieved by rest and is not directly caused by other conditions
Fibromyalgia	Characterized by widespread muscle pain. Symptoms may include insomnia, morning stiffness, headache, and memory problems
Functional gastrointestinal disorders	Conditions of chronic or recurrent symptoms related to any part of the gastrointestinal tract (irritable bowel syndrome, functional dyspepsia, and functional abdominal pain syndrome)
Undiagnosed illnesses	Symptoms that may include but are not limited to abnormal weight loss, fatigue, cardiovascular disease, muscle and joint pain, headache, menstrual disorders, neurological and psychological problems, skin conditions, respiratory disorders, and sleep disturbances

CFS, chronic fatigue syndrome; ME, myalgic encephalomyelitis.

SOURCE: Adapted from the U.S. Department of Veterans Affairs. (2019l). *Gulf War veterans' medically unexplained illnesses.* https://www.publichealth.va.gov/exposures/gulfwar/medically-unexplained-illness.asp.

health effects from participating in Project SHAD. A follow-up study published in 2016 revealed the same results (NASEM, 2016a). Even though studies have not yet supported a service connection, veterans should ensure that their family members know about their service if they participated in these experiments, and keep current with guidance from the VA.

MUSTARD GAS

Mustard gas was used as a chemical weapon in World Wars I and II and during the Iran-Iraq war in the 1980s. Some Operation Iraqi Freedom (OIF) veterans who demolished or handled explosive ordinances may have been exposed to mustard agents. In the 1940s, the DoD recruited "volunteer soldier" subjects for experiments using mustard agents to evaluate clothing, ointments, and equipment to protect American troops from mustard agent attacks. Nearly 60,000 military personnel were involved in a wide range of exposures; about 4,000 soldiers were subjected to severe, full-body exposures as a part of field exercises over contaminated ground areas (VA, 2019r). The VA has listed some conditions as "presumptive" meaning that it is presumed the disease is caused by exposure during military service (Box 5.6).

BOX 5.6

CONDITIONS CONSIDERED PRESUMPTIVE FOR EXPOSURE TO MUSTARD GAS

Eye conditions

- Chronic conjunctivitis
- Keratitis (inflammation of the cornea)
- Corneal opacities scar formation

Cancers

- Acute nonlymphocytic leukemia
- Nasopharyngeal cancer
- Laryngeal cancer
- Lung cancer (except mesothelioma)
- Squamous cell carcinoma of the skin

Pulmonary conditions

- Chronic laryngitis
- Bronchitis
- Emphysema
- Asthma
- Chronic obstructive pulmonary disease

SOURCE: Adapted from the U.S. Department of Veterans Affairs. (2019r). *Mustard gas.* https://www.publichealth.va.gov/exposures/mustardgas/index.asp

---

The VA conducted outreach efforts to identify veterans who participated in these tests to inform them about their benefits. It is not common for the military to continue treating veterans for service-related exposures after discharge, as typically the VA manages care of veterans, but for those who may have participated in research experiments from 1942 to 1975, the U.S. Army is providing medical care. Veterans should complete an application for medical care on the U.S. Army website for chemical or biological research programs which can be accessed at armymedicine.health.mil/CBTP.

WASTE INCINERATOR IN ATSUGI, JAPAN

From 1985 to 2001, personnel at Naval Air Facility (NAF) Atsugi in Atsugi, Japan may have been exposed to environmental contaminants from off-base waste incinerators (VA, 2019z). The Shinkampo Incinerator Complex was a combustion waste disposal site equipped with incinerators that burned up to 90 tons of industrial and medical waste daily. Emissions included chemicals and other particulate matter (PM). A private Japanese company owned and operated the business and when the U.S. Navy found a potential for increased health risks, they worked with the Japanese government to close the complex. The incinerator was shut down in May 2001. The long-term health effects could include a possible increase in the lifetime risk for cancer. Since the 1990s, the Navy has informed sailors and their families about the possible long-term health effects of living at Atsugi. Currently there is no definitive scientific evidence to show that living at NAF Atsugi while the incinerator operated has caused additional risk for disease (VA, 2019z).

EDGEWOOD/ABERDEEN EXPERIMENTS

From 1955 to 1975, the U.S. Army Chemical Corps conducted classified medical studies at Edgewood Arsenal, Maryland. The purpose was to evaluate the impact of low-dose chemical warfare agents on military personnel and to test protective clothing and pharmaceuticals. About 7,000 soldiers took part in these experiments that involved exposures to more than 250 different chemicals (VA, 2019j). The agents tested included chemical warfare agents and other agents such as inactive substances or placebos (saline) were also used (VA, 2019j):

- anticholinesterase nerve agents (e.g., sarin, common organophosphorus, and carbamate pesticides);
- mustard agents;
- nerve agent antidotes atropine and scopolamine;
  - nerve agent reactivators (2-pyridine aldoxime methyl chloride [2-PAM chloride]);
  - psychoactive agents (lysergic acid diethylamide [LSD], phenylcyclohexyl piperidine [PCP], cannabinoids);
- irritants and riot control agents; and
- alcohol and caffeine.

Long-term follow-up of the military personnel was not planned and a review of the potential for long-term health effects from these experiments did not find any significant long-term physical harm, except for some veterans who were exposed to larger doses of mustard agents (VA, 2019j).

CAMP LEJEUNE WATER CONTAMINATION

From the 1950s through the 1980s, persons at the U.S. Marine Corps Base Camp Lejeune, North Carolina, may have been unintentionally exposed to drinking water contaminated with industrial solvents, benzene, and other chemicals (VA, 2019d). In 2012 The Caring for Camp Lejeune Families Act was passed which makes any veteran who served on active duty at Camp Lejeune, North Carolina, for at least 30 days between January 1, 1957, and December 31, 1987, and their family members, eligible for hospital care and medical services through the VA for any of 15 listed cancers and other illnesses or conditions (H.R. 1627, 2012; Box 5.7).

BOX 5.7

CAMP LEJEUNE WATER CONTAMINATION QUALIFYING HEALTH CONDITIONS

- Esophageal cancer
- Breast cancer
- Kidney cancer
- Multiple myeloma
- Scleroderma
- Myelodysplastic syndromes
- Non-Hodgkin lymphoma
- Lung cancer
- Bladder cancer
- Leukemia
- Hepatic steatosis
- Miscarriage
- Neurobehavioral effects
- Female infertility
- Renal toxicity

SOURCE: Adapted from the U.S. Department of Veterans Affairs. (2019d). *Camp Lejeune: Past water contamination.* https://www.publichealth.va.gov/exposures/camp-lejeune/index.asp.

In addition to the qualifying conditions listed in Box 5.7, the VA has established a presumptive service connection for veterans exposed to contaminants in the water supply who later developed one of the following eight diseases (National Archives, 2017):

- adult leukemia,
- aplastic anemia and other myelodysplastic syndromes,
- bladder cancer,
- kidney cancer,
- liver cancer,
- multiple myeloma,
- non-Hodgkin lymphoma, and
- Parkinson's disease

Presently, these conditions are the only ones for which there is sufficient scientific and medical evidence to support the creation of presumptions; however, the Agency for Toxic Substances and Disease Registry (ATSDR) is conducting additional research of the Camp Lejeune service members to help further evaluate the incidence of cancer in this population (ATSDR, 2018). Thousands of veterans and their families served at Camp Lejeune during this time period and were potentially exposed to contaminated water, but many may not know about the exposure or risks.

This is one of the rare instances where not only the veteran but their family members may have been exposed to chemicals which could impact their health and may be eligible for care and compensation through the VA.

Gulf War

The Gulf War, also called Operation Desert Shield and Desert Storm was brief (1990–1991) and resulted in few injuries or deaths. On August 2, 1990, Iraqi forces, led by Saddam Hussein, invaded Kuwait. The UN told Iraq to peacefully withdraw troops by January 15, 1991, or face UN coalition forces. Saddam Hussein did not comply, and Operation Desert Storm began on January 17, 1991. The U.S.-led UN coalition had a great technological advantage in the sky and in February 1991, ground troops went into Kuwait and quickly overtook Iraqi forces. The Iraqi forces burned Kuwait's oil fields as they retreated. Although the Gulf War lasted less than 2 years, the Gulf War Era is still in effect for the purposes of VA benefits eligibility, which means anyone who served on active duty from August 2, 1990, to present is considered a Gulf War Era Veteran.

After serving in the Middle East in 1990–1991, approximately 25% to 32% of veterans began reporting a variety of unexplained health problems such as fatigue, headaches, cognitive dysfunction, musculoskeletal pain, and respiratory, gastrointestinal, and dermatologic complaints (White et al., 2016). This condition was named Gulf War illness (GWI), also known as Gulf War syndrome and chronic multisymptom illness (CMI). The VA refers to these illnesses as "CMI" and "Undiagnosed illnesses," as they prefer not to use the term "Gulf War syndrome" because the symptoms vary widely (VA, 2019l). However, most veterans will use the term GWI or syndrome.

The VA presumes certain chronic, unexplained symptoms existing for 6 months or more are related to Gulf War service without regard to cause (VA, 2019l). These "presumptive" illnesses must have appeared during active duty in the Southwest Asia theater of operations (geographical area in which active combat operations were conducted) or by December 31 of 2021. Illnesses related to Gulf War service are listed in Table 5.3.

Investigations of the health effects of past wars have been limited to hazards or health outcomes, such as infectious diseases, chemical hazards, and combat injuries. The Gulf War exposures involve many complex issues, such as exposure to multiple biological and chemical agents, limited exposure information, individual variability factors, and illnesses that are often nonspecific and lack defined medical diagnoses or treatment (NASEM, 2016b). Many of the exposures are not unique to the Gulf War, but military personnel may have been exposed to a variety of agents, at varying doses, and lengths of time (NASEM, 2016b).

The VA lists the following categories of exposure in Gulf War Veterans: vaccinations, oil well fires, DU, pyridostigmine bromide (PB), sand, dust and particulates, toxic embedded fragments pesticides, infectious disease, chemical agent resistant coating (CARC) paint, and heat injuries.

VACCINATIONS

Veterans who deployed during the Gulf War received the standard series of immunizations against infectious diseases provided to any U.S. citizen traveling to the Gulf (yellow fever, typhoid, cholera, hepatitis B, meningitis, whooping cough, polio, tetanus). In addition to the standard immunization approximately 150,000 troops received anthrax vaccinations and another 8,000 received botulinum toxoid (VA, 2019s). Unfortunately, medical records from the Gulf War have limited information on who, when, and what types of vaccines were administered; therefore, follow-up and surveillance of this group of veterans is challenging. Another consideration regarding vaccines is the fact that multiple vaccines may have been administrated together, but evidence is lacking to determine whether an association does or does not exist between multiple vaccinations and long-term adverse health effects (NASEM, 2016b).

OIL WELL FIRES

Between February and November 1991, Iraqi armed forces ignited over 750 oil well fires in Kuwait, producing dense clouds of soot, liquid, aerosols, and gases. Particles from oil well fires may cause skin irritation, runny nose, cough, shortness of breath, eye/nose/throat irritation, aggravation of sinus, and asthma conditions. Most of the irritation is temporary and resolves once the exposure is gone (VA, 2019y). Research has not provided evidence of long-term health problems from exposure to oil well fires at this time, but the VA has developed a registry for airborne hazards (Table 5.4) so veterans can keep updated.

DEPLETED URANIUM

The military began using DU on a large scale during the Gulf War. DU is used primarily in tank armor and some bullets (VA, 2019i). A bullet made with DU can penetrate the skin; however, it can also penetrate a vehicle, causing small pieces of DU to scatter and become embedded in muscle and soft tissue. Veterans exposed to DU in vehicles may inhale or swallow small airborne DU particles (VA, 2019i). The potential for health effects from internal exposure is related to the amount of DU that enters a person's body, as DU may remain in the body. High doses may affect the kidneys, but as of yet, no health problems associated with DU exposure have been found in veterans who were exposed to DU (McDiarmid et al., 2017). Researchers and clinicians continue to monitor the health of exposed veterans through the Depleted Uranium Follow-up Program (Table 5.4).

PYRIDOSTIGMINE BROMIDE

The 1991 Gulf War is the only conflict in which PB was widely used by military personnel. PB is an oral cholinesterase inhibitor tablet used in the treatment of myasthenia gravis orthostatic hypotension (NASEM, 2016b). PB tablets were provided to military personnel in the Gulf War to use as a prophylactic measure to protect against effects of possible cholinesterase-inhibiting nerve gas attacks. The theory behind the use of PB for prophylaxis is that by reversibly inhibiting a portion of the acetylcholine receptors in the body, a sufficient percentage of the receptors will be protected and will reactivate so as to permit survival in the case of a nerve gas exposure (NASEM, 2016b). Because PB was self-administered by veterans when they had concerns of exposure, it is difficult to determine the amount of PB ingested.

Surveys have reported approximately 50% of the Gulf War deployed personnel in the Army, Marine Corps, and Navy used PB tablets (NASEM, 2016b). Self-reported PB use has been identified as a significant risk factor for GWI (White et al., 2016), although the VA has concluded that the evidence does not support an association (VA, 2019l). Even though the VA currently does not conclusively state that PB exposure causes GWI, they do presume that certain medically unexplained illnesses are related to Gulf War service without regard to cause, therefore Gulf War veterans should report concerns to the VA. At a minimum, Gulf War veterans should enroll in the Gulf War Registry (Table 5.4), which allows the veteran and family members to be notified of updates to exposure-related issues.

SAND, DUST, AND PARTICULATES

Veterans who were deployed to the Persian Gulf, Afghanistan, and other dusty environments in the Gulf region were often exposed to sand, dust, pollution, and other airborne particles (VA, 2019v). PM air pollutants are a complex mixture of extremely small solid particles and liquid droplets in the air and, when breathed in, these particles can reach deep into the lungs and cause various health effects (U.S. Army Public Health Command [USAHPC], n.d.). These extremely small particles and liquid droplets are from natural and manmade sources and can include acids, chemicals, metals, soil, or dust. In the United States and other industrialized regions of the world, fossil fuel combustion and vehicle emissions are the primary sources of these pollutants, but in areas such as Southwest Asia, the PM levels are higher, and the sources of PM are different. In these areas the primary sources are short-term dust storms, dust from motor vehicle disturbances of the desert floor with levels often exceeding typical levels in the United States (as much as 10 times higher), and emissions from local industries near base camps and military operations such as burn pits which all may have increased the concentration of PMs and other toxic air pollutants (USAHPC, n.d.)

There are many variables which influence health outcomes including the size and chemical makeup of the PM, concentration levels, duration of exposures, and various human factors to include age, health status and existing medical conditions, and genetics (USAHPC, n.d.). These variables combined with scientific data gaps have limited the ability to estimate long-term health impacts on veterans.

TOXIC EMBEDDED FRAGMENTS

Some veterans of Operation Enduring Freedom (OEF), OIF, and Operation New Dawn (OND) have retained toxic embedded fragments (shrapnel) in their bodies after sustaining blast injuries (VA, 2019x). Shrapnel may have come from improvised explosive devices, bombs, mines, and shells. One of the main health concerns is the shrapnel may contain DU and the long-term effects are not yet completely understood.

The VA has created the Toxic Embedded Fragment Surveillance Center (TEFSC) to offer medical surveillance to veterans injured by a bullet (or other projectile), blast or explosion and who have retained embedded fragments from their injury. To document this, TEFSC created a registry of OEF, OIF, and OND veterans who have had a fragment removed or who still have a fragment(s) in their body (Table 5.4). Some of these veterans may use the VA for healthcare, but more often than not, veterans use civilian healthcare providers; therefore, it is important for nurses to assess veterans with shrapnel and encourage them to join the registry.

PESTICIDES

Pesticides were used in the 1990–1991 Gulf War and Post-9/11 conflicts to combat the endemic insect and rodent populations in Iraq, Afghanistan, and other Persian Gulf areas. The goal was to control insects that were vectors for infectious diseases such as leishmaniasis, malaria, and sand fly fever (NASEM, 2018a). Veterans may have used DEET on the skin as an insect repellant, worn permethrin-impregnated uniforms, slept under permethrin-treated bed nets or were exposed to area spraying. Various routes of exposure to pesticides includes dermal contact and inhalation and oral ingestion as a result of hand-to-mouth; the route of exposure can have significant implications for the toxicity of the pesticide. The VA evaluated pesticide exposure as a possible cause of Gulf War Veterans' chronic multi-symptomatic illnesses and concluded that research does not support an association currently (VA, 2019t).

INFECTIOUS DISEASES

The National Academies compiled a complete report which identified the infectious diseases diagnosed in Gulf War veterans (IOM, 2007). This chapter only discusses the diseases that the VA presumes are related to military service during the Gulf War from August 2, 1990, to present and in Afghanistan on or after September 19, 2001 (VA, 2019n).

Veterans may have contracted one of the diseases, but in order for them to receive disability compensation, they must have had the disease within the specified time frames noted by the VA and have a disability as a result of that disease. Most of the diseases listed require that the disease caused at least a 10% disability within 1 year from the date of military separation for a veteran to receive disability compensation.

The most common infectious diseases include malaria, brucellosis, campylobacter jejuni, coxiella burnetii (Q fever), and visceral leishmaniasis. Additionally, veterans may have been exposed to West Nile virus, mycobacterium tuberculosis, Salmonella and Shigella (VA, 2019n).

CHEMICAL AGENT RESISTANT COATING PAINT

CARC is a paint used on military vehicles to make metal surfaces highly resistant to corrosion and penetration of chemical agents. Inhaling CARC during the painting and drying process can be harmful.

Gulf War veterans who painted combat vehicles and equipment during their military service may have been exposed to CARC paint or fumes without adequate respiratory protection (VA, 2019e). CARC paint contains several chemical compounds that can be hazardous when inhaled or exposed to the skin and can cause itching and reddening of skin, burning sensation in throat and nose and watering of the eyes, cough, shortness of breath, pain during respiration, increased sputum production, and chest tightness, asthma and kidney damage (VA, 2019e).

HEAT INJURIES

Veterans serving in hot, desert climates, such as in Iraq and Afghanistan, may have suffered from heat injuries. These heat injuries include heat stroke, heat exhaustion, and sunburn. Veterans who have suffered from heat injuries during military service may be more susceptible to heat and more serious heat injuries in the future (VA, 2019m).

Iraq War

The Iraq War is also called OIF and OND and is categorized as the period from March 20, 2003 to December 15, 2014. Iraq War veterans may have been exposed to sand, dust, particulates, infectious diseases, toxic embedded fragments, DU, heat injuries (discussed under the "Gulf War" section), mefloquine, burn pits, sulfur fire, rabies, chromium, and chemical warfare agents (Figure 5.2).

MEFLOQUINE (LARIAM®)

Malaria is not a common disease in the United States, therefore military personnel deploying overseas were required to take anti-malarial medications. Mefloquine is an oral tablet taken once a week that can help prevent malaria and military personnel, including those serving in Iraq and Afghanistan, may

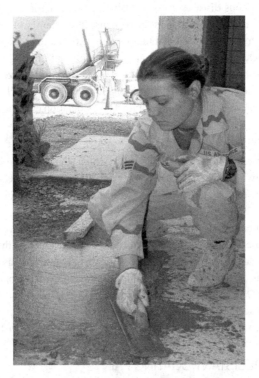

FIGURE 5.2 Sgt Angela Archer, USAF, carpenter/welder deployed in Iraq mixing and leveling concrete as part of her daily work activities.

have taken mefloquine as an antimalarial prophylaxis if they were unable to take other antimalarials such as doxycycline, atovaquone, and proguanil (VA, 2019p). The side effects of mefloquine are usually mild and may include nausea, vomiting, diarrhea, dizziness, difficulty sleeping, and bad dreams. More serious side effects can include mood changes, bad or vivid dreams, agitation, suicidal thoughts, and suicidal behavior.

Mefloquine was approved by the Food and Drug Administration (FDA) in May 1989 and in 2013, they issued a black box warning. The FDA black box warning noted that neurologic side effects can include dizziness, loss of balance, tinnitus, anxiety, paranoia, depression, or hallucinations (VA, 2019p). Neurologic or psychiatric side effects may occur at any time during drug use and may last for months to years after the drug is stopped. The VA is conducting a study on the long-term effects of antimalarial drugs.

BURN PITS

Burn pits were widely used as a method of solid waste disposal prior to 2010 at many OEF and OIF locations (Sharkey et al., 2014). Burning waste in open air pits can cause more pollution than if it were burned in an incinerator and the waste products at a deployment sites could have included numerous hazardous materials such as chemical, medical, food and human waste; unexploded ordinance; petroleum products; plastics and rubber. Incineration of these products and use of JP-8 jet fuel containing benzene, releases dangerous toxins which accumulate as measurable PM air pollution (Szema et al., 2017).

Military personnel who served in Iraq and Afghanistan were most likely exposed to burn pits. Although the long-term health effects are not known, the short-term effects such as eye and throat irritation, coughing and breathing difficulties, and throat burning are thought to be temporary and resolve once the exposure is eliminated. Currently the VA has not found enough evidence to say that there are long-term effects from burn pit exposure. The VA has established a voluntary registry (Table 5.4) to capture information regarding all potential exposures experienced by service members during deployment that may have possible impacts on future respiratory health.

CHROMIUM

During the spring and summer of 2003, about 830 service members guarded a water treatment facility in the Basrah oil fields at Qarmat Ali, Iraq. This facility was contaminated with sodium dichromate dust, which is a source of hexavalent chromium, a chemical that is known to cause cancer. Those assigned to the water treatment facility may have been exposed from breathing contaminated sodium dichromate dust. Prolonged exposure to breathing high concentrations of chromium over months or years is known to cause lung cancer, while exposure for short periods usually does not cause cancer (VA, 2019g). The symptoms associated with exposure to chromium include nasal irritations such as runny or itchy nose, sneezing, nosebleeds, nasal ulcers, and holes in the nasal septum. It also can cause respiratory problems such as asthma, skin irritation, and skin ulcers (VA, 2019g).

The VA developed a medical surveillance program for veterans who many have been exposed to hexavalent chromium at the Qarmat Ali Treatment Facility in Iraq. The program is provided free of charge or copay. Every 5 years after the initial exam, veterans will receive chest x-rays. Exam results will be tracked in VA's Gulf War Registry (Table 5.4). If any abnormalities are found, the veteran will be referred to the proper specialty service. Unfortunately, only an estimated 16% of those exposed are following up with the VA surveillance program (Ciminera et al., 2016); therefore, it is important that nurses are aware of the various surveillance programs and encourage veterans to enroll.

SULFUR FIRE

A fire that ignited in June 2003 at the Mishraq State Sulfur Mine Plant near Mosul, Iraq, burned for almost a month (VA, 2019w). Sulfur dioxide and hydrogen sulfide were released during the fire, and these gases can cause irritation of the nose and throat and eyes as well as coughing. A group of soldiers who were stationed in Iraq, most of whom had prolonged exposure to sulfur dioxide during the Mishraq Sulfur Mine fire, were evaluated for pulmonary symptoms in 2007. Many of these service members reported a significant change in their ability to run 2 miles on the Army Physical Fitness Test (VA, 2019w). The USAPHC (2012) is following soldiers exposed to the sulfur dioxide for long-term sequelae.

RABIES

Veterans of OEF, OIF, and OND who were bitten or exposed in some other way to the saliva of a warm-blooded animal while deployed, should be evaluated by a healthcare professional for the risk of rabies exposure. The risk of being exposed to rabies is much higher for veterans who served in parts of the world including Iraq and Afghanistan, where domestic animals are not vaccinated against rabies. A U.S. soldier who had served in Afghanistan died of rabies, so it is important for veterans who were bitten or had contact with the saliva from a warm-blooded animal such as a dog, cat, bat, fox, skunk, raccoon, mongoose, or jackal while deployed in the previous 18 months to seek medical care (VA, 2019u).

CHEMICAL WARFARE AGENTS

Veterans who demolished or handled explosive ordinances may have been exposed to warfare agents such as mustard agents or sarin (VA, 2019f). Some veterans have called the health consequences of chemical exposures in the Gulf war and other wars "toxic wounds" (White et al., 2016). The immediate symptoms and potential long-term health effects depend on the type of agent and the level of exposure:

- **Blister agents:** Long-term health effects are not expected after low level exposures that did not cause immediate symptoms or require medical attention, but higher-level exposures such as to the whole body or airways and lungs may result in cancers or other health problems.

- **Nerve agents (Sarin):** Long-term health effects are not expected after low level exposures with no or minimal symptoms (VA, 2019f).

There is no test currently available to confirm exposure after a few months (VA, 2019f).

Operation Enduring Freedom in Afghanistan

OEF is the name given to the war in Afghanistan, which began in October 7, 2001. OEF veterans may have been exposed to sand, dust, particulates, infectious diseases, toxic embedded fragments, mefloquine, burn pits, DU, heat injuries, and rabies (discussed in "Gulf War" and "Iraq War" sections). OEF may have also experienced cold injuries, (discussed in "Korea" section) and traumatic brain injury (TBI), which is an injury to the head caused by exposure to blast injuries and explosions that disrupts the normal functioning of the brain.

REGISTRIES

Veterans may be eligible to be included in registries specific to exposures. Registries are a way for veterans to voluntarily document their exposure experiences and health concerns through the use of web-based, self-reported questionnaires. The questionnaires may ask information such as deployment history and exposures, military occupational exposures, environmental exposures, air pollution, places lived, work history, home environment and hobbies, medical history, health concerns, and healthcare utilization (Sharkey et al., 2014). Although registries may not require medical evaluation for

TABLE 5.4 REGISTRIES FOR VETERANS

REGISTRY/RESOURCE	VETERANS WHO SHOULD REGISTER	WEBSITE
Agent Orange Registry	Veterans who served in Vietnam between 1962 and 1975; or in a unit in or near the Korean DMZ anytime between September 1, 1967 and August 31, 1971 or in Thailand February 28, 1961 and May 7, 1975	www.publichealth.va.gov/exposures/agentorange/benefits/registry-exam.asp
Airborne Hazards and Open Burn Pit Registry	OEF/OIF/OND/OFS veterans who have deployed to the Southwest Asia theater of operations on or after August 2, 1990 as well as those who have deployed to Afghanistan or Djibouti after September 11, 2001	veteran.mobilehealth.va.gov/AHBurnPitRegistry/#page/home
Gulf War Registry	Veterans who served in the Gulf during Operation Desert Shield, Operation Desert Storm, OIF, or OND	www.publichealth.va.gov/exposures/gulfwar/benefits/registry-exam.asp
Ionizing Radiation Registry	Veterans who had on-site participation in a test involving the atmospheric detonation of a nuclear device, whether or not the testing nation was the United States; or those who received nasopharyngeal (nose and throat) radium irradiation treatments while in on active duty; or involved in listed "radiation-risk activities"	www.publichealth.va.gov/exposures/radiation/benefits/registry-exam.asp
Depleted Uranium Follow-Up Program	Veterans who served in the Gulf War, Bosnia, OEF, OIF or OND	www.publichealth.va.gov/exposures/depleted_uranium/followup_program.asp
Toxic Embedded Fragment Surveillance Center	Veterans who served in OEF, OIF or OND. The Veteran must have, or likely have, an embedded fragment as the result of injury received while serving in an area of conflict	www.publichealth.va.gov/exposures/toxic_fragments/surv_center.asp
U.S. Army Chemical or Biological Research Program Participants	Veterans who served as a research subject in a U.S. Army chemical or biological substance testing program, including the receipt of medications or vaccines under the U.S. Army investigational drug review	armymedicine.health.mil/CBTP

DMZ, demilitarized zone; OEF, Operation Enduring Freedom; OFS, Operation Freedom's Sentinel; OIF, Operation Iraqi Freedom; OND, Operation New Dawn.

participation, some veterans will have the opportunity to request further medical assessment. The VA collects data and may contact veterans when new research is published or when benefits change. It is beneficial for veterans to sign up for the registries they qualify for in order for them to receive the most current information. Many veterans may not know about the registries as there is no requirement to sign up for the registry, so nurses can be a resource to inform veterans of these valuable benefits. Family members and caregivers should be aware of the registries, so they can encourage veterans to sign up and receive updates on potential exposures. Table 5.4 lists registry information.

NURSING INTERVENTIONS AND IMPLICATIONS

The U.S. Census Bureau (2018) estimates that in 2017, 18.2 million veterans are living in the United States. It bears noting that while many honorably discharged veterans are eligible for VA healthcare, approximately 24% utilize the VA for their healthcare (VA, 2017c). Recent policy changes within the VA system, namely the VA Mission Act of 2018, may potentially increase the number of veterans using non-VA providers for their care. This means that veterans are largely using civilian medical care facilities which supports the need for nurses and nurse educators to be versed in veteran-specific health issues.

Regardless of the location where veterans receive healthcare, nursing plays a vital role. Nurses are often the first contact for veterans, active duty members, and their support systems in the healthcare setting. Because of the important role of nurses, awareness of interventions and implications relating to this specific patient demographic is essential to achieve optimal care and to ensure that appropriate care is provided and referrals are made for military-related conditions.

Upon initial assessment of the individual, inquiring about military service is essential. The American Academy of Nursing (2014) suggested beginning every assessment with the question "Have you or someone close to you ever served in the military?" If the answer indicates military service, further exploration is necessary. Preliminary information can be gathered by use of the following questions:

- When did you serve?
- Which branch?
- What did you do while you were in the military?
- Were you assigned to a hostile or combative area?
- Did you experience enemy fire, see combat, or witness casualties?
- Were you wounded, injured, or hospitalized?
- Did you participate in any experimental projects or tests?
- Were you exposed to noise, chemicals, gases, demolition of munitions, pesticides, or other hazardous substances? (American Academy of Nursing, 2014).

Once preliminary information is gathered, the nurse should use the opportunity to more deeply explore any potential military related health concerns of the individual.

To assess hearing acuity/quality, the following questions are appropriate and helpful:

- What is/was your job in the military?
- Did you wear hearing protection devices? What type?
- Have you ever sustained an injury to your ears?
- How do you feel your quality of hearing is currently?
- Have you contacted your local Veterans Administration about your hearing quality?

While asking questions is very beneficial, performing a physical assessment and documenting findings may also identify hearing issues with emphasis on direct observation of the ear canal to visualize for the present of excessive cerebrum buildup and integrity of the tympanic membrane. Additionally, assessing the functionality of hearing assistive devices is important.

Military members and their families may have been knowingly or unknowingly exposed to hazardous exposures. By using current information on military service-related exposures, the assessment process may yield valuable information. Using information gathered from the initial assessment questions, the provider may consider asking focused occupational/environmental history questions as necessary, paying special attention to the chief complaint (or diagnosis) for clues suggesting a relationship to exposure and military service.

During the interview process questions regarding environmental exposures should focus on gathering more information to determine if an exposure occurred. Suggested questions may include the following:

- Do you suspect you may have been exposed to chemical, physical or biological agents during your military service?

- How long were you exposed?
- Are you concerned about the exposure? Can you tell me why/why not?
- Where were you exposed?
- When do you feel the exposure occurred?
- Who else may be exposed?
- Have you ever had a blood transfusion?
- Did you inject drugs into your body during your military service? Ever shared razors with another individual?
- Did you receive a tattoo/tattoos during your military service?

As with any health assessment, the importance of asking targeted questions can never be underestimated. In the case of a veteran or active duty individual, with a diagnosis of cancer or another condition linked to radiation exposure, specific and focused questions may offer valuable information. Questions specific to exposure may include the following examples:

- When and where did you serve in the military?
- What was your job in the military?
- To your knowledge, were you ever exposed to radiation in any form?
- Did you take any precautions to prevent or minimize the exposure?
- How were you exposed? Inhaled, on skin, swallowed, etc.
- Describe the exposure.
- What was the length of time of exposure?
- How concerned are you about the exposure?

Understanding veterans' responses and reactions to questions about their service is crucial. Some veterans may be very open and talk about their service, while others may avoid discussing details about their service. When discussing exposures, an appreciation that nurses may not have a thorough understanding of all the scientific data and medical knowledge regarding exposures is acceptable; however, at a minimum, nurses should have a basic understanding of exposures and know how to access resources for veterans and their families. Nurses can provide empathetic responses and verbally acknowledge and validate risk perceptions and emotions related to a health risk (Sharkey et al., 2014). The VA is a nationwide system and keeps up-to-date information on service-related exposures, so nurses should know the contact information for the closed VA hospital, clinic, or service center. Some veterans, especially Vietnam veterans, may have negative feelings about their service and harbor a distrustful opinion of the VA, so nurses should also be aware of other community-based veteran organizations and resources.

Education on the health concerns and needs of this population of patients is part of a holistic assessment. As nurses, it is a professional and ethical responsibility to explore and learn about those whom we care for. By attending educational conferences, in-services, and seeking out additional materials that address the health needs and challenges of veterans, Active Duty members and their families/support system, nurses can offer quality care to individuals. The ability to identify the health concerns of this demographic will greatly assist in facilitating a partnership to improve patient satisfaction, outcomes, and quality of life.

IMPLICATIONS FOR NURSING EDUCATION AND PRACTICE

Curricular instruction that includes discussion of occupational/environmental exposures of veterans and active duty personnel offers the learner expanded knowledge on the potential hazards of exposure.

Available resources for occupational/environmental exposures, for use in nursing education, are valuable in teaching this subject to students. Through teaching the exposure hazards of military service, the goal is to enable the nursing student to perform a focused patient history along with an exposure assessment as a means to identify possible health concerns that were not previously considered. Acquisition of this knowledge may identify symptoms or concerns at an early stage where treatment may be optimized, and patient health is benefited. In the end, the nursing student is offered knowledge that is useful in many care delivery venues.

Nursing education must also recognize that veterans are separating from the military at increasing numbers. Zogas (2017) projected that nearly 4.3 million Post-9/11 service members will have separated from the military between 2003 and 2019. As veterans transition from military service to higher education, nursing faculty must recognize that student veterans may experience physical, emotional, and mental health challenges. Challenges for veterans may include the effects of TBI, posttraumatic stress disorder, or combat-related injuries which present as impairment of mobility, hearing, visual acuity, or speech. In order to maximize the education experience of student veterans, nursing education should acclimate the learning environment and content delivery to meet the needs of the learners through innovative and adaptive methods. Student veterans should be encouraged to visit the disability services office as they may qualify for accommodations such as recording lectures, sitting in the front of the classroom, note takers, or extra time for examinations.

FUTURE RESEARCH PRIORITIES

In order to gain knowledge on the effects of exposures, research is necessary. As the veteran population continues to diversify and age, physiological changes may occur that may render/impede the delivery of complete and comprehensive healthcare to this demographic of patients and their families; especially in terms of the long-term effects of environmental and occupational exposures related to military service:

- investigation/exploration into the claims of generational health concerns of Agent Orange,
- patient and family lived experience with an Agent Orange related illness,
- long-term health effects of environmental and occupational exposures in OIF/OEF/OND veterans,
- the impact of veteran exposure assessment questions in non-VA settings, and
- best practices for including veteran centric content in nursing curricula.

CONCLUSION

Military service-related health concerns tend to be assimilated to combat. While this connection is commonly recognized, former and current military members may have been exposed to lesser known health hazards. Exposure to noise, extreme temperatures, ionized radiation, chemicals, and pesticides also possess concerns for individuals. Heathcare providers may not be aware of these numerous sources and the potential health concerns they possess. In order to predict, identify, and treat the potentially harmful effects of exposures, it is critical for providers to possess knowledge of the various sources which may negatively impact health.

RESOURCES

CATEGORY	RESOURCE	WEBSITE
General assessment of veterans and their support systems	American Academy of Nursing	www.haveyoueverserved.com
	Military Health History Pocket Card for Health Professions Trainees and Clinicians	www.va.gov/OAA/pocketcard
Veterans Affairs	Environmental Exposure Assessment (General)	www.publichealth.va.gov/exposures/providers/exposure-assessment.asp
	Director of Environmental Health Coordinators by State	www.publichealth.va.gov/exposures/coordinators.asp
Noise	Centers for Disease Control and Prevention	www.cdc.gov/nceh/hearing_loss
Radiation	U.S. Department of Veterans Affairs	www.publichealth.va.gov/exposures/radiation/sources/index.asp
	National Cancer Benefits Center	https://www.publichealth.va.gov/exposures/radiation/how-va-confirms-exposure.asp www.cancerbenefits.com/?gclid=EAIaIQobChMIiKei6c2y5AIVh56fCh3VnwHSEAMYASAAEgL_zPD_BwE
Agent Orange	Agent Orange Registry Exam	www.publichealth.va.gov/exposures/agentorange/benefits/registry-exam.asp
	Department of Veterans Affairs – Agent Orange	www.publichealth.va.gov/exposures/agentorange www.vets.gov/disability-benefits/conditions/exposure-to-hazardous-materials/agent-orange
	Vietnam Veterans of America	vva.org/what-we-do/outreach-programs/agent-orange
Liver flukes	Cholangiocarcinma Foundation	cholangiocarcinoma.org/vietnam-veterans
	U.S. Department of Veterans Affairs	www.publichealth.va.gov/exposures/infectious-diseases/cholangiocarcinoma.asp
Hepatitis C	U.S. Department of Veterans Affairs	www.hepatitis.va.gov/policy/military-blood-exposures.asp
	HCVets	www.hcvets.com
All	National Academies of Sciences, Engineering, and Medicine.	The National Academies (formerly IOM) has over 120 evidence reviews, reports on military exposures for all war eras and other exposures
	Veterans	https://www.nap.edu/search/?rpp=20&ft=1&term=veterans+exposures

REFERENCES

The complete reference list for this chapter appears in the digital version of the chapter, accessible at https://connect.springerpub.com/content/book/978-0-8261-3597-1/chapter/ch05

Recommended Readings and Web Resources

Grassman, D. L. (2011). Peace at last, stories of hope and healing for veterans and their families. Vandamere Press. ISBN 978-0-918339-72-0

Martini, E. A. (2012). *Agent Orange: History, science, and the politics of uncertainty*. University of Massachusetts Press.

Wilcox. F. A. (2011). *Waiting for an army to die: The tragedy of Agent Orange* (2nd ed.). Seven Locks Press.

Burn pits 360. https://www.burnpits360.org/

We honor veterans. https://www.wehonorveterans.org/

Opus Peace Soul Injury. https://opuspeace.org/

National League of Nursing. *Veteran unfolding case studies*. http://www.nln.org/professional-development-programs/teaching-resources/veterans-ace-v

PHYSICAL INJURIES COMMON TO MILITARY AND VETERAN POPULATIONS

KELLY L. DYAR

I'm a little wounded but I'm not slain; I will lay me down to bleed awhile, then I'll rise and fight with you again.

Thomas Dryden

KEY TERMS

veterans	multi-limb trauma
Gulf War illness	spinal cord injury
traumatic brain injury	pain
tinnitus and hearing loss	

INTRODUCTION

Veterans may experience complex health problems as a result of their time in military service. Such health concerns can include physical sequelae of training and time in service regardless of deployment status. These health problems may include Gulf War illness (GWI), orthopedic problems, neurological injuries, or chronic pain. Many of these diagnoses will be comorbid, meaning the veteran may experience more than one service-related diagnosis, or the service-related diagnosis may occur concurrently with other health problems that are unrelated to service. Many of these diagnoses may also intersect with mental health issues such as posttraumatic stress disorder (PTSD). Caregivers of veterans with ongoing health problems may also experience health challenges. This chapter provides a background to understanding health problems experienced by veterans as well as describes each healthcare topic. Each of these complex medical issues has implications for nursing practice and education. Research implications are also noted.

BACKGROUND

Many members of the U.S. military have served in various roles at assorted military installations, both stateside and overseas. A military installation is a location at which the military member is assigned

---

The complete reference list for this chapter appears in the digital version of the chapter, accessible at https://connect.springerpub.com/content/book/978-0-8261-3597-1/chapter/ch06

for duty, and these installations may include a deployment into a combat area. A large number of military personnel will separate from the military with one or more health needs. Some of these health problems will resolve quickly, while others may be permanent or persistent, becoming a chronic concern that requires ongoing management. Further, some injuries could lead to temporary or permanent disability. Military service includes risk for injury regardless of whether the member deploys or serves in a combat situation.

Risk for Injury

Military service is demanding in many ways, whether the service occurs during training, regular duties, or deployment. As a result of the physical demands of military service, there is potential for injury due to the highly athletic nature of preparing for and remaining fit for duty. Members of the military are described as tactical athletes. Tactical athletes are those who are in a profession, such as the military, in which there are requirements to maintain physical fitness and performance standards related to the work; such requirements are necessary to ensure readiness to perform job tasks (Sefton & Burkhardt, 2016).

Training, both initial and ongoing, has the potential to cause physical stress that can have a lasting impact on the body of the military member. For example, training often includes rigorous physical activity to prepare military members to pass the physical fitness test (PFT), which includes tasks such as running, performing push-ups, and sit-ups (Anderson et al., 2015). These activities can result in stress on the joints with the potential of causing long-term damage. Training also may include walking, hiking, or marching long distances, often while carrying large amounts of equipment. Such an exercise is typically referred to as a ruck march (Smith, 2019), and the added weight of equipment can put additional stress on the body, especially the weight-bearing joints. The job classification of a military member, known as a military occupational specialty (MOS), may also require extensive weapons training. Exposure to the noise from firing weapons has the potential to result in hearing damage or loss.

The primary injury types experienced during military training and service are those classified as musculoskeletal. The U.S. Department of Defense (DoD) produces an annual report on the health of the U.S. military force. The 2018 Health of the Force Report describes both acute and cumulative traumatic injuries, reporting 305 acute injuries per 1,000 service members and 988 cumulative traumatic injuries per 1,000 service members with female service members having a higher overall injury rate (DoD, 2018). The most common acute injuries reported are sprains and strains, typically in the lower body. For cumulative injuries, the lower body is also most affected, specifically the lumbar spine region followed by knee and lower limb, ankle and foot, and shoulder. Inflammation and pain are the most common complaints for the cumulative injuries at a rate of 86.6% (DoD, 2018). There is also a high incidence of stress fractures in recruits. Recruits are those who are new to the military and are undergoing initial training. This incidence does have gender differences as male recruits experienced stress fractures at a rate of 19.3/1,000 while women experienced these at a rate of 79.9/1,000 (Lovalekar et al., 2016).

The risk of injury may be associated with MOS. Anderson et al. (2015) described MOS based on physical demands, noting a military rating system that ranged from very heavy physical demand to light physical demand. Those with a MOS rated as having a very heavy physical demand may be required to lift and carry weights of greater than 100 pounds while those with a light rating may only be occasionally required to lift and carry up to 20 pounds. Further, Lovalekar et al. (2016) explored the rates of musculoskeletal injuries in the Army's 101st Airborne (Air Assault) Division. This Army unit may perform airborne jumps but typically does not engage in high altitude parachute jumps (Lovalekar et al., 2016). Despite this, there were 29.5 injuries per 100 subjects/year, with the majority being lower extremity, ankle, and knee injuries. These were associated most often with running or direct trauma that occurred during regular physical training, including during parachute jumps from a stationary tower or an aircraft. The use of a parachute ankle brace was shown to be an effective way of reducing ankle injury (Lovalekar et al., 2016). Anderson et al. (2015) found that a higher risk of injury among

U.S. Army soldiers was among those in a chemical, explosives, and ammunition/infantry job or to an armor/infantry position. Risk of injury was also found to be associated with ages between 21 to 29 years, cigarette smoking, poor PFT run scores, and being overweight or obese (Anderson et al., 2015).

Hearing loss and heat illnesses are additional health problems that may occur during training or job performance. According to Guard Your Health (2015), hearing loss is an increasing concern in the U.S. military, potentially as a result of failure to use hearing protection. Additionally, noise levels that are continual can be a factor in hearing loss. As an example, military members may travel in convoys over great distances and lengthy periods. Per Guard Your Health (2015), the engine noise in a convoy lasting 4 hours can damage hearing the same way as an explosion. Heat illnesses occur when the body's core temperature exceeds the body's ability to self-regulate; these disorders include heat exhaustion, which is less severe, and heat stroke, which is potentially life-threatening (Armed Forces Health Surveillance Branch [AFHSB], 2019). According to the AFHSB, the rates of heat illnesses have increased 18.7% from 2016 to 2018, and the risk is highest during training. Those at greatest risk are males who are less than 20 years of age, are Asian/Pacific Islanders, and are in the Army or Marines. Further, those who are in a combat specialty are at the greatest risk.

The physical challenges experienced by military service members may result in an injury that gives rise to claims for compensation or care from the U.S. Department of Veterans Affairs (VA) upon separation from service. Compensation may be requested for service-connected disabilities arising from or aggravated by injuries, diseases, or events that occurred during military service (VA, 2019a). Veterans may be eligible to receive such compensation when they served under conditions other than dishonorable, and the disability is not the result of the veteran's misconduct. The VA may provide additional compensation if the disability is severe enough to confine the veteran to their home, require help from others, or have resulted in anatomical loss or loss of use of an extremity or reproductive organ (VA, 2019a). In the 2018 Annual Benefits Report to Congress, the VA provided information on the most common reasons for disability compensation with over 25 million disabilities reported (Table 6.1).

GULF WAR ILLNESS

The Gulf War era began in early 1991 and included Desert Storm and Desert Shield. During this time, there were over 2 million members of the U.S. military, with almost 700,000 deploying into

TABLE 6.1 MOST PREVALENT SERVICE-CONNECTED DISABILITIES REPORTED FOR 2018

DISABILITY	NUMBER
Tinnitus	1,971,201
Hearing loss	1,228,936
Posttraumatic stress disorder	1,039,794
Scars, general	1,036,677
Limitation of flexion, knee	10,210,281
Lumbosacral or cervical strain	989,835
Paralysis of the sciatic nerve	781,178
Limitation of motion of the ankle	636,178
Migraine	548,999
Degenerative arthritis of the spine	505,553
Total number of most prevalent disabilities	9,760,307
Total number of disabilities	25,127,129

SOURCE: From the U.S. Department of Veterans Affairs. (2019a). *Compensation.* https://www.benefits.va.gov/REPORTS/abr/docs/2019-compensation.pdf

the Persian Gulf area (VA, 2017). Following the return home, estimates indicate up to 33% of these veterans are experiencing a set of multiple symptoms that has a profound effect on daily functioning (National Academies of Sciences, Engineering, and Medicine [NASEM], 2016).

There are multiple manifestations of GWI that encompass sets of symptoms. These sets of symptoms have come to be known as GWI with Table 6.2 providing several definitions for GWI. Although the definitions vary slightly, there are some common themes related to fatigue, mood, pain symptoms, neurological and cognitive symptoms, and visceral/somatic symptoms including gastrointestinal, respiratory, and skin symptoms.

There has been much debate related to GWI, including disagreements over prevalence of symptoms and causation. Many veterans have had VA benefits claims denied with accusations of psychosomatic illness or that the symptoms are related to mental health concerns (Conard & Armstrong, 2019). As a result of the pervasive belief that symptoms may be psychological, veterans receive referrals for mental healthcare rather than having a full evaluation and subsequent treatment for their symptoms.

TABLE 6.2 DEFINITIONS OF GULF WAR ILLNESS

DEFINING ENTITY	DEFINITION
Centers for Disease Control and Prevention	One or more symptoms from at least two of the following categories: • fatigue • mood and cognition with symptoms of feeling depressed, difficulty in remembering or concentrating, feeling moody or anxious, difficulty finding words, difficulty sleeping • musculoskeletal symptoms lasting 6 or more months with varying severity; symptoms include joint pain or stiffness or muscle pain (Fukuda et al., 1998)
Kansas definition	Developed by Steele (2000), this definition requires symptoms to be present in three of six domains, which include: • fatigue and sleep problems • pain symptoms • neurological, cognitive, or mood symptoms • gastrointestinal symptoms • respiratory symptoms • skin symptoms
Haley definition	Characterized by the presence of three major syndromes: • impaired cognition including problems of attention, memory, and reasoning and insomnia, depression, daytime sleepiness, and headaches • confusion-ataxia including problems with thinking, disorientation, problems with balance, vertigo, and impotence • arthromyoneuropathy, including joint and muscle pains, muscle fatigue, difficulty lifting, and paresthesia of the extremities (Haley et al., 1997)
VA	Referred to as CMIs rather than GWI, this is a cluster of medically unexplained and chronic symptoms experienced by Gulf War veterans and includes: • fatigue • headaches • joint pain • indigestion • insomnia • dizziness • respiratory disorders • memory problems (VA, 2018)

CMI, chronic multisymptom illness; GWI, Gulf War illness; VA, U.S. Department of Veterans Affairs.

To aid in evaluation of symptoms, the VA now offers a GWI registry. This registry is a free service and begins with a comprehensive health exam to determine if the veteran is experiencing any long-term health effects as a result of environmental exposures occurring during time in service (VA, 2015). The exam does not require enrollment in VA benefits and does not satisfy the requirements for determining disability (VA, 2015). Those who served in the Gulf area during multiple conflicts are eligible for the exam, which the veteran can schedule by contacting a VA Environmental Health Coordinator. The veteran can initiate contact through the VA website at www.publichealth.va.gov/exposures/gulf-war/benefits/registry-exam.asp. With the potential environmental exposures resulting in health problems, the VA has also made available an Airborne Hazards and Open Burn Pit Registry (VA, 2015). There are currently over 180,000 registered. Veterans can join the registry through a website at www.publichealth.va.gov/exposures/burnpits/registry.asp.

In 2016, NASEM released an update on the health effects of serving in the Gulf War. Although there was no unifying pathophysiologic reason presented for GWI, there was acknowledgment in the report that those deployed to the Gulf War region have increased risk for PTSD, chronic fatigue syndrome, functional gastrointestinal conditions, generalized anxiety disorder, and GWI. Further, there was some limited and suggestive evidence that amyotrophic lateral sclerosis is associated with deployment during the Gulf War (NASEM, 2016). To date, no one causation or pathophysiology has been identified yet several causes have been hypothesized.

Causation of Gulf War Illness

Determination of causation has been challenging due to difficulties in recovering records; documenting frequency, intensity, and duration of exposures; and the lack of data describing contact. Despite this difficulty, several proposed causes include exposure to chemicals such as pesticides, chemical and biological warfare agents, and multiple mandatory vaccinations. Chen et al. (2017) offered a theory that mitochondrial DNA damage is a potential cause of GWI as veterans with GWI were found to have more significant mitochondrial dysfunction, and this dysfunction may be the result of the multiple environmental exposures during deployment. Of the veterans studied, 76% were exposed to pyridostigmine bromide (PB), and almost 67% were exposed to pesticides. An anticholinergic, PB was administered to military personnel as a prophylactic treatment for chemical warfare exposure. Chen et al. (2017) noted that the mitochondrial damage is irreversible and therefore might explain the persistence of the symptoms.

Mawson and Croft (2018) also considered exposure to chemical and environmental agents yet focused more on the multiple vaccinations required during this era, noting that GWI is also present in some veterans who did not deploy yet received the multiple mandatory vaccines. In veterans with GWI, Mawson and Croft (2018) noted that there was also an accompanying liver dysfunction and thus proposed that the liver dysfunction and GWI symptoms may be the result of the dumping of vitamin A following concurrent administration of multiple vaccines. Immune dysfunction and chronic inflammation may also play a role as one study demonstrated elevated levels of c-reactive protein, leptin, and brain-derived neurotrophic factor in deployed Gulf War veterans (Johnson et al., 2016).

Despite the lack of a clearly identified pathophysiology and a universally accepted definition, GWI symptoms are real, and veterans are experiencing multiple effects, especially related to cognitive function. Memory deficits have been noted in those with GWI including significantly decreased performance with attention and executive function, visuospatial skills, and learning and memory (Chao, 2017; Janulewicz et al., 2017). Tremors were present in approximately 26% of those with GWI, and subsequent evaluation indicated brain atrophy was present; this atrophy was consistent with exposure to organic solvents (Christova et al., 2017). Falvo et al. (2018) noted a decrease in cerebrovascular flow with a concurrent decrease in autonomic function in those with GWI.

ORTHOPEDIC ISSUES AND LIMB TRAUMA

As previously discussed, members of the military may experience musculoskeletal injuries during physical training, MOS-specific training, or conducting job-related duties, including while on deployment. Orthopedic issues can include osteoarthritis, osteopenia and osteoporosis, and limb trauma.

Orthopedic Issues

Osteoarthritis is an orthopedic issue experienced by some veterans. Rivera et al. (2016) reported that arthritis is the most common reason members of the military receive a medical discharge and is among the most common causes for treatment in VA facilities. Approximately 12% of veterans of Operation Enduring Freedom (OEF) and Operation Iraqi Freedom (OIF) have osteoarthritis, a rate that is greater than in the general population (Rivera et al., 2016). Further, these authors found that arthritis was associated with comorbidities relevant to cardiovascular health. These comorbid diagnoses included diabetes mellitus, hyperlipidemia, hypertension, and obesity. Additional comorbid conditions identified were mental health diagnoses including PTSD, depression, anxiety, and substance abuse (Rivera et al., 2016). In an earlier study, Scher et al. (2009) found that women military members had higher incidence rates of hip osteoarthritis when compared to males. Rates were also increased in those who were Black, junior and senior enlisted, senior officer, and in the Navy, Army, or Marines.

Another orthopedic challenge experienced by veterans is that of osteopenia and osteoporosis, sometimes complicated by or revealed through a low-trauma fracture. However, of note is that treatment for osteoporosis among veterans may be less than sufficient. One reason for this may be that osteoporosis and osteopenia are frequently seen as a disease affecting females. Thus, male veterans may not be screened or treated for this metabolic disorder with orthopedic implications. In one study, less than 24% of veterans received appropriate evaluation or treatment for osteoporosis within 6 months of having experienced a low-trauma fracture (Lee et al., 2014). This finding prompted an intervention to initiate an osteoporosis electronic consult (E-consult) program. In this predominately male population, the E-consult recommended treatment with bisphosphonates for 29% of the patients; providers responded by prescribing these medications for only 57% of those for whom this treatment was recommended. In 58% of the patients, the E-consults recommended bone density assessments. Among those assessed, 23% revealed osteoporosis and 39% indicated osteopenia (Lee et al., 2014). As a result of the screening, 56% started treatment with calcium and vitamin D therapy or medications to treat or prevent osteoporosis. Additional patients were referred for follow-up and management through the bone clinic (Lee et al., 2014). As osteoporosis and osteopenia have been noted in veterans, including those who are male, care should include screening for these disorders regardless of gender, especially when a fracture is present.

Limb Trauma

Limb trauma, including amputation, has been described as a signature injury of modern war (Edwards et al., 2014). As early as World War I, physicians and surgeons identified the severity of injury and pain associated with limb trauma (Edwards et al., 2014). While the injuries to limbs during earlier battles resulted from gunshots and shrapnel or fragments from munitions, the more recent injuries are more likely to be due to blasts or fragments resulting from improvised explosive devices (Edwards et al., 2014). Despite the differences in causation, the effects remain similar and continue to include peripheral nerve damage.

In wars of the past, such as World War I, most who experienced a battlefield limb injury, especially those requiring amputation, had a lower likelihood of survival. However, with current advances in battlefield surgical care, it is likely that nurses will see more patients who not only survived the initial injury but survived without amputation either on the battlefield or in a surgical suite. Debridement of wounds is becoming the preference with an emphasis on limb and length preservation (Edwards et al., 2014). Further, primary amputation, which is amputation that typically occurs on the battlefield, is discouraged and is recommended only when the limb injury results in questionable survivability (Edwards et al., 2014). Once the service member has arrived for surgical care, amputation should occur only with the agreement of two surgeons and the anesthesiologist (Edwards et al., 2014). Following amputation, the new priority becomes rehabilitation and maintenance of function of the remaining or replacement limb. Despite such advances, pain during the immediate time to surgery and the postoperative period is a challenge. Many service members will continue to experience pain following surgical recovery, with some studies indicating that chronic pain can last for over 25 years (Bhatnagar et al., 2015).

With many members of the military experiencing more than one deployment, the risk of battlefield injury increases. Although battlefield amputation was common during earlier wars (Edwards et al., 2014), advances in protective body armor and battlefield treatment has resulted in fewer surgeries at the point of combat or injury; survival rates have also improved with some estimates of survival following battlefield injury as high as 90% (Bhatnagar et al., 2015; Gallagher & Sandbrink, 2019; Szuflita et al., 2016). Along with increased survival rates, there are higher rates of PTSD, traumatic brain injury (TBI), and multi-limb trauma (MLT) requiring amputation or reconstruction.

In 2010 and 2011, over 300 amputations annually resulted from injuries sustained due to combat injury (Bhatnagar et al., 2015). Such injuries reasonably require extensive surgical repair along with lengthy intensive physical rehabilitation and restoration that include orthotics and prosthetics. Rehabilitation can take anywhere from 9 to 15 months on average. Further, veterans may require up to three prosthetics, including basic devices to allow simple ambulation and have an approximate cost of $10,000. Others may require prosthetics for specialized activities or to allow computer guidance; these devices may cost more than $30,000 (Bhatnagar et al., 2015).

MLT, including those resulting in amputation, can be complicated by additional injuries. In veterans with comorbid diagnoses of PTSD, TBI, or substance abuse, recovery from limb trauma was extended and more complicated, perhaps as a result of decreased or altered coping skills (Bhatnagar et al., 2015). For those experiencing MLT with or without amputation, costs for treatment were increased with these additional diagnoses of PTSD, TBI, or substance abuse due to extended rehabilitation, and increased use of psychiatric and pharmacy services (Bhatnagar et al., 2015). In their study, Bhatnagar et al. (2015) made a discovery related to those who had experienced bilateral lower limb amputation. Such veterans had the lowest prevalence of PTSD and also experienced lower costs related to psychiatric care despite having received higher injury severity scores (ISSs). An ISS is calculated to assess the combined effects of injuries in those who have experienced multiple injuries and has been shown to correlate with mortality and morbidity (Agency for Clinical Innovation, 2019). This score includes ratings from six regions of the body, including head or neck, face, chest, abdomen, extremities or pelvic girdle, and external body. These veterans also were more likely to have experienced their injuries during more recent conflicts. This finding perhaps indicates that care is advancing, especially related to a focus on the reduction of developing PTSD. Of note is that one medical management advance was earlier administration of morphine or sedation during battlefield injury management and the inclusion of earlier and more intensive psychiatric treatment and psychological support for those sustaining such injuries as a result of combat (Bhatanagar et al., 2014). As a result, those with bilateral lower-limb amputations, who were most likely to receive sedation in the field and more intensive psychiatric therapy and support, may be less likely to experience PTSD symptomatology, despite the severity of their injuries. This field treatment and psychiatric support could reduce the sequelae that may result from experiencing PTSD.

MLT and amputation previously would have been treated only by exogenous prosthetics and would likely have resulted in immediate medical discharge from military service. The current advances in care and evaluation of fitness for duty have resulted in change. One new approach, used for transfemoral amputation, is known as osseointegrated reconstruction. In this approach, surgeons implant a device into the remaining femoral bone tissue (Al Muderis et al., 2018). The implanted device provides the hinge joint previously present in the knee. This approach allows for a more normal range of movement, including that of the hip, which can improve function. Improved function is essential as most who experience an amputation will take over a year to return to work, and over 90% of those experiencing a transfemoral amputation will become wheelchair bound.

Al Muderis et al. (2018) followed 37 people who underwent the osseointegration surgery and found that they had significant improvement in all outcome measures when comparing pre-operative to post-operative ratings. In this group, 12 patients were confined to a wheelchair before surgery and were thus unable to be tested on the Six-Minute Walk Test (6MWT) and the Timed Up and Go (TUG) test. The 6MWT is an assessment of functional capacity and evaluates the distance someone can quickly walk on a hard, flat surface, such as a hallway, in 6 minutes (American Thoracic Society, 2002). As such, this assessment provides information on all systems used during ambulation, including cardiovascular, pulmonary, neurological, and musculoskeletal systems. The TUG test is an assessment of a patient's mobility and risk of falling. In this assessment, the patient begins in a seated position and is asked to stand up from the chair, walk to a line 10 feet away, turn, walk back to the chair, and sit. Those who take more than 12 seconds to complete the test are at increased risk of falling (Centers for Disease Control and Prevention [CDC], 2017a). Following surgery, however, all experienced improvement and were able to complete both the 6MWT and the TUG test (Al Muderis et al., 2018).

In the current military experience, having an amputation no longer means medical discharge and return to civilian status. However, rates of return to duty (RTD) remain low. Hurley et al. (2015) explored military records of those who had experienced an amputation as a result of a combat injury. Of those identified, only 2% (16 service members) were found to be fit for duty and able to return to their preinjury role. Further, only 11% (103 service members) were allowed to continue on active duty; however, these military members returned to a less physically demanding role, and 56% were identified as fully disabled. Those who returned to duty in any capacity did have a lower ISS than others.

Over time and despite improvements in care and rehabilitation, very few service members with amputations will return to active duty; many will be diagnosed with multiple conditions that contribute to a high level of disability (Hurley et al., 2015). To determine the degree of fitness, the military uses a disability evaluation system for determining the disability level resulting from a service-related injury (DoD, 2014). This system includes the Physical Evaluation Board Liaison Officer (PEBLO) to determine the level of function and disability that results from a severe injury. The PEBLO are non-medical case managers who guide injured service members through the disability process, including the process to determine whether an injured member of the military can RTD (Hurley et al., 2015; DoD, 2014). From the evaluation, the PEBLO can determine the dispensation of the service member. Such determinations include if the service member has recovered enough to continue serving on active duty status, be placed on a temporary disabled retired list and allowed additional time to recover, permanently retired, or separated from service with severance pay without disability pay (Hurley et al., 2015). If the service member is considered recovered and able to continue as active duty, a further determination will include whether the individual is fit to return to full duty, eligible to continue on active duty in a limited capacity, or continue but assigned to a new MOS (Hurley et al., 2015). The PEBLO assigns a disability rating; those ratings greater than 75 are considered to be fully disabled and eligible to receive the maximum amount of disability pay.

Although the study by Hurley et al. (2015) revealed that few who experience an amputation during combat will return to their role as a member of the military in any capacity, the findings can provide guidance for the treatment and rehabilitation priorities while also setting expectations following a combat-related amputation. Further, rates of return to duty vary between the branches of service, perhaps due, in part, to the larger numbers of amputations occurring among Army soldiers and Marines as compared to Air Force or Naval members. Service members in the Marine Corps or in the Navy are less likely to be able to RTD in any capacity, while those in the Air Force are more likely to be found fit for RTD (Hurley et al., 2015).

NEUROLOGICAL INJURIES

Military service, including combat deployments, have the potential of exposing the military member to situations in which neurological injury or permanent damage can occur. There is the potential for spinal cord injury (SCI), TBI, and auditory or visual disturbances which may occur as a result of or separate from TBI.

Spinal Cord Injury

According to a 2013 Spotlight, the VA provides care to approximately 26% of people with a SCI in the United States. Providing care to approximately 27,000 people with SCI each year, the VA claims to be the largest provider of SCI care in the world (VA, 2019b). SCI is more prevalent among veterans who served in Iraq or Afghanistan than those in prior wars with most injuries occurring during combat. Most SCIs sustained in combat are due to blast injuries causing blunt trauma while non-combat injuries resulted from falls, machinery, or sports (Szuflita et al., 2016). Combat-related SCI began to increase in the early 2000s, with injuries increasing from 38% in 2003 to 80% in 2007 (Szuflita et al., 2016). Despite advancements in body armor and field treatment, blast injuries likely cause more damage than penetrating injuries due to most occurring while the military member is seated inside armored vehicles. These injuries tend to be polytraumatic, more severe, and include multiple levels of spinal damage and injury (Szuflita et al., 2016).

Although many veterans with SCI will seek ongoing care through the VA health system, every acute care VA hospital does not have a SCI center or long-term care facility. For this reason, veterans with SCI in those geographic areas could access care through a civilian health agency or system. In addition to the immobility that may result, veterans with SCI may also experience urologic challenges. Neurogenic bladder is a primary challenge and is present in almost 83% of veterans with SCI. Neurogenic bladder can occur from failure to store urine due to muscle and sphincter resistance, failure to empty urine, or lack of the bladder muscle coordinating with the sphincter to relax, causing incomplete emptying (Rabadi & Astor, 2015).

A higher-level injury is associated with neurogenic bladder and the occurrence of more frequent urinary tract infections (UTIs). Those veterans with recurring UTI were more likely to have renal atrophy and hydronephrosis. Bladder training can aid in this as can encouraging adequate fluid intake of 1.5 to 2 L per day so that urinary flow is sufficient (Rabadi & Astor, 2015). For those with neurogenic bladder, treatment may include intermittent bladder catheterization, use of an external (condom), indwelling, or supra-pubic catheter, and good personal hygiene. Hygiene includes replacing any indwelling or supra-pubic catheters and the collection system every 28 days (Rabadi & Astor, 2015). Among veterans with SCI and neurogenic bladder, clean intermittent catheterization was the most frequently used bladder program and was shown to decrease occurrence of UTIs (Rabadi & Astor, 2015).

Depression has been associated with SCI in both non-veteran and veteran populations. Risk factors for depression among those with SCI include shorter time since injury, a higher level of injury, younger age, female gender, less than a high school degree, marital separation or divorce, unemployment, pain, and substance abuse (Wilson et al., 2018). Among veterans with SCI, almost 41% had been diagnosed with depression; a rate greater than in the general population. Additionally, female veterans were more likely to have higher rates of lifetime depression diagnoses than men, while among male veterans, bodily pain was a significant predictor of depressive symptoms and diagnosis (Wilson et al., 2018).

The level and completeness of injury may also be a factor in depressive symptoms or diagnosis. SCI is rated by the Asia Impairment Scale (AIS) with a rating of D indicating spinal cord damage that is least complete; thus, those with an AIS-D rating retain more functional abilities and are more likely to be ambulatory (Ames et al., 2017). However, those with an AIS-D rating experienced higher self-reported depressive symptoms, higher pain, and lower subjective quality of life (Ames et al., 2017). One hypothesis for this is that those with incomplete injuries often receive less support; the injury may not be visible thus the fatigue and frustration felt may be overlooked. Assessments of veterans with SCI should include assessment and evaluation for depressive symptoms along with quality of life assessment, including exploration of somatic symptoms, especially pain. Recreation including adaptive sports tailored to the interests and abilities of the veteran with SCI has been shown to improve quality of life (Mulhollon & Casey, 2016).

Another concern for the veteran with SCI is related to survival following a cardiac arrest as differences in survival rates have been documented in veterans with SCI who experience an in-hospital cardiac arrest. Among the general population, the survival rate following in-hospital cardiac arrest ranges from 0% to 44%, with a mean survival rate ranging from 15% to 20% (Caruso et al., 2014). However, in a study of 36 male veterans with SCI who experienced cardiac arrest while hospitalized, only two survived to discharge, resulting in a post-cardiac arrest survival rate of only 5.5% (Caruso et al., 2014). These findings indicate that veterans with SCI may have a worse outlook when cardiac arrest occurs within an acute illness context. Caruso et al. (2014) suggested this reduced survival rate may be due to comorbidities among those with SCI that may worsen the prognosis following cardiac arrest. These comorbidities included chronic kidney disease, cardiac ischemia that is without symptoms, or presence of pressure ulcers (Caruso et al., 2014). SCI patients are considered to be a high-risk population; thus, advance care planning should include educating veterans with SCI on decisions that may be required during an acute illness.

Traumatic Brain Injury

TBI as a result of war is increasing. Similar to limb trauma, TBI has been labeled as a signature injury of OIF and OEF. Since 2000 the U.S. military has recorded almost 350,000 diagnoses of TBI; most are considered to be mild (Cooper et al., 2014; O'Neil et al., 2017; Uchendu et al., 2016). TBI can occur when there is a physical force against the head, resulting in neuropathology; such injury can result from minor injuries such as lacerations or from major injuries that could include decapitation (Marshall et al., 2012).

The pathophysiology of TBI is a direct result of tissue damage occurring from macroscopic and cellular changes within the brain. The location and the severity of the damage will determine the sequelae of the injury, with the treatment focus being that of minimizing a secondary injury to the brain (Marshall et al., 2012). As many TBIs result from blast injuries, acceleration-deceleration injury is the most frequent concern. In these injuries, there is acceleration, or movement, of the brain toward the skull, resulting in the impact of brain tissue against the hard and rough internal surface of the skull (Marshall et al., 2012). As a result of this, the brain then rapidly moves in the opposite direction, causing the deceleration injury. In some cases that are most severe, the brain may rotate on the brainstem causing a diffuse axonal injury (Marshall et al., 2012).

Uchendu et al. (2016) described TBI as altered brain function or other evidence of pathology of the brain that has resulted from an external force; impairments in cognitive, physical, or psychosocial functioning may be temporary or permanent. Veterans deployed in support of both OEF and OIF have a higher proportion of head and neck injuries compared to those who served in prior eras (Amara et al., 2014). This increase in head and neck injuries is likely due to the increased use of explosives such as roadside bombs, mines, and improvised explosive devices. Further, TBI may be undiagnosed or have a delayed diagnosis due to other more obvious or critical injuries. Personnel may also be reluctant to report symptoms of TBI due to having been in a combat setting, lack of obvious injury, or feeling that seeking help is an indication of weakness (Amara et al., 2014; Gallagher & Azuma, 2018).

Although women veterans experience deployment-related TBI less frequently than men, data suggest that approximately 11% of women veterans have a probable TBI, and symptoms have been significant (Amara et al., 2014). Due to the risk of TBI, VA personnel are prompted by the electronic medical record to screen all OEF/OIF veterans for TBI. The screening includes exposure to events increasing risk of TBI, symptoms occurring after the event, new symptoms or symptoms that worsened after the event, and current symptoms (Amara et al., 2014). When a veteran responds positively to one or more problems, they are considered positive for TBI and offered a referral for a more thorough evaluation and assessment.

For most who have experienced a TBI, clinical recovery may occur within the days to weeks following the injury. However, many will continue to experience persistent symptoms for months and years. Symptoms may be cognitive and reduce functional ability and include headache, light sensitivity, depressed mood, and reduced attention (Jurick et al., 2016; O'Neil et al., 2017). TBI can be described as mild or causing post-concussive symptoms and may affect vision and hearing.

MILD TRAUMATIC BRAIN INJURY AND POST-CONCUSSIVE SYNDROME

A diagnosis of mild traumatic brain injury (mTBI) occurs when there has been an initial impairment in sensorium for 30 minutes or less; this mild impairment can be when the individual becomes unconscious or has altered consciousness (Uchendu et al., 2016). The International Statistical Classification of Diseases, 10th edition provides criteria for post-concussive syndrome which has been adopted by the VA (O'Neil et al., 2017). This adoption may result in better diagnosis and follow-up care. Diagnosis requires a history of brain injury, usually with loss of consciousness, and the development of symptoms from at least three of six categories. The symptoms must last for at least 4 weeks after the injury. The symptom categories range from headache to fear of permanent brain damage (Box 6.1).

BOX 6.1

ICD-10 CATEGORIES FOR POST-CONCUSSIVE SYNDROME

Headache, dizziness, malaise, fatigue, noise intolerance
Irritability, depression, anxiety, emotional lability
Subjective complaints of concentration or memory difficulty
Insomnia
Reduced alcohol tolerance
Preoccupation with these symptoms and fear of permanent brain damage

ICD-10, International Statistical Classification of Diseases, 10th edition.

The long-term effects of a single or multiple mTBI are unclear; however, there is a potential connection between multiple concussions or mTBI and neurodegeneration, such as has been described as chronic traumatic encephalopathy (CTE; Uchendu et al., 2016). Because members of the military are at risk for multiple types of TBI, CTE is a risk that may result in multiple mood disorders along with neuropsychiatric and cognitive impairment (Uchendu et al., 2016).

TBI affects many aspects of a veteran's life, including satisfaction with life (SWL). Seidl et al. (2015) found that symptoms of TBI were significantly related to SWL. Specifically, headache impact, pain interference, sleep quality, posttraumatic stress symptom severity, and social support were related to SWL. Interestingly, when adjusting for posttraumatic stress severity as a covariate, only sleep quality and social support remained significantly associated with SWL. For this reason, the treatment of posttraumatic stress symptoms in those with TBI is imperative, as is maximizing sleep quality and social support. PTSD can add to the somatic effects of an mTBI. Dizziness and postural instability can occur and be a lingering component of post-concussive syndrome; these complaints can worsen when there is presence of PTSD (Wares et al., 2015).

AUDITORY AND VISUAL DISTURBANCES

Auditory dysfunction and disturbances can occur as a component or result of TBI. Auditory problems may be present even when hearing is clinically normal. In one study, participants who experienced a TBI as a result of a blast injury self-reported experiencing auditory problems in situations in which it would be difficult to listen, such as when there was background noise, long conversations, fast speech, and during telephone conversations (Saunders et al., 2015). Further, the participants had deficits related to tasks rather than global hearing deficits; this may indicate that the problem following a blast injury is damage to processing in the central auditory system rather than the structures of the ear.

Gallun et al. (2016) followed up on the original study, which included participants who had experienced high-intensity blasts and a control group which was similar in age and hearing abilities but had not sustained a blast injury. The findings of the subsequent study indicated that those who had experienced a blast injury continued to perform abnormally on task-specific measures, reinforcing that peripheral hearing loss is not present, yet there is a problem with central auditory processing.

Acoustic trauma, with or without TBI, is also a risk for those who are members of the military or work in a military setting (Moring et al., 2018). Such trauma can occur as a result of the firing of mortar rounds, gunfire in a combat or training setting, exposure to engine noise during transport or convoys, or from blasts that may occur from a myriad of reasons. One symptom that may occur as a result of auditory trauma is tinnitus, which can present in multiple ways such as ringing, buzzing, or rushing sounds (Moring et al., 2018). Alone, tinnitus can be bothersome but can also result in a lack of pleasure in experiences, anxiety, sensitivity to some sounds or frequencies, depression, and insomnia (Moring et al., 2018). Thus, tinnitus may contribute to TBI symptom severity or may be exacerbated by the presence of TBI. Moring et al. (2018) also described a relationship between tinnitus and PTSD, both of which are most frequently the result of exposure to explosions. As there is some association between TBI and PTSD, the additional presence of tinnitus may be an additional risk to the veteran's overall sense of well-being.

Visual challenges may also arise from TBI and may be short-term or long-term. Magone et al. (2014) performed a retrospective case series in patients who had experienced mTBI for more than 12 months. The participants had not experienced an eye injury. During the blast, most veterans in the study (71%) had lost consciousness, and most (68%) were moved by the explosion from their position in which they were located before the blast. The majority experienced visual problems including photophobia, or light sensitivity, and difficulty reading. Those diagnosed with more than one TBI experienced more visual complaints. Those who were asymptomatic had experienced the TBI in the more distant past, perhaps indicating that elapsed time since injury may improve vision.

Similarly, Goodrich et al. (2014) explored the overlapping symptoms of visual disturbances, TBI, and PTSD. TBI alone can result in visual changes yet before this study PTSD and vision changes had not been explored. A retrospective review explored patients with TBI and found that no significant differences in vision were noted for those with TBI with or without PTSD. Despite this, those with PTSD self-reported more visual disturbances than those without (Goodrich et al., 2014). The chief complaints were light sensitivity and reading problems. As a result, patients who have a diagnosis of TBI and PTSD may struggle more with visual symptoms.

One way in which veterans who have experienced blast-related mTBI are finding support is through goal management training. Goal management training is an intervention focused on developing and enhancing metacognition that helps improve executive function (Waid-Ebbs et al., 2014). In this approach, veterans learn self-regulation to identify when errors in processing occur and then implement strategies to reduce these errors. When an error occurs, the veteran may be prompted to stop and consider what they are doing, define a goal, list steps, learn steps, and check to see if they are proceeding as planned.

PAIN

Many veterans are living with some degree of chronic pain. This pain often fits within what is known as the polytrauma triad, which includes TBI, a mental health diagnosis, and pain (Gallagher &

Sandbrink, 2019). Improvements in battlefield medicine resulting in increased survival rates and decreased mortality means many veterans come home with complex health needs that require management and treatment. Within the polytrauma triad, pain has an effect upon the well-being of the veteran that cannot be overlooked. For example, injury resulting in pain may likely have occurred in the context of a combat situation, incorporating both physical and psychological components. When chronic pain results, the neurological system encodes the pain such that it is difficult to separate it from the psychological sequelae (Gallagher & Sandbrink, 2019). As a result, stress and PTSD symptoms can trigger or increase the severity of pain while the pain itself may result in increased stress and PTSD symptoms. Estimates indicate that as many as 49% of patients with chronic pain also have a diagnosis of PTSD (Outcalt, Ang et al., 2014). TBI also is associated with increased pain, especially following exposure to blasts from explosive devices (Stratton et al., 2014). As a result, veterans who have a diagnosis which includes all legs of the polytrauma triad should be carefully evaluated and referred for treatment of all three disorders.

Some estimates indicate that over half of those returning from Iraq or Afghanistan experience chronic pain; approximately 47% reported mild pain while another 28% reported their pain as moderate to severe (Legarreta et al., 2016; Matthias et al., 2014). Veterans with chronic pain may experience a phenomenon known as pain catastrophizing. Pain catastrophizing is ruminating or often thinking about the pain, magnifying pain sensations, or feeling helpless about pain (Outcalt, Ang et al., 2014). Veterans living with persistent or chronic pain have described living with the pain as "a burden on my soul" (Matthias et al., 2014, p. 27) with a range of emotions including feelings of hopelessness, anger, and fear of worsening pain. In the study by Matthias et al. (2014), veterans felt that talking about pain could be helpful yet sometimes they avoided talking with others about their pain. This avoidance was due to a feeling that providers and others lack an understanding of their pain experience. While social support was effective, veteran peers offering support may also be helpful. The experience of chronic pain in the presence of PTSD has resulted in OIF/OEF veterans describing higher pain severity, greater disability related to pain, increased pain interference, increase affective distress, and more maladaptive pain cognitions such as catastrophizing (Outcalt, Ang et al., 2014).

Among veterans with pain, comorbidities outside of the polytrauma triad may worsen the pain, especially a diagnosis of overweight or obesity. The CDC (2017b) defines normal weight as having a body mass index (BMI) between 18.5 to 25 while overweight is a BMI of 25 to less than 30. Obesity is present when the BMI is greater than 30. Higgins et al. (2016) found that almost 77% of veterans in the VA system were overweight or obese and that there was a significantly higher rate of low back pain among veterans as compared with non-veterans. When pain was comorbid with a diagnosis of overweight or obesity, there was an increased risk of experiencing pain with the presence of obesity predicting the progression of pain; the presence of obesity was compounded by the individual avoiding physical activity due to the pain. This presence of pain then complicated management of other chronic conditions, leading to poorer healthcare outcomes (Higgins et al., 2016).

In addition to obesity and overweight being a comorbidity for pain, pain among veterans has also been shown to have gender and racial differences and may be affected by the level of education and service branch. Higgins et al. (2014) reported that those experiencing chronic pain were more likely to be Black, female, enlisted and on active duty, in the Army, and have a high school education or less. Further, Higgins and colleagues noted those with mental health disorders, including mood disorders, PTSD, substance use, and anxiety along with a history of TBI or a diagnosis of overweight or obesity were more likely to experience persistent pain. Cichowski et al. (2017) noted that women veterans who had experienced military sexual trauma (MST) were more likely to experience chronic pain compared to those without a history of such trauma. Such pain conditions were widespread and could include irritable bowel syndrome and other abdominal pain, back pain, fibromyalgia, and headaches. Driscoll et al. (2015) echoed these findings in that, as compared to male veterans, women veterans reporting chronic pain had lower levels of combat exposure yet greater reports of childhood interpersonal trauma and MST.

Some outcomes, however, are positively associated with being of female gender. In a study by Olivia et al. (2015), female veterans in the VA system were more likely to receive care aligned with chronic pain guidelines. This care included receiving appropriate mental health assessment, rehabilitation, and pharmacy reconciliation. However, one negative outcome reported in this study was that women received more sedative medication prescriptions, which did not follow the guidelines. In another study focused on veterans who participated in chronic pain rehabilitation with an interdisciplinary perspective, female veterans were younger and less likely to be White and with a partner or married; they also tended to report pain of shorter duration and were less likely to be prescribed opioids (Murphy et al., 2016). These females also did not maintain gains in pain intensity or sleep disturbances after opioid cessation as compared to the gains experienced by males.

Differences related to race and pain have been described related to outcomes, opioid treatment, and beliefs related to complementary and alternative therapies. In a retrospective review of VA medical records data, Burgess et al. (2016) found no significant association between race and pain interfering with functioning or the perceived effectiveness of pain treatment. Interestingly, having an opioid prescription was not associated with whether patients perceived their treatment was effective. Goldstein et al. (2015) explored the beliefs and interests of inner-city veterans related to complementary and alternative medicines (CAMs). Interest in CAMs was high overall, with interest being strongly associated with African American veterans.

Veterans with pain seek care for pain and other diagnoses. Those who have pain and an additional diagnosis, especially for mental health problems, are more likely to need more care. For example, in one study, veterans who had a diagnosis of pain and PTSD (pain + PTSD) sought care from multiple departments more frequently than those diagnosed only with pain or only with PTSD (Outcalt, Yu et al., 2014). Interestingly, those with pain + PTSD sought primary care 7% more often than those only diagnosed with pain, and almost 50% more often than those only diagnosed with PTSD. This finding reinforces that the combination of pain and PTSD is a complex issue that may have additive effects on the veteran's health. Another factor affecting pain may be use of tobacco. Volkman et al. (2015) found that among those who were current smokers or had smoked previously, the pain was more likely to be reported as moderate to severe.

The response to pain by the veteran may be affected by what some describe as a military mindset. This military mindset, a form of stoicism, may be the result of the acculturation that occurs during military service and arises from the training and expectations of military service. Military training includes setting aside pain and other personal concerns so individual members can complete challenging tasks and the mission can be accomplished (Grigorescu, 2009). The resulting stoicism may result in controlling and suppressing, or hiding, emotions and feelings, including those of pain (Elliott, 2017; Grigorescu, 2009). As a result of this stoicism, the veteran experiencing pain may seem to withdraw and might feel as if the pain is something to be endured through using their military training and experience (Elliott, 2017).

CAREGIVERS OF VETERANS

Caregivers of veterans also experience challenges, including what has been called a chronic multi-symptom illness (CMI) and mental health symptoms. Blanchard et al. (2017) used retrospective data to explore whether spouses of Gulf War era veterans also experienced CMI diagnosis or symptoms. In comparing data between spouses of those who had been deployed and those who had not, results indicated that CMI prevalence was 19.5% in those who had deployed and 17.3% in those who had not. A CMI diagnosis was more likely when the veteran spouse also was diagnosed with GWI; however, deployment was not found to be a predictor of CMI. Despite this finding, it was also noted that spouses of veterans who had GWI reported worse physical and mental functioning.

Saban et al. (2016) also reported that caregivers of veterans experienced higher levels of symptoms that can decrease quality of life. These symptoms included fatigue and disturbed sleep, decreased self-esteem, and financial difficulties. In another study focused on health-related quality of life, caregivers of veterans with TBI most frequently discussed social and emotional health with physical health being discussed least frequently (Carlozzi et al., 2016). Further, the participants described anger over difficulties accessing healthcare, suppressing emotions even when they are struggling, and hypervigilance over their behavior so as not to upset their veteran partner. Social health was impacted related to loss of employment and thus experiencing financial changes and through changes in relationships (Carlozzi et al., 2016). Emotional health was impacted due to caregiver strain, depression, anxiety, and even feelings of loss (Carlozzi et al., 2016). Physical health, although minimally discussed, included difficulties maintaining personal health behaviors and care, sleep disturbances, and changes in intimate relationships (Carlozzi et al., 2016). The needs of veterans who sustained injuries, both physical and mental, can be complex and challenging. Griffin et al. (2017) found that the intensity of care that was needed was associated with increased caregiver burden and poor mental health of the caregiver. Thus, it is important to consider the needs of caregivers along with the needs of veterans, including connecting caregivers with sources of support.

IMPLICATIONS FOR NURSING EDUCATION AND PRACTICE

Veterans may experience complex health concerns that will benefit from nursing care. Rather than assuming a veteran has a health concern or need related to military service, nurses should complete a thorough health history and assessment to gather information. Nurses in clinical practice can increase their knowledge and understanding of the health concerns of veterans in order to be prepared to perform a high-quality assessment and form a comprehensive and appropriate plan of care. Creation of plans of care for veterans should consider the influence of health concerns on daily functioning. Nurse educators can also increase their knowledge and understanding of these issues to prepare future or practicing nurses on how best to care for military personnel, veterans, and their caregivers.

Implications for Practice

One way of exploring whether a patient is a veteran is by asking what is known as the universal question. According to Cipriano (2014), fewer than one third of veterans will seek care within the VA health system; thus, nurses in the civilian sector must be prepared to inquire about military service as part of a complete history and assessment. This universal question is worded as "Have you ever served in the military?" and should be asked of all adult patients to help identify any risks of illness or injury as a result of time spent in military service (American Academy of Nursing, n.d.; Cipriano, 2014). Nurses can also obtain pocket cards, posters, and patient reminder cards through this web link. Asking this question can aid nurses in the identification of veterans and provide an opening to have a conversation to explore any health issues that the veteran might be experiencing. Nurses can provide a holistic approach by being open to hearing what the veteran has to say and share.

Once the universal question has been asked and the patient has identified as a veteran, questions about military service can guide the remainder of the nursing assessment. The Military Health History Pocket Card (www.va.gov/oaa/pocketcard) can be downloaded onto a mobile device to guide the assessment based on the veteran's time in service. As care managers and advocates, nurses can then recommend and guide an interprofessional approach to care to evaluate and treat all symptoms (Conard & Armstrong, 2019; Fox et al., 2018). As some health problems have comorbidities, careful exploration can aid the nurse in determining the full effects of a health condition. Such determination may then assist the nurse in forming a plan that will be comprehensive, interdisciplinary, and appropriate for management of the veteran's conditions.

GULF WAR ILLNESS AND TRAUMATIC BRAIN INJURY IMPLICATIONS

Those with a diagnosis of GWI may experience an array of symptoms. Nurses should not assume that the symptoms are psychosomatic or that the symptoms and syndrome are not real. Veterans who have this diagnosis may be reluctant to discuss their symptoms as there is controversy regarding the causation, diagnosis, and treatment (Conard & Armstrong, 2019). Mental health problems may be a confounding and compounding factor for veterans with GWI; therefore, it is also imperative to evaluate and treat mental health issues.

Both GWI and TBI may result in cognitive difficulties or dysfunction. The nursing assessment should thus include an evaluation of memory and the presence of tremors that might affect the ability to complete psychomotor tasks such as activities of daily living or self-administration of medications, especially medications that are injected and might require greater manual dexterity or the ability to read the small print on syringes. When the nurse notes memory impairment or cognitive dysfunction, teaching should be tailored to the needs and abilities of the veteran. It may be helpful to provide education in multiple formats both to meet the learning preferences and needs of the veteran as well as enhance learning and comprehension. Using the teach-back method can help ensure that the veteran understood the information. The teach-back method is a closed-loop form of communication in which the nurse evaluates teaching. In using this technique, the nurse provides a demonstration or explanation and then asks the patient to "teach-back" through either a return explanation or demonstration (Ayzengart, 2017).

Balance may also be affected in those with GWI or TBI. Those with GWI may have decreased cerebrovascular flow and may experience autonomic dysfunction; these changes have the potential to affect balance. In veterans with TBI, balance may be reduced, especially when PTSD is a comorbid condition (Wares et al., 2015). Therefore, a thorough assessment should include an assessment of balance, including observing gait and the ability to stand with and without assistance. Nurses should provide assistance with ambulation when the assessment indicates there is an increased risk of falls or injury. Further assessment may also include obtaining orthostatic blood pressure measurements to identify drops in blood pressure that could increase fall risk.

A diagnosis of PTSD often accompanies a diagnosis of TBI (Wheeler & Puskar, 2015). Therefore, nurses should advocate for coordinated care that addresses both diagnoses effectively. Nonpharmacologic care for PTSD may include cognitive processing therapy and prolonged exposure therapy (Wheeler & Puskar, 2015). These therapies may be equally effective, and treatment adherence tends to be high. Although mental health providers, including mental health nurse practitioners, provide both therapies, nurses can provide information on these therapies and support veterans who are engaged in these forms of treatment.

ORTHOPEDIC IMPLICATIONS

Veterans may be at risk for osteoarthritis, osteopenia, or osteoporosis. Assessment of veterans should include risk factors and symptoms for each of these. Nurses can advocate for screening for any patient who has risk factors for these disease processes, regardless of gender or current or prior military service. Following any fracture, nurses should ask about factors contributing to the injury, especially when the fracture is the result of a low-trauma incident. Nurses can advocate for their patients by requesting or recommending bone density studies. When such studies indicate the presence of osteopenia or osteoporosis, nurses can then request or recommend treatment following current treatment guidelines and recommendations. Such care would include providing proper education to the patient and aiding in arranging follow-up care and treatment. When studies do not indicate the presence of decreased bone density, education can include osteoporosis prevention.

Next, nurses should not presume a limb trauma or amputation is the result of military service. Such trauma may be the result of a motor vehicle crash or other trauma, injury, or disease. Many modern prosthetic devices, especially those for lower limbs, are of such high quality that gait may not be impaired or altered. Part of the assessment of patients experiencing MLT, including amputation, should include observing the gait and the ability to safely perform necessary tasks including activities of daily living. When an amputation is present, assessment of the stump should be performed to identify any areas of redness or irritation. This assessment should consider the potential for tissue breakdown or pressure injury or ulcer. If there is any indication of a poor fit, the nurse should work with the interprofessional rehabilitation team for improved fit or even advocate for a replacement prosthetic. Nursing care would also include notifying the provider of the assessment findings and consider referral to a wound care nurse. Emphasis should be on the abilities of the veteran rather than limitations. However, careful assessment will include psychological effects and symptoms to make the appropriate referrals needed.

As limb trauma and amputation often result in significant pain that may become chronic, a thorough pain assessment is warranted. A pain assessment should include what helps the pain improve and the veteran's target or acceptable pain level. Careful assessment can help identify whether the veteran is experiencing ongoing sensations that are considered forms of post-amputation pain. These sensations fall into three categories including phantom sensations, phantom limb pain, or residual limb pain (Potter et al., 2009). Between 90% to 98% of those with a limb amputation experience some type of phantom sensation or limb pain; these sensations can be brief or become chronic (Malchow et al., 2009). The mechanism of injury may help determine the type of sensation or pain experienced following amputation and limb restoration. For example, in those who experienced a traumatic amputation, such as a grenade exploding in the hand, phantom pain may be more likely to occur, possibly due to neuroma development (Malchow et al., 2009). See Table 6.3 for descriptions of the types of pain the veteran may experience (Edwards et al., 2014; Potter et al., 2009).

Treatment for limb trauma or amputation pain would be individualized depending upon the type and severity of pain. Understanding the differences in types of pain following limb trauma or amputation can aid the nurse is making recommendations for appropriate treatment. Such treatment may be interdisciplinary and could involve the use of complementary therapies. The formation of neuromas, which are bundles of severed nerve fibers that continue to transmit pain signals, may be treated through surgical excision; however, such removal has not been shown to offer significant improvement of the pain (Malchow et al., 2009). Physical therapy, along with anesthesiology and surgery, may

TABLE 6.3 DESCRIPTIONS OF TYPES OF LIMB TRAUMA PAIN

TYPE OF PAIN	DESCRIPTION
Residual limb pain	Pain that is spontaneous and may be ongoing or intermittent. This pain can also be elicited and is perceived as originating to the residual limb and includes the stump. The pain is unrelated to the amputation and arises from other injuries to tissue such as nerve or tissue damage above the level of the amputation
Phantom sensation	Any feeling that the amputated limb remains. This sensation is most often non-painful but can include pain and sensations felt within the limb. May include tingling, itching, pins and needles, or numbness. Additional sensations may include feeling as if there is a ring or sock present on the missing limb
Phantom limb pain	Spontaneous pain that can be ongoing or intermittent. This pain can also be elicited and is perceived as pain that is in the missing limb. The quality of pain varies but is often described as burning or throbbing and can be a mild ache to excruciating and intolerable pain that can often be localized

SOURCES: From Edwards, D. S., Mayhew, E. R., & Rice, A. S. (2014). "Domed to go in company with miserable pain": Surgical recognition and treatment of amputation-related pain on the Western Front during World War 1. *Lancet, 384* (9955), 1715–1719. https://doi.org/10.1016/S0140-673614)61643-3; Potter, B. K., Granville, R. R., Bagg, M. R., Forsberg, J. A., Hayda, R. A., Keeling, J. J., Shrout, J. A., Ficke, J. R., Doukas, W. C., Shawen, S. B., & Smith, D. G. (2009). Special surgical considerations for the combat casualty with limb loss. In P. F. Pasquina & R. A. Cooper (Eds.), *Care of the combat amputee* (pp. 153–190). Office of the Surgeon General at TMM Publications.

be able to aid in the management of the pain resulting from amputation. Treatments have included transcutaneous electrical nerve stimulation, tightly fitting sheaths or socks, botulinum toxin injections, nerve blocks, acupuncture, and nonsteroidal anti-inflammatory medications (Malchow et al., 2009). Additional pharmacotherapy may include acetaminophen, tricyclic antidepressants and anticonvulsants such as gabapentin, or low-dose ketamine when tricyclic antidepressants and opioid therapy have failed (Malchow et al., 2009).

NEUROLOGICAL IMPLICATIONS

One role for nurses and nurse educators is that of being an advocate. Veterans with SCI will possibly experience multiple challenges including physical and psychological challenges. Those veterans with a less severe or incomplete injury may experience less support perhaps as a result of the injury being less visible. Those with an SCI as a result of military service are allowed an annual examination; nurses can inquire if this has occurred regularly and can serve as an advocate to arrange the examination when it is past due. Becoming familiar with local VA services and hospitals is imperative to aid in making referrals or connections to appropriate and adequate treatment.

Assessment should include the level and context of the injury to determine if concurrent polytrauma may contribute to additional injuries or complications that continue to require evaluation, treatment, or management. Nurses should evaluate for physical limitations, maintaining an interdisciplinary mindset to engage rehabilitation specialists for provision of assistive devices. Referrals to adaptive recreation or sports may be warranted and appreciated. As there is a risk of pressure injury or ulcer related to impaired mobility resulting from SCI, nursing assessment should include a thorough skin assessment. If there is any indication of tissue breakdown or pressure injury, the provider should be notified and a referral should be made to a wound care nurse. With the risk of urologic complications, include an assessment of voiding patterns, methods, and presence of urinary or bowel incontinence. When incontinence is present, appropriate nursing care should be incorporated to minimize skin breakdown. Finally, provide teaching for proper personal hygiene or bladder and bowel training as part of the education plan.

Nurses can also become engaged in caring for veterans with SCI through affiliation with the Paralyzed Veterans of America (PVA). The PVA, through a nurse-led team, makes site visits to the 31 VA SCI units and long-term care centers to observe for adherence to quality standards and to advocate for consistency with identified directives and standards (Groth, 2018). Nurses can periodically review information published by the PVA to remain current with knowledge or volunteer to serve on a site visit team. Table 6.4 provides additional resources for nurses caring for veterans with an SCI.

As there is a risk of both auditory and visual changes in those who have experienced a TBI, nurses should be prepared to assess hearing and vision. This assessment may include recommending or advocating for a full auditory and vision evaluation. Patients with TBI with auditory problems may struggle

TABLE 6.4 RESOURCES FOR VETERANS WITH SPINAL CORD INJURY

RESOURCE	WEB LINK
U.S. Department of Veterans Affairs Spinal Cord Injuries and Disorders System of Care	www.sci.va.gov/index.asp
Paralyzed Veterans of America	www.pva.org/
Christopher & Dana Reeve Foundation	www.christopherreeve.org/living-with-paralysis
Military.com	www.military.com/benefits/veterans-health-care/veterans-with-spinal-cord-injury-disorders.html
Imperial County VA and Spinal Cord Injury Resources	imperial.networkofcare.org/veterans/library/article.aspx?id=1687

VA, U.S. Department of Veterans Affairs.

to hear well during lengthy or telephone conversations or with the presence of background noise. Minimize sounds and distractions in the room and present information in smaller segments. Carefully complete any teaching or information-gathering via telephone to make sure the veteran can hear and comprehend the information. In all interactions with a veteran with auditory complaints, using a teach-back approach could help the nurse evaluate if the information was understood and comprehended.

TBI may also result in visual problems, especially photophobia. As a result, nurses should assess for the presence of photophobia. If this is present, then a comfortable lighting level should be provided. When more light is needed, such as for procedural tasks in which the nurse may need brighter light, provide a way for the veteran to cover the eyes or otherwise block the light to avoid causing pain from photophobia. When teaching requires visual engagement of printed material or educational material, such as syringes or other items for learning self-care, lighting should be adequate to enhance vision yet not trigger pain from photophobia. Printed materials should be clear and of a font size that is sufficient for reading. Finally, a thorough assessment should include asking if any visual or auditory corrective devices are used and making sure that these are available and worn during conversations.

PAIN IMPLICATIONS

Nurses should remain up to date regarding current trends and practices related to pain management and care. Pain is considered to be a comorbid problem among veterans, mostly due to the causes of pain being polytrauma or complicated by PTSD or TBI (Kerns & Heapy, 2016). Treatment of pain is complex, and the rising awareness of opioid misuse and abuse may complicate the care plan; providers may be reluctant to prescribe opioids even when this is the best way to manage the veteran's pain. There has been limited research related to pain among veterans; however, a renewed focus on this topic has resulted in additional evidence to support care and treatment in multiple ways, including with opioids and other analgesics as well as with nonpharmacologic measures.

Awareness of VA guidelines on pain management with opioids is crucial as the nurse can make recommendations for treatment or management as well as advocate for appropriate interventions. The VA guidelines for pain management have been recently updated with the guidelines categorized as opioids for the management of chronic non-cancer pain. These updated guidelines include multiple algorithms, including determining when an opioid prescription is appropriate, treating patients with opioids, tapering and discontinuing opioids, and caring for those on opioids (VA and DoD, 2017). Nurses can access the full guidelines at https://www.healthquality.va.gov/guidelines/Pain/cot/VADoDOTCPG022717.pdf. A strength of the revised guidelines is that the panel tasked with the revisions included veterans. This inclusion of veterans allowed insights into the complex and often perplexing issue of chronic pain among veterans and their perspective on issues related to the management of chronic pain (McLellan, 2017). The new guidelines are comprehensive and include requiring the prescribing provider to acknowledge and consider upper dosing thresholds, drug-to-drug interactions, treatment contracts, appropriate and regular monitoring of the overall health of the patient, and finally active monitoring of all patients for well-known risks of misuse of and addiction to opioids prior to prescribing (McLellan, 2017). Providers must also monitor patients throughout their treatment for potential change in risk for abuse status.

When caring for those with chronic pain who are taking opioids, nurses must also consider the barriers and facilitators of pain management. Veteran patients have described their pain as having an uncontrollable impact on their life as they struggled to access care. This description included frustrations with the VA healthcare system and feelings that they were poorly supported and felt isolated (Simmonds et al., 2015). As a result of these feelings, veterans did not use an interdisciplinary care team and the multiple modes of treatment that may have been beneficial.

Access to care is one challenge to address for veterans living with persistent or chronic pain. The VA implemented a telementoring program that incorporates distance technologies such as video-conferencing to connect patients with providers of care (Carey et al., 2016; Frank et al., 2015). This novel approach allows those with geographic barriers to interact with and be evaluated by pain specialists. Through this approach, there was increased use of services and the initiation of non-opioid medications.

Telementoring falls within the VA's Extension for Community Healthcare Outcomes (ECHO) program and specifically is housed within the Specialty Care Access Network (SCAN) that includes multiple specialties. In the SCAN-ECHO program, veterans in remote and medically underserved areas access care through telehealth, often meeting with numerous providers for disease management (VA, 2012). Assessment of the veteran with pain, whether acute or chronic, should include any barriers to care that may be present. When the barriers include geography or other reasons for decreased ability to access care, nurses can make referrals or inquiries as to whether the veteran may qualify for enrollment in the SCAN-ECHO program. As this is a multispecialty program and pain is often a comorbidity with other diagnoses, this may be an appropriate way to engage the veteran in care that addresses all the presenting issues and challenges.

Nurses should complete an in-depth pain assessment for the veteran reporting pain. Such assessment must include the cause of the pain along with how the veteran manages the pain, including what is most effective. Pain management may consist of therapies that are non-medical or nonpharmacologic. In one study, veterans felt that they had better pain outcomes when they participated in regular exercise and their depression was treated with antidepressants; a concern of re-injury was present and should be explored (King et al., 2015). Pain management may include behavioral therapy, including use of cognitive behavioral therapy (CBT). Veterans enrolled in one study using CBT reported improvement in thinking about pain and also had a decrease in disability due to pain and less distress related to pain (Stratton et al., 2015).

The findings of these pain management studies are supported in a study by Edmond et al. (2018). In this study, 22.6% of patients used psychological or behavioral therapies to manage pain, over 50% used some type of movement including exercise, and 51.7% used manual therapies such as chiropractic care, massage, acupressure, or acupuncture. Those veterans who were more highly educated or had worse mental health symptoms were more likely to use psychological or behavioral therapies while those who were female or using non-opioid pain medications were more likely to use exercise or movement therapies. Non-White veterans with higher education levels were more likely to use manual therapies. Nurses can share with patients that some veterans have found relief and improved pain outcomes when using nonpharmacologic treatments.

Nonpharmacologic therapies for pain can include peer support, CBT, and massage. As previously discussed, veterans appreciate social support from family and friends but felt that peer support might be beneficial. Matthias et al. (2015) explored the use of peer support for veterans with chronic musculoskeletal pain. After 4 months of having biweekly conversations with a peer coach, the veterans enrolled in the study expressed improvement in pain including improved self-efficacy and pain centrality or negative thoughts about pain.

CBT has been used effectively for pain management. Carmody et al. (2013) focused on CBT for older veterans with the therapy delivered via phone. The study followed patients randomized to either receive telephone-delivered education on pain or telephone-delivered CBT. Although the study found no differences in pain outcomes between the groups, there was a significant increase in the participant's physical and mental health, a reduction in overall pain, and depressive symptoms. The patients also experienced a reduction in dwelling on thoughts of pain. Therefore, offering patients pain education or referring for CBT may be warranted.

Fletcher et al. (2016) explored the perceptions of veterans receiving massage and found that the use of massage was perceived to be an effective way to manage and reduce chronic pain. The veterans also felt that their mobility increased, and they used less opioid medication. However, the veterans also reported that there was difficulty in accessing complementary therapies such as massage due to the limited number of practitioners within the VA system. Further, cost issues were a problem as fees are often high and may not be reimbursed by the VA when the veteran seeks care outside the system.

The data from these studies support the use of nonpharmacologic methods providing some relief from chronic pain. Providing education on complementary and alternative therapies for veterans to explore for treatment or management of pain should be a priority of care. Additionally, nursing needs to advocate for ways to minimize the barriers to access to these alternative strategies for these patients.

SLEEP IMPLICATIONS

Sleep may also be affected in veterans experiencing health problems. Pain, PTSD, and GWI may affect sleep with veterans with GWI describing sleep as nonrestorative (Chao et al., 2016). Chao et al. (2016) also found that there was higher risk for sleep apnea among those with GWI and there was also greater insomnia severity. Taking opioids may worsen the risk of sleep apnea and sleep latency, which is the time it takes to fall asleep (Morasco et al., 2014). Nursing care should include assessment of sleep quality as well as teaching and promoting sleep hygiene. For the hospitalized veteran, promotion of good sleep hygiene can include limiting noise and interruptions during optimal sleep hours. Referrals to a sleep clinic may be appropriate, especially when assessment indicates symptoms of sleep apnea. Care following a diagnosis of sleep apnea may include monitoring respiratory function during sleep, including monitoring oxygen saturation levels. Nurses should provide the prescribed treatment for sleep apnea, which may include continuous positive airway pressure equipment.

CAREGIVER IMPLICATIONS

Caregivers of veterans may also require support from nurses. As previously discussed, caregivers of veterans with GWI may have higher rates of similar chronic multisymptom illnesses, and the caregiver burden may be higher when the physical and other support needs of the veteran are greater. Given the caregiver burden along with the risk of mental or physical problems to the caregiver, nurses must include caregiver assessment in interactions with veterans and their families. Such assessment must include consideration of resources that may improve access to care for the veteran and caregiver along with resources to reduce the burden of care. Nursing care may include arranging homecare services, including respite care. Children living in the home of a veteran requiring a caregiver may also be affected, and thus nurses should consider their needs as well when arranging or referring for care.

Many of these healthcare issues experienced by veterans may be compounded by the presence of PTSD or other mental health problems or diagnoses. The polytrauma triad of PTSD, TBI, and chronic pain has been significantly associated with an increased risk of suicide ideation and attempt; ideation risk is significantly increased with the comorbid presence of depression or substance abuse (Finley et al., 2015). Nursing care should include screening for suicide risk, especially in patients who have diagnoses consistent with the polytrauma triad. When suicide risk is present, appropriate notifications and referrals should be made. Patients with pain and PTSD have been shown to have lower rates of mental health visits than those without pain (Outcalt et al., 2016). For patients with these diagnoses, nurses can facilitate access to mental healthcare services when needed.

Cole et al. (2015) reported that patients with mTBI, PTSD, and psychiatric symptoms responded positively to a mindfulness-based stress reduction intervention, including an increase in attention immediately after participating in the mindfulness exercise; this improvement in attention was sustained 3 months later as was reduction in PTSD symptomatology. Nurses in clinical settings and nurse educators can inform and educate veterans on mindfulness and make referrals to appropriate resources. Improving attention and decreasing PTSD symptoms can be beneficial for any veteran whether in a healthcare or academic setting.

Implications for Nursing Education

Nurse educators should familiarize themselves with issues that may impact the functional ability of veterans, including ways to support the veteran in self-management and care. A recent increase in literature indicates growing interest in issues experienced by military service members and veterans. As a result, there is increasing information available to nurse educators that can be useful for personal knowledge and to provide accurate, current content. Remaining current by exploring the literature related to military members and veterans is one way in which nurse educators can maintain current knowledge of the topic. Academic nurse educators can also build connections with campus resources that serve student veterans as well as invite student veterans to share their experiences with faculty and students. Nurse educators working in acute care and community-based agencies can also build connections with veteran's resources in the community. These connections may include building relationships with local VA facilities or inviting veterans to be members of advisory committees that may guide development of content and policies affecting the care of veterans.

Academic nurse educators also must consider how best to support student veterans who may present with complex health needs. Student veterans have expressed that they do not wish to be treated differently yet want their service experience and history to be respected and appreciated (Dyar & Brown, 2019). A component of respecting and appreciating such experiences can include having a conversation with the student veteran about needs and preferences that may enhance learning, including within the clinical setting. Dyar and Brown (2019) also found that student veterans prefer hands-on learning in which they can apply what they have learned. As a result, learning in the clinical setting is preferred and enjoyed. Student veterans may have impaired sleep; therefore, one conversation that nurse educators can have is discussing available options for clinical placement. For example, a student veteran may prefer a clinical assignment that begins later in the day, such as an evening shift, so that sleep can be extended and enhanced by not having to arrive early for a day shift assignment.

Student veterans with limb trauma may present with missing or prosthetic limbs, which would be considered an orthopedic disability. Horkey (2019) found that nurse faculty felt they lacked resources and experienced barriers in providing clinical accommodations for students with orthopedic disabilities. One key barrier was not the university but instead was the clinical setting. Further, the faculty perceived the student's ability to be engaged in the accommodations process to be helpful (Horkey, 2019). Therefore, nurse faculty can serve as an advocate for the student veteran requiring any accommodations, including in clinical agencies, by being informed and knowledgeable about policies and resources at their university as well as the clinical agency. Nurse educators should talk with the student veteran about their needs, with a focus on abilities and what they can do rather than focusing on what they cannot.

Academic nurse educators must also consider the implications for a student who is a veteran with chronic or persistent pain. Pain, and the accompanying comorbidities, may affect attention span and concentration. Anxiety and restlessness may be an accompanying symptom of pain; therefore, a student veteran experiencing pain may have difficulty sitting for long periods, such as in a classroom lecture-type setting. Faculty must consider allowing freedom to move when movement might alleviate pain or address anxiety or restlessness.

Cognitive implications of TBI, including potential visual and auditory difficulties are another consideration for nurse educators whether working in academic or professional development settings. TBI, with or without auditory problems, can affect the attention span and the ability to process information delivered through a learning situation that is lengthy, rapid-paced, and complex such as traditional lectures (Jurick et al., 2016; O'Neil et al., 2017). Visual challenges may result in difficulty reading items such as textbooks or journal articles that may have smaller fonts. Presentation slides should follow best practices and limit the amount of information on each slide. Black font that is of adequate size is preferable. Although faculty cannot adjust for font size in a textbook or other scholarly sources, printed materials for student use should be of an adequate font size for ease of reading and comprehension.

If academic nurse educators note learning deficits in the student veteran, make appropriate referrals to campus resources for evaluation of a possible disability and potential accommodations for learning, assessment, and evaluation. When a student veteran receives accommodations, it is both a legal and ethical imperative to comply with the designated accommodations. Academic nurse educators must be aware of and familiar with institutional policies related to providing students with academic accommodations and should consider whether it might be appropriate to refer a student veteran for evaluation to receive such services. With the granting of accommodations, compliance is imperative as these are federally mandated. However, the nurse educator can incorporate best practices in teaching that would benefit all students, including the student veteran with challenges as a result of TBI. For example, lecture-style teaching can be broken into smaller chunks of information, allowing time for interactive learning and movement. Making sure volume levels are adequate, including using a microphone when needed, will aid all students in hearing the information presented. Allowing students to record lectures can provide the opportunity for review of the material after class ends.

Many nursing programs and healthcare agencies require drug screening as part of the clinical placement process. Opioids may be part of the veteran's pain management protocol; thus, a student treated with opioids may screen positive for opioid use. Nurse faculty should be aware of and adhere to institutional policies and procedures for responding to a positive screen. While protecting the safety of patients is imperative, it may also be appropriate to advocate for the student veteran with a valid opiate prescription. Being an advocate includes protecting patient safety; thus, in the event a veteran on prescribed opiates demonstrates any signs of impairment in the clinical setting, the nurse educator must follow appropriate institutional policies related to relieving the veteran of their patient assignment.

FUTURE RESEARCH PRIORITIES

Multiple areas related to veterans offer opportunities for nursing research. The majority of the research described in this chapter was conducted by physicians or other researchers; few studies originated with or included nurses as part of the research team. Nurses can advocate for veterans by joining a research team or conducting studies with a greater focus on the nursing care needs of veterans who are experiencing any of the described complex health problems. Likewise, nursing research could explore the needs of caregivers of veterans to identify ways in which nurses can support caregivers. Nursing education research could explore identification of learning preferences and best practices for teaching veterans with various health needs. This research could focus on examining education in a healthcare or academic setting. Finally, research could also focus on identifying knowledge levels of nurses and nurse educators to identify areas where their education is needed to improve nursing care.

CONCLUSION

Veterans, whether they deployed or not, may experience one or more health challenges. Many such challenges will be comorbid with one or more diagnoses often occurring along with mental health issues. These complex issues require ongoing and collaborative management and care. Nurses can be an integral part of the interdisciplinary care team and need to take the role of advocate for veterans and their caregivers. Academic nurse educators must consider potential health challenges experienced by student veterans and also advocate for and provide the best teaching practices to support and enhance learning. Lastly, to advance the science of nursing, nurses need to be involved in nursing research related to uncovering and supporting the healthcare needs of veterans both in its delivery and support for learning.

REFERENCES

The complete reference list for this chapter appears in the digital version of the chapter, accessible at https://connect.springerpub.com/content/book/978-0-8261-3597-1/chapter/ch06

MENTAL HEALTH CONCERNS IN MILITARY AND VETERAN POPULATIONS

RICHARD J. WESTPHAL | SEAN P. CONVOY

Civilian society prizes individual freedom. … The warrior culture, on the other hand, values cohesion and obedience. The soldier or sailor is not free to do whatever he wants. He serves; he is bound to perform his duty.

Steven Pressfield, The Warrior Ethos

KEY TERMS

military personnel	mental disorders
military ethos	burnout
psychological stress	grief
stress injuries/disorders	moral injury

INTRODUCTION

The goal of this chapter is to summarize those psychiatric disorders commonly seen among veterans in both student and client roles and to assist educators to integrate knowledge about veteran mental health concerns into educator and clinical faculty roles. This chapter is intended to challenge educators to operate from within their educator role by developing a necessary context to educate veterans who may be struggling emotionally, behaviorally, and psychologically. Additionally, this chapter provides insights for faculty who are preparing students to work with veterans as patients and clients. That being said, this chapter provides the reader with a composite picture of Global War on Terrorism (GWOT) veteran, common mental health concerns affecting veterans, a military centric stress first aid framework from which to assess and respond to crisis, and two vignettes designed to apply the introduced concepts.

BACKGROUND

The demands of preparing to serve in combat and live within the military ethos are sources of strengths and vulnerabilities for veterans. This chapter addresses an overview of mental health issues that are associated with military service. The psychological impact, both positive and negative, of

---

The complete reference list for this chapter appears in the digital version of the chapter, accessible at https://connect.springerpub.com/content/book/978-0-8261-3597-1/chapter/ch07

military service is as old as military service itself. The terms and concepts used to describe the impact of the military ethos are linked to the language and values of each era. A military era is usually defined by the major deployment of military personnel in a particular time frame, such as, Vietnam Era, Gulf War era, or the GWOT (Torreon, 2018). Within the eras are wars and operations, such as Operation Enduring Freedom (OEF) in Afghanistan and Operation Iraqi Freedom (OIF) in Iraq. The GWOT officially began on September 11, 2001 (Torreon, 2018) and continues to the writing of this chapter with a shift in focus from direct combat missions to support and training in often dangerous areas of the world. The generation of students who are entering college currently represent an American generation whose adolescence and young adulthood has been influenced, and arguably, defined by military culture and war. As of 2018, over 2.77 million women and men have served in the GWOT in over 5.4 million deployments with the majority of those members no longer on active duty and qualifying for government healthcare and education benefits (Wenger et al., 2018).

Each military era has health risks and concerns that are associated with the exposures related to the confluence of geography, technology of war, and available healthcare (U.S. Department of Veterans Affairs [VA], 2019). All veterans of all eras have common risks related to noise exposure ranging from military equipment and weapons that can impact hearing and psychologically traumatic exposures that can impact long-term psychological health. The World War II and Korean War veteran exposures include mustard gas with respiratory injury, extreme cold with long-term peripheral neuropathy, and ionizing radiation from nuclear tests. Chemical exposures to Agent Orange (a toxic defoliant) and hepatitis C were additional signature exposures for the Vietnam veteran cohort that results in higher rates of cancer and liver disease. The Vietnam veteran cohort was the first veteran group where the diagnosis of posttraumatic stress disorder (PTSD) was officially recognized and acknowledged for its long-term impact on mental health. The Gulf War was unique for a particular cluster of toxic exposures of external chemical insults—oil fires, chemical and biological weapons, and pesticides; combined with various forms of prophylaxis for viruses and endemic diseases that are associated with atypical immune disorders.

In particular, the Post-9/11 cohort of veterans have unique healthcare needs and concerns (Waszak & Holmes, 2017). The physical and mental healthcare needs are related to a range of exposures that included toxic burn pits, depleted uranium ammunition, physical trauma of combat and work accidents that included a high rate of extremity and traumatic brain injuries, and exposure to potentially injurious stressors. The intense psychosocial stressors associated with military service in the Post-9/11 era can result in depression, anxiety, sleep disorders, suicidal ideation, substance abuse, military sexual trauma, and PTSD (Tanielian & Jaycox, 2008; Trivedi et al., 2015; Waszak & Holmes, 2017). While the Post-9/11 veterans have the highest rate of veteran disability of any previous cohort they also have the lowest rate of engagement with Veterans Health Services (National Center for Veterans Analysis and Statistics, 2018) that further increases the likelihood of a student veteran that has a mental health concern and may not be connected with needed clinical or social supports. It is important to highlight that while approximately 20% of Post-9/11 veterans screen positive for PTSD or Depressive Disorders (Tanielian & Jaycox, 2008) 80% do not have PTSD or depression. Given the collective trauma exposure of this cohort it will be important for educators not to assume that a veteran has a mental health concern or that responses to current academic and life stressors are necessarily related to the veteran's military service.

The role of *educators* is used broadly in this chapter to refer to any member of the academic community—faculty, instructors, counselors, support staff, and so on—who would interact with a student veteran. Each member of the education team has opportunities to significantly influence the experience of the student veteran. The term *veteran* in this chapter refers to all service members who qualified for veteran educational benefits after separation from military service. The cultural focus for this chapter is the GWOT Post-9/11 era of military service as an era shaped by terror attacks within the United States, an all-volunteer force serving without conscription, and a society that acknowledged that service members who participated in combat would be changed by that experience. The GWOT era veterans are those who are most likely to use veteran's benefits to attend college or enroll in second degree programs for a career change. It is important to note that not all veterans that serve during a combat era were deployed to combat.

MILITARY CULTURE AND ETHOS

All veterans have experienced enculturation to the military ethos and will have varying degrees to which they incorporate that ethos into their personal identity. Military culture includes both overt and implicit concepts that create structure and expectations for service members and their families. The overt symbols of military culture include items such as uniforms, rank structure, military units, unit and personal awards or ribbons, and protocols. Implicit symbols include values associated with being a member within the military such as oath of enlistment or commissioning, mottos and logos associated with each military command, or the military ethos.

The military ethos comprises guiding beliefs and values (Table 7.1) that can be sources of strengths and vulnerabilities for veterans' mental health and transitions into occupational and academic settings (VA, 2014, Module 1). The guiding beliefs and values associated with the military ethos have deeper meaning for most service members and are more enduring than the cultural artifacts of military service, such as uniforms, base locations, or military equipment; or the memories of military service. The miltiary ethos for most veterans and their families provides a touch stone of values that is used unconsciously and conciously to evaluate life choices. For some veterans and family members the military ethos becomes a permanent part of their self-identity and is a dominant lens for their world view. There is variability in the extent that veterans will embrace the military ethos and it is important that educators and clinicians assess the potential impact of military service by asking, "What does being a veteran mean to you?"

Military ethos can influence both the academic and mental health experiences of student veterans as a lens that filters the view of self, others, organizational rules, and symptom experience. It is important for educators to reflect on military ethos traits identified in Table 7.1 and the implications

TABLE 7.1 MILITARY ETHOS STRENGTHS AND VULNERABILITIES

STRENGTH	TRAIT	VULNERABILITY
Placing the welfare of others above one's own welfare	Selflessness	Not seeking help for health problems because personal health is not a priority
Commitment to accomplishing missions and protecting comrades in arms	Loyalty	Survivor guilt and complicated bereavement after losing friends
Toughness and ability to endure hardships without complaint	Stoicism	Not acknowledging significant symptoms and suffering after returning home
Following an internal moral compass to choose "right" over "wrong"	Moral Code	Feeling frustrated and betrayed when others fail to follow a moral code
Meaning and purpose when defending societal values	Social Order	Loss of meaning or betrayal when rejected by society
Becoming the best and most effective professional possible	Excellence	Feeling ashamed of (or not acknowledging) imperfections

SOURCE: From the Department of Veteran Affairs. (2014). *Military culture: Core competencies for healthcare professionals.* http://www.deploymentpsych.org/military-culture, Module 1.

for student behaviors. For example, student veterans may feel comfortable with challenging group assignments (selflessness), immerse themselves in a project with no complaint (stoicism), and often take a leader role within the group (social order). Simultaneously, they may be less likely to ask for help or clarification of an assignment (selflessness), have low tolerance for the complaints of peers about how much other work they have to complete (stoicism), and may stifle the contributions of team members in order to get the project done on time (social order). An example of the military ethos at an individual level may include the student veteran expecting that the syllabus clearly defines the assignment expectations (social order), grading is equally applied across all the faculty that are supporting a course (moral code), and all students will be held accountable for academic and personal behavior (excellence).

The military ethos has been identified as a confounding variable for mental illness stigma and not seeking care (Hoge et al., 2004); stress injuries such as complicated grief, chronic post traumatic stress, and moral injury (Litz et al., 2009; Stein et al., 2012); and reduced efficacy of standardized treatments for PTSD (Bradley et al., 2005). Help-seeking and the use of academic or student health services may be difficult for the student veteran with either service or student related psychological challenges.

MENTAL HEALTH CONCERNS

Mental health concerns related to the veteran experience is much broader than a clinical focus on mental disorders. The clinical model of stress exposure focuses on traumatic events related to life threat, severe injury, or sexual assault, and how these events lead to disorder and mental illness. Advances and innovations in healthcare often occur during war. The ongoing Post-9/11 medical research has been notable for advancements in what have been called the invisible wounds of war: traumatic brain and stress injuries (Tanielian & Jaycox, 2008). In particular, there has been significant knowledge developed regarding the psychosocial impact of acute and chronic stress, new models for understanding resilience and stress injuries, and innovative interventions ranging from stress first-aid through treatment for stress-related disorders (Figley & Nash, 2007; Koffman et al., 2011; Litz et al., 2016; Whybrow et al., 2013).

Each of the military branches developed stress recognition models to account for service members who showed functional changes in behavior that were anticipated reactions to high stress events and should not be considered as disorders. Most Post-9/11 veterans have had specific awareness and intervention training regarding stress reactions and strategies to support individual and peer resilience. It is useful for educators to expand their view of mental health concerns related to student veterans across a continuum of stress reactions and disorders. Gained understanding can be further used by educators to support student nurses who may encounter patients experiencing stress responses in clinical settings.

The stress continuum model was developed by the Department of the Navy in 2007 as an visual tool to promote understanding that there is a range of stress responses, to shift the policies and training from mental disorders to psychological health, and to develop interventions that would support service members who were injured but not disordered (Combat and Operational Stress Control, 2016). The stress continuum uses a color schema of green, yellow, orange, and red as visual cues for four stress zones (Exhibit 7.1). The stress continuum uses a cultural heuristic that is used by most industrialized societies. Green lights to represent that objects are working well, yellow or amber lights to warn of change, and red to indicate problems or to stop. The stress continuum is used as a metaphor for individual stress responses that considers a range from resilience through illness or disorder. The stress continuum labels the stress zones as Ready, Reacting, Injured, and Ill (Combat and Operational Stress Control, 2016).

EXHIBIT 7.1

STRESS CONTINUUM MODEL

READY (Green)	REACTING (Yellow)	INJURED (Orange)	ILL (Red)
DEFINITION ✧ Adaptive coping ✧ Effective functioning ✧ Wellbeing	**DEFINITION** ✧ Mild and transient distress or impairment	**DEFINITION** ✧ More severe and persistent distress or loss of function **Types** ✧ Wear and tear ✧ Loss ✧ Life threat ✧ Moral injury	**DEFINITION** ✧ Clinical mental disorder ✧ Unhealed stress injury **TYPES** ✧ PTSD ✧ Depression ✧ Anxiety ✧ Substance abuse
FEATURES ✧ In control ✧ Calm and steady ✧ Getting the job done ✧ Playing ✧ Sense of humor ✧ Sleeping enough ✧ Ethical and moral behavior	**FEATURES** ✧ Anxious ✧ Irritable, angry ✧ Worrying ✧ Cutting corners ✧ Poor sleep ✧ Poor mental focus ✧ Social Isolation ✧ Too loud or hyperactive	**FEATURES** ✧ Loss of control ✧ Impaired sleep ✧ Panic or rage ✧ Apathy ✧ Shame or guilt	**FEATURES** ✧ Symptoms persist and worsen over time ✧ Severe distress or social or occupational impairment

PTSD, posttraumatic stress disorder.

SOURCE: Adapted from Combat and Operational Stress Control. (2016). *Marine corps combat development command.* MCTP 3-30E/NTTP 1-15M. https://www.marines.mil/News/Publications/MCPEL/Electronic-Library-Display/Article/899535

The stress continuum model uses a conservation of resources framework for understanding sources of resilience and how people transition between the stress zones. In Hobfoll's (1989) Conservation of Resources model, the psychosocial impact of stress and coping can be understood as an active process of using resources to cope with demands. There are two major strategies that people use to adjust to immediate stressors. One is to reduce the stress or exposure to the stressor. The other way is to increase resources to compensate for the additional demands that coping with the stressor requires. From a conservation of resource perspective, people develop and conserve resources that are used for coping and meeting changing demands. Over time and through life experiences people invest in a reserve of coping resources (objects, conditions, personal characteristics, and energies; Hobfoll, 1989). Hobfoll (2012) used the concept of a *resource caravan* that includes interrelated personal, material, and social resources that are developed slowly over time and provides a collective resource buffer against stress demands.

The *Ready Zone* (green) represents those who have been able to develop a robust resource caravan and have a greater capacity to respond to stress events. While the student veteran may have unique vulnerabilities, they also have unique resource caravans that support resilience. For example, many student veterans' resource caravans may include objects (e.g., house, car, job skills), conditions (e.g., education tuition benefits, established interpersonal relationships, social supports outside of the student role), personal characteristics (e.g., expanded world-view, self-efficacy, resilience building life-experiences), and energies (e.g., time to dedicate to student role, veteran's education stipend, first-aid or medical knowledge and skills).

The *Reacting Zone* (yellow) include physical and psychological reactions to an immediate stressor related to the fight, flight, or freeze response. *Yellow zone* reactions are transient and resolve quickly when the stressor is reduced or removed. The *Injured Zone* (orange) is characterized by a change in behavior and role functions that often require the use of coping caravan resources to mitigate distress.

Orange zone stress injuries are not transient and have their origins in exposures to trauma and life threat, loss and bereavement, long-term stress exposure that results in burnout, and unresolved moral and ethical conflicts. A peer support Stress First Aid intervention can be used by peers and family members to augment coping resources for those that present with stress injury behaviors (Combat and Operational Stress Control, 2016; Watson et al., 2013; Westphal & Convoy, 2015).

The *Ill Zone* (red) includes the stress related mental disorders. These are conditions that exceed normal resource caravan capacity and require professional intervention or long-term augmentation with symptom management strategies (e.g., ongoing therapy, medications, lifestyle changes) to reduce symptoms. The remainder of this chapter focuses on the mental health concerns of stress injuries and mental disorders.

Stress Injury

Service members are exposed to multiple stress experiences throughout their military service. Military training represents a designed strategy of systematically moving military members from the *Ready Zone* (green) into the *Reacting Zone* (yellow). This process of stress exposure and recovery is a form of stress inoculation that can promote resilience (Ashokan et al., 2016). The process of planned transition from *Ready* to *Reacting* stress with reflecting and confidence building is common in nursing education and clinical simulation as well as military training simulation. When working with student veterans it is important to keep in mind that echoes from past experiences that are present in nursing education may act as triggers to stress injuries. Similar to physical injuries that leave a scar, psychological injuries can leave an emotional scar that is often experienced as an echo of past events that intrude into the present.

Stress injury is defined as a "severe and persistent distress or loss of functioning caused by disruptions to the integrity of the brain, mind, or spirit after exposure to overwhelming stressors" (Combat and Operational Stress Control, 2016, pp. 1–3). The brain, mind, and spirit elements of the definition are important for understanding the injury that is associated with toxic or chronic stress exposure. The brain hypothesis of injury presents the potential for stress injury to disrupt neurons and receptors in regions of the brain responsible for memory processing, modulation of the fear response, spatial orientation, response to social cues, attention and concentration, and problem-solving (Gao et al., 2014; Krishnamurthy & Laskowitz, 2016; McEwen et al., 2016). The mind hypothesis presents the potential for impairment in social, psychological, and interpersonal functioning that contributes to adverse psychosocial outcomes, impaired problem-solving, and diminished self-efficacy (Hobfoll, 2012; Lazarus, 2013; Wilkinson et al., 2017). The spirit domain identifies the role that moral distress, guilt, and shame can have on self-identity, beliefs, and moral/ethical decisions (Farnsworth et al., 2017; Litz et al., 2016).

Veterans and students can experience a wide range of stress exposures before, during, and following nursing education. Most of these *Yellow Zone* stressors are of limited duration and do not cause functional impairment. Typical Yellow Zone stressors in the academic experience include the expected demands of exams, writing papers, preparing for clinical or practicum rotations, participating in student activities, and time management of multiple courses. There are four sources of stress experience that do have the potential to evoke *Orange Zone* stress injury responses that result in impaired role function and increased demand on coping resources: Loss, Wear and Tear, Trauma/Life Threat, and Inner Conflict (Figure 7.1; Combat and Operational Stress Control, 2016). Knowledge related to the four sources of stress injury as individual and cumulative sources of stress can assist faculty in understanding student and client behaviors that result in impaired function and increased coping demands.

LOSS/GRIEF

Loss is the experience of separating from a person, a cherished object, or a belief before being ready to let go and grief is the reaction to that loss (Walter & McCoyd, 2016). Loss is a component of many assessment items, both adverse and positive, used in stressful life events research (Holmes & Rahe, 1967;

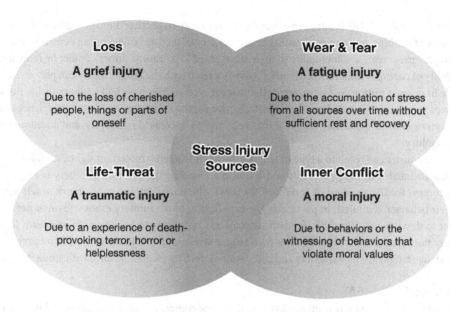

FIGURE 7.1 Four Sources of Stress Injury in the Orange Zone.

Spurgeon et al., 2001). From a resource caravan perspective, loss as a stress injury experience usually entails significant demands to two or more of a person's stress caravan resources (objects, conditions, personal characteristics, and energies) that require choices in order to conserve the remaining resources.

The sudden death of a cherished person is an example of a prototypical stress injury; a change in functional ability without a mental disorder. With a few words—often an incomplete sentence-a person comes to realize that an important person has died. Immediately, there is a change in behavior and affect. There is an observable change in physical presentation, voice, ability to process information, and the relationship to others. Social rituals and supports related to loss and grief are additional resources available to the bereaved. The activation of coping resources for the person or family is intended to help them process the grief and regain temporarily lost functional abilities. The loss experience has left a fundamental life experience, a stress injury scar, which can be triggered by sights, sounds, smells, or a memory that may produce future stress injury reactions.

People with loss (grief) injuries are often provided time, resources, and social space for recovery. There is the expectation that grief reactions are temporary (*Orange Zone* Injured) and that with support they will be able to return to full capabilities (*Green Zone* Ready). It is not uncommon for Post-9/11 veterans to have personal experience with a close friend or a peer who has died in combat or in military training. The relationship between military team members is not like a relationship with a coworker outside of the military. The military ethos binds team members closer together than most people can imagine. As it relates to intensity of military kinship, those who have worn the uniform require no explanation. As it relates to those who have not, no explanation is likely possible. The loss of a teammate in a cohesive unit is as powerful as the loss of a spouse or cherished family member. Academic activities or assignments that engage students in recalling loss experiences can evoke the echoes of a loss/grief injury and bring the emotions and thoughts of the event into the academic experience.

WEAR AND TEAR/BURNOUT

The experience of extended exposure to chronic low intensity stressors—such as occupational stress, long-term health challenges, sleep deprivation, and strained social relationships-consumes coping resources (Staal, 2004). Nursing, as a profession, recognizes this type of stress injury as burnout

(Todaro-Franceschi, 2019). From a conservation of resources perspective, the expenditures of resources, income, relationships, and personal resilience are not replenished as fast as coping demands. A fatigue stress injury may create a vulnerability to toxic stressors of loss, trauma, inner conflict by reducing the availability of coping resources. The resource loss associated with the fatigue injury can play an important role in delayed responses. For example, the student veteran may have had a traumatic life threat or loss event years in the past and has developed effective coping strategies. Academic experiences in the classroom or clinical space may trigger intrusive thoughts, increased irritability, and additional signs of stress injury.

Fatigue injuries can result in a type of scar, a scar that is triggered by certain sights, sounds, or experiences associated with the past events and result in a response that appears to others as exaggerated or out context for the situation. It is difficult for those who have a fatigue stress injury to self-identify that their behavior is injured. In particular, the expectation of the military ethos will often negate any attempt to develop self-care skills. Student veterans are very likely to be externally and team focused and may not recognize the signs of their own fatigue stress injury. Educators need to be prepared to acknowledge fatigue injury behaviors and discuss sleep, rest, life/school balance with student veterans.

TRAUMA/LIFE THREAT

The Life Threat source of stress injury is one of the more commonly known sources and is frequently associated with PTSD. Similar to Acute Stress Disorder, there tends to be identifiable events where a person was exposed to actual or threatened death, serious injury, or sexual violence where the exposure could be direct, witnessing, or learning about exposure of a significant other (American Psychiatric Association, 2013). The resource caravan plays an important role in the experience of potential life threat. Trauma can manifest differently in relation to a host of endogenous and exogenous variables. People with prior trauma experiences can range from those who are trauma naïve to those with significant trauma exposures. The trauma naïve person, with limited life experience, may experience helplessness and victimization that result in profound unpleasant autonomic arousal and stress behaviors. Conversely, those who train, simulate, and experience life threat and intense trauma as a chosen career are rarely surprised or experience helplessness in a trauma exposure.

The trauma naïve and trauma experienced individuals have very different resource caravans for engaging and navigating life threat and trauma stress. For example, the dark humor of coping used by experienced trauma nurses and veterans may be perceived as inappropriate and insensitive by the less experienced. The trauma experienced person will often move toward a threat and will use autonomic arousal as a source of energy. Veterans often have training or experience that include real or simulated trauma. One of the goals of military training is to prepare individuals to respond to perceived threats by moving toward (and through) the threat as a team. Veteran nursing students who served as Medics or Hospital Corpsmen may have trauma experiences that are unimaginable even in an urban trauma center.

It is important to recognize that there is no immunity to stress injury. Each individual has a point where traumatic stress demands will exceed their coping resources with a resulting stress injury. Full appreciation of this reality is destigmatizing in nature and should be restated for effect. In trauma, the exposure is a potentially injurious event and the functional impairment related to the exposure is the injury. Human resilience in the face of trauma is significant. The percent of people who develop PTSD is low compared to the number exposed to significant trauma and life threat (Schnurr, 2014). Pietrzak et al. (2012) reported that of police officers who responded to the 9/11 World Trade Center attack, 5.4% had full PTSD and 15.4% had subsyndromal (stress injury) symptoms, and nearly 80% did not have PTSD or trauma stress injury symptoms.

Not all student veterans who experienced combat or military training trauma will develop trauma stress injury or PTSD. There is, however, a dose–response relationship between the number of exposures and development of stress injury or PTSD symptoms. It is important for educators not to assume that a traumatic exposure may be the most problematic experience the student has. Similarly, educators need to be aware that a trauma exposure in the course of nursing education may be the accumulative load that results in a trauma stress injury response.

INNER CONFLICT/MORAL INJURY

The inner conflict source of stress injury represents moral ethical dilemma and moral distress. Inner conflict as a moral injury is defined as, "perpetrating, failing to prevent, bearing witness to, or learning about acts that transgress deeply held moral beliefs and expectations" (Litz et al., 2009, p. 700). The process of trying to live up to the ideals of the military ethos and the challenging reality of combat and disaster experiences lay the foundation of inner conflict for veterans. Inner conflict and moral injury increase the demands on moral, ethical, and existential resources. Moral injury occurs when individuals are unable to separate the implications of an event from their own identity. Poor integration of the moral and ethical challenge into a refined self-identity leads to guilt, shame, persistent psychological distress, and avoidance of potential triggers (Litz et al., 2009).

The characteristics of moral injury are also known as acts of commission—doing something that violates beliefs; omission—not doing something that one should have and bearing witness—observing or being part of a group that acted in violation of beliefs. The living by a moral code that is part of the military ethos contributes to the vulnerability of developing a moral injury. How the veteran reconciles the inner conflict influences whether or not the conflict becomes a moral injury. Loss, Wear and Tear, and Life Threat are predominately external experiences that place direct demand on coping resources. Moral injury increases the demand on existential, ethical, and spiritual resources.

One of the challenges for veterans with moral injury is to navigate the redefinition of self: Who am I now that I have had these experiences and how do I make amends for my transgressions? Student veterans with a moral injury are not likely to share those experiences with non-student veteran peers or educators. It is challenging for educators to recognize the presence of moral injury because the injured person is often not willing to talk about the experience. The words that student veterans may use that indicate the presence of moral injury are "could've, should've, ought'of, if only."

Most student veterans have sufficient coping resources and skills to address one or two potentially injurious experiences at a time. Student veterans' capacity for resilience and the depth of the coping caravans will often exceed the resources of their non-veteran peers. It is important for educators to recognize that the sources of stress injury are not mutually exclusive. There are times when life events, academic demands, and current non-academic stressors overlap, and the additional coping demands could result in a stress injury (see Case Study 7.1).

CASE STUDY 7.1 VETERAN INTEGRATION INTO A NURSING COHORT

Kendal is a 29-year-old veteran who is in the second semester of an intensive entry-level master's degree clinical nurse leader (CNL) program. Kendal served for 4 years in the Army as a heavy equipment operator and mechanic with one Operation Enduring Freedom deployment without combat exposure. During military service, Kendal started taking college courses that were offered on base and online. After service release, Kendal joined a local fire and emergency services station, completed the Emergency Medical Technician-I and II certifications, and completed a bachelor of arts degree through online studies. Kendal's experience in pre-hospital care and working as a member of the healthcare team led to the commitment to enroll in the intensive CNL program. The CNL cohort has 50 students with a broad range of first degrees, the average age is 25 years old, 96% female, with two veterans, and four military spouses. The CNL program uses many group learning activities and simulation experiences. During the second semester of CNL education, the cohort carries 14 semester credits across five courses that include Research and Evidence-Based Practice, Pharmacology, Introduction to Nursing Leadership, Medical-Surgical Nursing Clinical, and the Psychiatric Clinical.

Two of Kendal's classmates approached course faculty during week three of the semester requesting to be assigned to another group. They verbalized personal discomfort with Kendal's over-bearing, intrusive, and verbally aggressive behavior. Faculty observed Kendal to commonly embrace the student leader role, was not always prepared for class discussions, and often used military or fire service examples and language in class and in writing assignments. Upon initial consideration, the faculty assessed none of Kendal's reported behavior crossed a threshold that required direct intervention. The faculty member provided guidance to the students for addressing communication issues within the group and encouraged them to be assertive with each other. The faculty member also looked for an opportunity to have a dialogue with Kendal. That opportunity became available later that week following an exam. Kendal had a low score on the exam and the faculty member used the opportunity to discuss study strategies and to assess Kendal's view of the small group process. In this discussion the faculty member learned about Kendal's military experience. Kendal reported that everything is going well, apologized for the low score and promised to work harder, and thought the group was prepared for completing the next small group assignment.

One of the two students who originally requested to be re-assigned scheduled an office-hours meeting with the faculty member the next week and tearfully insisted that she needed to be moved. She stated that she did not feel safe working with Kendal. When the faculty member assessed the specific concerns of the student it became clear that the student had significant prior trauma experience and that Kendal was triggering those trauma memories. The faculty member assisted the distressed student to have a Counseling and Psychological Services assessment and re-assigned that student to a different group. The faculty member did a follow-up with the group to discuss shifting the group membership and assess the group's progress. In that meeting Kendal stated, "It's too bad that Sue could not suck it up and do the work. Now we will need to carry her load. I am sure that this team can get it done on time though." Most of the group members had heard Sue's concerns previously and expressed support for Sue. Kendal quickly tried to move the conversation to task assignments and timelines.

Kendal had a low score on the mid-term exam and the faculty member scheduled a meeting to review Kendal's academic deficiency, discuss a remediation plan, and to assess other factors that may be impacting Kendal's performance. Before the mid-term performance meeting, the faculty member learned from other CNL faculty that Kendal was doing extremely well in the clinical courses and showing skills that were at the top of the class but was struggling in the other didactic course. Initially, Kendal was respectful and apologetic for not doing better and promised to double efforts in this course. There was a change in behavior when the faculty asked what specific changes Kendal was planning to implement. Kendal shifted in the chair, sat upright, facial affect was neutral with gaze straight without making eye contact, and the voice was calm and precise. Kendal stated, "I take full responsibility for my actions. I can shift more study time to your course. I will do better on the next exam." The faculty member chose to change the direction of the dialogue and used a three-question assessment to better understand Kendal as a student and a person. The three questions that the faculty member used were, "Since starting the CNL program, what are your greatest challenges or frustrations? What are your greatest successes or rewards? What does it mean to you to be a nurse?"

Kendal paused, took a deep breath, and physically relaxed a little. Kendal initially discussed how different the CNL courses were from any previous college courses. Historically, Kendal found classes to be rather easy and did well on most tests with minimal study time. Kendal was finding the amount of assignments, mixed with clinical demands, working part-time, and trying to meet family needs was overwhelming. Kendal paused and apologized for complaining. The faculty member acknowledged how challenging the program was and invited Kendal to continue. Kendal expressed the frustration of not fitting in with the other CNL students. In particular, Kendal was particularly bothered by several behaviors. Kendal found many classmates to be self-absorbed mostly interested in themselves or their phones, were only willing do enough to get by and not their best work, complained about insignificant issues, and did not follow-through on their assigned small group tasks. The faculty asked for clarification about the disconnect between Kendal's expectations and experience. Kendal used examples from the Army and Fire Service as to how teams should work together and personal responsibility.

The faculty then was able to get Kendal to focus on study skills and making plans for success in the course and program. Kendal clearly expressed a commitment to the clinical course expectations, that *real* nurses needed to know how to take care of patients, and that the majority of effort needed to go to clinical preparation. When discussing managing multiple course demands, Kendal talked about mission and accident scene triage and that most of the effort needs to go to that which is most important and that the lesser priorities will be addressed later. The faculty used that opportunity to expand the dialogue about the complexities of nursing decision-making and the need to balance many competing demands and engaging the education support team to help develop a more balanced approach to both the clinical and didactic challenges in the program. It was clear to the faculty that Kendal was going to need more support than this one mid-term review. Part of the academic remediation plan included referral to the CNL academic support staff, a follow-up meeting to discuss the small group communication process, as leader led versus team negotiated, and the development of a study plan that would balance time across the five courses.

Case Study Review Questions

As the faculty member:

1. What Military Ethos Traits from Table 7.1 are present in the case study?
2. What stress zones from Exhibit 7.1 are present in the case study?
3. What educator's behaviors were effective or ineffective?
4. What other resources would the educator or student need to be successful?

Understanding that student veterans can have a stress injury that is showing some functional impairment can create opportunities for professional nursing development as well as mentoring and advising challenges. It is also important for educators to understand that the student veteran may have a mental disorder and can also experience a stress injury that is not directly related to that disorder. For many students, the challenges of pursuing a professional degree in nursing can be the primary exposure to potentially injurious experiences.

Mental Health Implications for Clinical Practice

One of the most important clinical steps in caring for a veteran is to ask, "Have you ever served in the military?" ("Have You Ever Served in the Military?," 2019). This assessment step is crucial as many veterans will not disclose their military history unless asked. The follow-up assessment would include time frame and branch of service to further establish rapport and to begin the dialogue about the veteran's current health issues and their military service. A second level of assessment would be to assess for the presence of the four sources of stress injury in relation to the veteran's current concerns. It is important to recognize that the mental health concerns associated with stress injuries can add to the complexity of symptom presentation and ability of the veteran to engage in care. For example, the factors related to each of the stress injuries presented earlier in this chapter would be applicable to formulating assessment and plans of care for the veteran patient. For example, a veteran with a trauma exposure stress injury could have sources of resilience or vulnerability that would be relevant to cardiac rehabilitation, initiating chemotherapy for cancer treatment, or addressing trust with the healthcare team. The stress injuries in particular can be related to an accumulative exposure of stressors. For some veterans, the symptoms or conditions that necessitated acute care may be part of a stress load that exceeds the capacity of their resource caravan and that overload would be an important factor in developing the nursing plan of care.

MENTAL DISORDER CONCERNS

While the recent incidence and prevalence of mental disorders are higher among military service members and veterans as compared to their civilian counterparts (Kessler et al., 2014), this statistical reality should not incline educators to dramatically change their tactics, techniques, and procedures in the classroom setting. Likely influenced by comparable doses of stigma, fear and media mischaracterization, the general public has arguably become overly sensitized to the presence of mental disorders yielding an all too commonly tone-deaf response that interferes with understanding the nuances of the veteran experience. It is for this reason that we will deemphasize formal psychiatric disorders as given in the *Diagnostic and Statistical Manual of Mental Disorders*, Fifth Edition (*DSM-5*; American Psychiatric Association [APA], 2013) disorders in lieu of the easier to understand symptoms that define them. Extrapolated from the work of Trivedi et al. (2015), Table 7.2 offers a list of the most common psychiatric disorder categories seen among military service members followed by symptom summaries, actual *DSM-5* diagnosis (APA, 2013) and student exemplars that contextualize the condition within the academic setting.

While the psychiatric conditions listed in Table 7.2 are not comprehensive, they are generally representative of what can be expected among some percentage of veterans entering the academic setting. As it relates to the trauma and stressor related diagnostic category, educators should not assume that all veterans have encountered clinically significant trauma. Moreover, it would also be equally unwise to assume that the trauma veterans encounter is always combat related. Koola et al. (2013) examined the prevalence of childhood physical and sexual abuse amongst psychiatrically hospitalized veterans finding a prevalence rate of 19.4%. According to the U.S. Department of Veterans Affairs (VA, 2019), one in four women and one in 100 men endorse to Veterans Health Administration providers having encountered military sexual trauma while on active duty. As previously established, trauma can have varied etiologies. The more chronic expressions of trauma disorders are commonly born of multiple trauma encounters manifesting over the life span. The more complex expressions of traumatic disorders are commonly associated with early exposure to trauma.

While there are variations in treatment for traumatic disorders based upon etiology, acuity, chronicity, and comorbidity, such nuances are not relevant to the educator and consequently this chapter. The educator need not apply a clinical lens but rather be sensitive to the potential for veterans to present with varied psychiatric symptoms that may require intervention and accommodations. Those who chronically struggle with trauma develop strategies to navigate their daily environment. While these strategies vary from healthy to unhealthy, the educator best serves the veteran through equal doses of consistency, reliability, and unconditional positive regard. The educator needs to resist the urge to be a voyeur of the veteran's trauma. While the instinct to listen and engage veteran trauma is earnestly intended, it is nonetheless unwise to cross over the line demarcating educator and clinician. The best practice is to not solicit details about a veteran's trauma but, in the right setting, be receptive to listening and connect the veteran with formal mental health services. Regularly working with veterans that have encountered trauma can be vicariously traumatizing. It is for this reason that faculty leadership should regularly monitor the vicarious load of trauma encountered by their educator team and staff to provide additional support services to them as indicated.

As it relates to the depressive and anxiety disorder diagnostic categories, research published in 2015 suggests veterans were no more likely to have depressive disorders than non-veterans (Gould et al., 2015). Notwithstanding, national prevalence rates of major depression are estimated to be 7% with a 1.5 to 3.0 odds increase for women (APA, 2013). As it relates to the anxiety disorder diagnostic category, cross-sectional research conducted among four Veterans Affairs Medical Centers yielded that 12% of participants met diagnostic criteria for Generalized Anxiety Disorder (Milanak et al., 2013). Likewise, rates of diagnosable anxiety disorders among active duty military service members have increased 450% between the years of 2000 and 2015 (Armed Forces Health Surveillance Center, 2013). While there is

TABLE 7.2 COMMON VETERAN SYMPTOMS AND DISORDERS

SYMPTOM SUMMARIES	*DSM-5* DISORDERS	STUDENT EXEMPLAR
Trauma and Stressor Related Disorder		
A constellation of **trauma-based symptoms** (e.g., intrusion, increased arousal, alterations in cognition and mood, and avoidance) that range from mild to severe and acute to chronic in response to traumatic event(s), real or perceived	Acute stress disorder Posttraumatic stress disorder	A military veteran that encountered MST during active duty who struggles with flashbacks and hypervigilance while participating in practical skills testing with peers and faculty during a health assessment course
Depressive Disorder		
A constellation of **depressive symptoms** (e.g., depressed mood, anhedonia, weight/appetite changes, sleep disturbance, psychomotor dysregulation, fatigue, anergia, guilt, impaired concentration and suicidal thoughts) that range from mild to severe and acute to chronic	Major depressive disorder Dysthymic disorder Substance/medication induced depressive disorder Depressive disorder due to another medical condition	A military veteran medically separated for major depressive disorder who continues to struggle with insomnia, cognitive delay and impaired concentration that is negatively influencing test performance and classroom attendance
Anxiety Disorder		
A constellation of **anxiety-based symptoms** (e.g., anxious mood, ruminative worry, impaired concentration, panic attack, phobic reactions, social anxiety, sleep disturbance, irritability and restlessness) that range from mild to severe and acute to chronic	Specific phobia Social anxiety disorder Panic disorder Generalized anxiety disorder Substance/medication induced anxiety disorder Anxiety disorder due to another medical condition	A military veteran who struggles with perseverated worry over course assignments and faculty's presumed satisfaction with their work performance to such a point that it negatively impairs sleep, self-care, academic and social functioning
Substance Use Disorder		
A constellation of specific **substance-related symptoms** (e.g., increased tolerance, persistent desire to consume substance, cravings, withdrawal and functional impairment) that range from mild to severe and acute to chronic	Alcohol use disorder Caffeine related disorder Cannabis use disorder Opioid related disorder Sedative, hypnotic, or anxiolytic related disorder Stimulant related disorder Tobacco related disorder	A military veteran who reports a 10+ year habit of alcohol binge drinking that contributed to their precipitous service release who is now struggling with academic functioning during clinical nursing rotations due to the same behavior
Neurocognitive Disorder		
A constellation of **cognitive deficits** associated with attention, executive function, learning, memory, language, perceptual-motor or social cognition that range from mild to severe and acute to chronic	Neurocognitive disorder, secondary to traumatic brain injury	A military veteran who was medically retired after having incurred traumatic brain injury secondary to a concussive blast from a roadside bomb who continues to struggle with acquired and sustained attention as well as frustration intolerance in large classroom settings

DSM-5, Diagnostic and statistical manual of mental disorders (5th ed.); MST, military sexual trauma.

compelling evidence to suggest that both depression and anxiety disorders are heritable conditions, the science is also declarative about the relative influence that stress exposure has upon both its acuity and chronicity. It is for this reason that veterans appear to be particularly vulnerable. While the symptoms that constitute depression and anxiety are varied, their functional impact is consistent. The expressions of depression and anxiety can be generally classified into three domains of affective (e.g., problems with emotional regulation), cognitive (e.g., problems with executive functioning), and physiologic (e.g., problems with physiologic and somatic reactivity) symptoms. Educators encountering veterans struggling with depression and anxiety can anticipate these types of symptoms particularly during periods of increased stress during the semester or program of study.

According to the Substance Abuse and Mental Health Services Administration (SAMHSA, 2015), one in every 15 veterans struggle with a substance use disorder. The most common forms of substance-related problems seen among the veteran population revolve around binge drinking and tobacco use (Teeters et al., 2017). Seal et al. (2011) noted that the unique constellation of environmental stressors common to service (i.e., deployment, combat exposure, and redeployment) appear be linked with an increased risk for the development of a substance use disorder. Nursing programs across the country have clearly defined standards as it relates to substance misuse. While no special allowances should be made for veterans, there may be value in seeing substance misuse as a warning sign of an unaddressed mental disorder. The nursing profession has a well-established history of identifying and treating impaired nurse providers (National Council of State Boards of Nursing, 2011). Applying the same line of reasoning, schools of nursing are encouraged to explore strategies to get student veterans connected with services as opposed to a default disenrollment.

As it relates the neurocognitive disorder diagnostic category, a study of Post-9/11 military veterans established that 17.3% met diagnostic criteria for traumatic brain injury (TBI) during their period of military service (Lindquist et al., 2017). Swanson et al. (2017) identified statistically significant reductions in quality of life, cognition and emotional functioning among veterans diagnosed with TBI. More disturbing, Shura et al. (2019) identified that veterans who have incurred TBI are approximately twice as likely to have reported recent suicidal ideations. TBI is diagnostically scaled from *mild* to *moderate* to *severe*. While those with *severe* expressions of TBI are likely less inclined to matriculate into secondary education, those with *mild* to *moderate* expressions of TBI will do so more commonly. *Mild* to *moderate* TBI all too commonly goes undetected and undiagnosed both during and following military service.

General recognition of TBI related symptoms commonly defaults to the acute impact of *coup contrecoup* injuries where damage to the brain occurs at both the point of impact and opposite side of the brain associated with the abrupt deceleration of the brain. What has been less understood but arguably more contributory to the long-term sequelae of TBI is the associated diffuse axonal injury (DAI) that follows the acute injury secondary to uncontrolled inflammation. DAI is recognized as the principal factor that determines morbidity, mortality, and functional impact with TBI (Vieira et al., 2016). Considering the cognitive and emotional excrescences of TBI, these symptoms can translate to low academic performance, cognitive rigidity, and inappropriate behavior. While it is not realistic to expect the educator to assess for the presence of TBI in their student veterans, it is important to remain vigilant for the signs and symptoms and encourage the veteran to seek care when it is suspected.

High-Risk, High-Volume, and Problem-Prone Scenarios

While the previously mentioned disorders will likely represent the majority of veteran psychiatric presentations nurse educators will encounter in the academic and clinical practice setting, the authors would be remiss if we did not discuss other possible clinical presentations. As presented in Table 7.3, some symptoms can be classified as either *high-risk*, *high-volume*, or *problem-prone*. Educators are encouraged to work with their faculty leadership to operationalize strategies to navigate these types of encounters and coordinate care to a healthcare provider.

TABLE 7.3 SYMPTOM RISK CONSIDERATIONS

SYMPTOM STATES RELEVANT TO MILITARY SERVICE MEMBERS AND VETERANS		
High-Risk	High-Volume	Problem-Prone
Active psychosis Active mania Active substance intoxication Active substance withdrawal Active suicidal ideations Active homicidal ideation	Adjustment reaction Stress reaction/injury Co-occurring medical – psychiatric disorder Subclinical symptoms	Dual diagnosis conditions Substance use disorder Personality disorder

HIGH-RISK SYMPTOMS

High-risk situations are associated with the presence of symptoms suggestive of serious mental illness and acute risk. Psychotic thought and behavior are generally defined by the presence of hallucinations, delusions, disorganized speech and behavior. Manic thought and behavior are generally defined by a decreased need for sleep, racing thoughts, distractibility, increased goal orientation, psychomotor agitation, and impulsivity. Active substance intoxication and withdrawal will be defined by the substance used. Lastly, suicidal and homicidal ideations are hopefully self-evident *high-risk* situations. In dealing with high-risk situations, faculty and staff are encouraged to recognize the risk to client and staff safety and coordinate with support resources expeditiously to increase safety while remaining engaged with the client (Combat and Operational Stress Control, 2016).

HIGH-VOLUME SYMPTOMS

High-volume situations are commonly expressed in the form of adjustment related problems during matriculation, periods of high stress throughout the course of study like clinical rotations, and upon graduation. By the nature of their service, many veterans have been stress-sensitized and consequently can react (or overreact) to that which is unfamiliar, unanticipated, or perceived as illogical. For example, the earnest educator that changes a critical element of a course syllabus without communicating said change or does not follow up with a student request as promised may receive a reaction disproportionate to the situation. Given the nature of military service, some percentage of student veterans will present with co-occurring medical problems (e.g., chronic orthopedic pain, limb amputation, hazardous chemical exposure sequelae) that can inform and be informed by co-occurring psychiatric illness (Olenick et al., 2015). Lastly and arguably most commonly, veterans can present with symptoms that, while below the clinical threshold for formal psychiatric diagnosis, such as stress injuries, can prove to be mildly to moderately functionally impairing. Using a heuristic known to nursing, subclinical psychiatric symptoms are analogous to the insensible loss of fluid that nurses are unable to calculate on an intake and output record. Over time, these losses can accumulate but are more commonly not recognized until a clinical threshold is exceeded.

PROBLEM-PRONE SYMPTOMS

Problem-prone situations can be expressed in the form of a dual diagnosis presentation where the veteran is experiencing problems with both a psychiatric condition (e.g., PTSD, major depressive disorder, generalized anxiety disorder) alongside a substance use disorder (e.g., alcohol use disorder, cannabis use disorder, or tobacco use disorder). These scenarios are problem prone due to their complex nature as the symptoms from each clinical problem have the tendency to negatively reinforce the other. Lastly, some veterans will present with symptoms suggestive of a personality disorder. By definition, personality disorders are not a product of military service but rather the result of a lifelong set of experiences and patterns of behavior. The presence of a personality disorder is a risk factor for other psychiatric and medical conditions (Quirk et al., 2016).

TABLE 7.4 EDUCATOR AND CLINICAL ROLES

CHARACTERISTIC	EDUCATOR ROLE	CLINICAL ROLE
Goal	Student learning Nursing competency Role acquisition	Target symptom improvement Improved functional capacity Patient self-determination
Length	Course or program length	Duration of therapeutic relationship
Content	Student learning objectives	Patient clinical needs
Responsibility	Mutual; educator > student	Mutual; clinician > patient
Compensation	Altruism, pay, recognition	Altruism, pay, recognition

Mental Disorder Implications for Clinical Practice

The principal goal of this chapter is to foster greater understanding of the student veteran in healthcare education and offer culturally sensitive strategies that can support all involved through the educational process. Notwithstanding, there is indication to briefly speak to some clinical practice implications given the fact that educators and students will likely be interacting with veterans in the clinical practice setting. Many of the principles offered in this chapter can generally apply to the clinical support of veterans. It is critical for the educator to be sensitive to their role as they alternate between educator and clinician roles. The primary differences between the educator and clinical role are captured in Table 7.4. As this chapter has thus far principally focused on the educator role, we will now spend some time exploring the clinician role.

As it relates to the delivery of care, nursing practice does not appreciably change when one compares veteran and non-veteran (Box 7.1). This is best understood by differentiating the "what" and the "how." The "what" is associated with *what* nurses do in the clinical role. Nurses deliver evidence-based nursing care. The "how" is associated with *how* nurses do what they do in the clinical role. Nurses regularly and dynamically apply evidence-based nursing care strategies through the prism of any number of social, cultural, and religious variations. In kind, nurses working with veterans in the clinical role will best serve their patients by first developing the requisite knowledge, skills, and attitudes (KSA) associated with evidence-based nursing practice. Over one's nursing career, the KSA becomes more refined upon exposure to diverse populations and settings.

IMPLICATIONS FOR NURSING EDUCATION AND PRACTICE

Not unlike their civilian counterparts, the matriculating military veteran with psychiatric symptoms can struggle amid the fast paced, multitasking, socially demanding setting of nursing and the allied health professions. While definite progress with stigma has been made in the military over the past two decades, there remains numerous barriers to care that send mixed messages regarding tolerance of mental illness in uniform (Ben-Zeev et al., 2012). Military enculturation in uniform will influence the military veteran out of uniform. Military service entry training aspires to intentionally strip new accessions of their civilian identities and replace them with a set of utilitarian, mission-minded edicts defined by *always placing the mission first, never accepting defeat, never quitting,* and *never leaving a fallen comrade behind* (Parson et al., 2013). These aspirational values, while absolute in nature, afford veterans the facility to do exceptional things under extraordinary circumstances. Regrettably, these aspirational values also foment psychiatric symptoms in and out of uniform due to their overly idealistic nature. It is for these reasons that military veterans entering nursing school will likely fully embrace the servant nature of nursing but will also struggle with finding the balance between service to others and self.

BOX 7.1

CLINICIAN GUIDING PRINCIPLES FOR WORKING WITH VETERANS

PRACTICES FOR WORKING WITH VETERANS IN THE CLINICAL SETTING

1. Be patient and let the veteran determine the degree and pace of self-disclosure

2. Veterans have been socialized to be assertive (sometimes referred to as "straight shooters"). Consequently, you can best utilize your time by asking the "difficult" questions about self- and other-directed violence in a straightforward manner

3. Anticipate and assess for the presence of commonly co-occurring general medical problems (e.g., traumatic brain injury, orthopedic problems, endocrine related disorders) that can further complicate the clinical picture

4. Ensure a comprehensive substance usage history has been collected and consequently factored into the clinical decision-making process

5. Take additional time and effort to research the veteran's military occupational specialty as doing so can illuminate potential sources of trauma and available support systems

6. Assess if the veteran has been formally evaluated by the Department of Veteran Affairs for a disability rating

7. Encourage veterans to augment their plan of care by (re)connecting with veteran peers they have past served with

8. Do not assume all forms of trauma exposure are military sourced. Augment nursing assessment by administering the Adverse Childhood Events Scale that is open source available via the Centers for Disease Control and Prevention website

9. Veterans have been trained to perform extraordinary tasks under extraordinary circumstances. They develop these skills through a pattern of serial exposure. Consequently, veterans will respond best when given anticipatory guidance about the plan of care

10. Recognize that veteran mental healthcare is complicated by stigma. Take the necessary effort to assess how mental illness stigma can be reinforced, either intentionally or unintentionally, in your care area and change the messaging. Consider these two resources as a starting point for learning more about professional practice roles and working with veterans (deploymentpsych.org/military-culture and www.medalofhonorspeakout.org)

Educators working with student veterans in the academic setting must be mindful of their role function and limitations. While the line between educator and clinician can significantly overlap in the Venn diagram of education, educators are strongly encouraged to steer clear of this line with student veterans in particular. Influenced by stigma, some student veterans may seek out educators for psychological support as opposed to engaging the formal mental healthcare delivery system. In this instance, educators may be unwittingly enabling student veterans to not engage formal care as they attempt to meet their short-term needs in an unofficial clinical capacity. Scenarios like this are rife with risk and limited reward. Educators best serve student veterans and their institutions by being able to recognize high-risk, high-volume and problem-prone mental health problems in their students and know how to connect them with the right services in an expeditious manner. In this regard, educators should be less the resource and more the resource liaison.

CASE STUDY 7.2 ACTIVATION OF SUICIDAL IDEATION

Jamie is a veteran nursing student, with prior service experience as a combat medic, currently navigating the second year of nursing school. Academically speaking, Jamie's grades are near the top of the class. Interpersonally speaking, Jamie's behavior is avoidant, passive, and stoic. While Jamie takes great effort to meaningfully engage in the obligatory aspects of group work, faculty recognize that doing so takes much effort on Jamie's part. Jamie politely keeps peers at a distance and Jamie's peer group generally honors the unspoken boundary.

Jamie is taking four credits of health assessment this semester. Three credits are didactic, and one credit is fulfilled through a skills lab involving online test trainers, manekins, student peers and standardized patients. Faculty recognize Jamie has become progressively more distracted and socially uncomfortable over the semester. During skills lab, Jamie is last to arrive and first to leave the classroom setting. Jamie regularly looks disheveled, sleep deprived, and despite the winter weather is visibly diaphoretic and sweat stained by the end of each class. Jamie has reluctantly partnered with Reginald for skills practice and testing since the beginning of the semester. In preparation for a final summative health assessment skills test, the cohort of students procured the skills lab for a marathon 4-hour health assessment practice session ahead of the next day final exam. During the practice session, Jamie and Reginald awkwardly struggled through the primary and secondary health assessment process several times. Approximately one hour into the practice session Jamie abruptly ran out of the lab without explanation.

The student class leader quickly reached out to the course faculty, Dr. Johnson, via a text message verbalizing concern for Jamie and the abrupt nature of the departure. Dr. Johnson immediately went to the skills lab to collect more information, speaking to both the class leader and Reginald. Dr. Johnson asked if anyone had been able to contact Jamie. Regrettably, no student had Jamie's phone number and denied having any virtual contact via social media. Dr. Johnson returned to her office, attempted to call Jamie via cell phone and informed her department chair of the situation. Thereafter, Dr. Johnson walked through the building eventually finding Jamie in a bathroom stall with one hand stuffed in a backpack and the other leaning against the dividing section of the bathroom stall. Upon finding Jamie, Dr. Johnson stepped back from the bathroom stall door and slowly brought her open hands into full view. Recognizing Jamie's hand concealed in the backpack, she calmly asked if Jamie was okay. Jamie's head moved slowly to the left and right. Dr. Johnson asked if Jamie was feeling safe. Again, Jamie's head moved slowly to the left and right. The class student leader then entered the bathroom and Dr. Johnson asked her to notify another faculty member of where they were. Dr. Johnson verbalized concern with Jamie's hand concealed in the backpack and slowly reached out her left hand to guide Jamie's right hand out of the backpack and then out of the bathroom stall. Dr. Johnson then asked if she could take Jamie's backpack. Jamie tearfully honored the request. Dr. Johnson then escorted Jamie to her office. Upon arrival, both were met by the Department Chair. After verifying Jamie was not carrying a weapon, Dr. Johnson shared with Jamie what she was seeing in terms of behavior, verbalized her concern for Jamie's well-being, and encouraged Jamie to be willing to accept care. This request was also tearfully honored. Jamie was escorted to the Counseling and Psychological Services (CAPS) office and emergently evaluated by one of the on-call counselors.

The nature of trauma suggests that those who struggle with it are commonly triggered by present oriented sensory stimuli that resemble the historical index trauma(s). This is why some veterans who experience direct combat struggle with loud sounds in unfamiliar environments. This is why some veterans cannot tolerate familiar smells of charred meat or the noxious smell of diesel fuel. This is why some veterans cannot enter a department store without establishing an exit strategy. This is why some veterans cannot tolerate physical intimacy without emotionally dysregulating.

Jamie experienced a military sexual trauma encounter while deployed to Afghanistan in 2010. Jamie did not disclose it to anyone, prior to or following service release. After leaving the military,

Jamie dramatically redefined physical and emotional boundaries with others. Jamie's encounters with Reginald in simulation apparently exceeded this new boundary set. Anticipating having to engage Reginald during each skills lab over the course of the semester was proving to be progressively more activating and triggering. Driven by a strong sense of obligation, Jamie suffered in silence during the semester despite the simulation labs deleterious impact on symptoms and functioning. The yellow zone stress associated with the student role requirement during physical health assessment class illuminated an orange zone injury revealing clinically significant symptoms that required intervention.

As it relates to the interaction with Jamie, Dr. Johnson made wise choices consistent with her role as an educator. She remained calm, communicated with leadership, assessed for imminent safety, and connected Jamie with same-day crisis intervention services. Dr. Johnson didn't ask probing questions about what presumably triggered Jamie nor did she physically violate Jamie's boundaries. Dr. Johnson acted in accordance with her role by not operating as the mental health resource but rather a mental health resources liaison.

Applying the lens of prevention, there were missed opportunities to assist Jamie before the crisis. An educator's first priority in the academic setting is to foster a sense of inclusivity and community. Early efforts to foster mutually tolerable levels of community can translate to peer support which could have provided Jamie with some degree of social ballast—an augmented resource caravan—to navigate the triggering events. Educators recognizing the early warning signs (e.g., behaviorally avoidant, disheveled, sleep deprived, and diaphoretic) and inquiring as to how Jamie is doing earlier in the semester could have created an opportunity for an earlier CAPS referral. In no small part due to the military ethos, mental illness stigma, and other recognized barriers to care, veterans reluctantly and ambivalently engage mental health service long after their symptoms and functioning are impaired. Educators working with veterans must recognize this tendency and be assertive when it comes to such matters.

Case Study Review Questions

As the faculty member:

1. What Military Ethos Traits from Table 7.2 are present in the case study?
2. What stress zones from Figure 7.1 are present in the case study?
3. What educator's behaviors were effective or ineffective?
4. What other resources would the educator or student need to be successful?

Box 7.2 provides a set of guiding principles that educators can use to create an academic environment that is both sensitive to the unique needs of student veterans but also recognizes the role limitations of educators whose principle priority is to teach and not therapize.

FUTURE RESEARCH PRIORITIES

There is a gap in the body of knowledge regarding the educational and occupational experience across the stress continuum. This gap is represented by a need to test a theoretical framework, the need for stress injury sensitive outcomes, and testing of peer support strategies for stress injury mitigation. The Stress Continuum and Stress First Aid model represent a middle range theory about stress injuries within an occupational or academic context. As a middle range theory, the concepts are well defined, operational, and can lead to practical practice applications. Opportunities for research in an academic setting would include the use of a longitudinal cohort design that follows a group of students across a program of study. The process of learning nursing skills and the transformation of a personal identity into a professional identity has exposures to all four sources of stress injury. Questions about the types

BOX 7.2

EDUCATOR GUIDING PRINCIPLES FOR WORKING WITH VETERANS

PRACTICES FOR WORKING WITH VETERANS IN THE CLASSROOM SETTING	
Helpful	**Unhelpful**
1. Encourage students with documented disabilities who have the potential to impact educational achievement to contact their school's Office of Accommodation	1. Do not solicit veteran trauma encounters
2. Encourage the veteran who is struggling to pursue an evaluation for accommodations	2. Resist the urge to compare service experiences/pedigree with veterans
3. Meet regularly with the veteran to discuss strategies for success and lessons learned	3. Do not assume that all veterans have post traumatic stress disorder
4. Be both clear and explicit with academic performance expectations	4. Among those veterans that have encountered trauma, do not assume it is always etiologically combat in nature
5. Provide anticipatory guidance about significant changes to course delivery and program of study	5. Do not rationalize evidence of substance abuse; take action
6. Connect the student with local veteran support service resources to develop an organic support system	6. Resist the urge to step outside the academic role by delivering psychosocial support
7. Monitor the relative load of vicarious trauma that educators carry in support of the student veteran	
8. Remain vigilant for the potential of implicit bias that can subsume the student veteran-educator relationship	
9. Obtain military culture competency training	

and patterns of stress exposures in relation to course scheduling and educational transformation would provide knowledge about risk factors, timing of high-stress evolutions, and opportunities to mitigate unnecessary stress while maintaining motivation and building self-efficacy.

There is a need for developing and testing stress injury sensitive outcomes. The dominant framework for researching occupational stress usually starts with assumptions about event exposure and clinical levels of impairment. Common outcome measures include clinical scales for PTSD, anxiety, depression, and substance dependence. The use of clinical scales designed to identify and measure dysfunction will bias results with low instrument sensitivity for pre-clinical symptoms or over report clinical impairment. Additionally, one of the first symptoms of a stress injury is a reduced ability to recognize our own stress level. Self-report scales of stress levels will often produce under reporting of symptoms. Peer assessment and objective measures for stress injury versus disorders need to be developed.

The third area for future research is in the testing of peer support strategies for health professional students and workers. Peer support in the first responder and health professions culture needs to reflect and respect the micro-cultures of teams and clinical units. Some teams may benefit from a formal structure of asking the three questions about challenges, successes, and meaning. Other teams may benefit from the "Orange Zone Huddle" for spontaneous and fluid peer support. Other teams may need both. Implementation studies need to evaluate the different processes of peer support and the characteristics of the strengths and limitations of peer support in the context of the team and micro-culture. An additional element of peer support and stress mitigation interventions is to evaluate the impact of the interventions on student self-efficacy, retention, and licensure pass rates. In the work environment, outcome measures should consider absenteeism, retention, and engagement. Ultimately, future research that expands knowledge of understanding regarding occupational well-being, recognition and mitigation of stress injuries, and strengthening a future work force is needed to shape the educational and occupational future.

CONCLUSION

Every war has produced the need to integrate the human cost of armed conflict back into society as a whole. By and large, this effort is notable for short-lived fanfare and platitudes with a predictable and rapid disenfranchisement of the veteran. Throughout nursing history, in response to alarming levels of social need, leaders such as Nightingale, Breckinridge, Barton, and Wald ushered in critical social and professional transformation. Our generation stands at the precipice of social need with an opportunity to once again integrate the human cost of war back into society. Veterans that choose a second career of service in nursing bring with them a unique set of strengths, vulnerabilities, opportunities, and challenges. In most cases, the vulnerabilities and challenges can be effectively reduced, or in certain cases completely mitigated, provided all involved leverage equal doses of consistency, reliability, and unconditional positive regard. What has been offered in this chapter aspired to provide educators with a knowledge set designed to integrate the veteran into the next generation of nurses.

REFERENCES

The complete reference list for this chapter appears in the digital version of the chapter, accessible at https://connect.springerpub.com/content/book/978-0-8261-3597-1/chapter/ch07

RESOURCES

www.va.gov/health/
www.mentalhealth.va.gov
deploymentpsych.org/military-culture
www.medalofhonorspeakout.org
www.samhsa.gov/smvf-ta-center

ADVOCACY FOR RESERVE/ NATIONAL GUARD PERSONNEL, MILITARY WOMEN, LGBT, AND PRIVATE MILITARY CONTRACTORS

MICHAEL J. KELLER | PATRICIA L. CONARD | MYRNA L. ARMSTRONG

If our hopes of building a better and safer world are to become more than wishful thinking, we will need the engagement of [many different types of military] volunteers more than ever.

Kofi Annan, Ghana, co-recipient of the 2001 Nobel Peace Prize

KEY TERMS

Reservists	posttraumatic stress disorder (PTSD)
National Guard	Gulf War illness
lesbian	chronic multisymptom illness
gay	suicide
bisexual	MST
transgender	military women
private military contractors	military sexual trauma (MST)
defense contractors	

INTRODUCTION

As the Iraq and Afghanistan War veteran population now exceeds 2.5 million, awareness of significant groups of service members of the total Armed Forces milieu is important. Four diverse groups, within and surrounding military environments, are examined in this chapter. The Reserve and National Guard component (RC), military women, and the LGBT community are actively within the service. Private military contractors (PMCs) are the fourth group; they are civilians that provide services to the military while employed by agencies or businesses outside the military sector. Health outcomes following

The complete reference list for this chapter appears in the digital version of the chapter, accessible at https://connect.springerpub.com/content/book/978-0-8261-3597-1/chapter/ch08

military and combat-zone experiences for these groups present both civilian and veteran healthcare providers with significant challenges. With less attention on these groups in the published literature and changes in demographic trends within the military, nurses and healthcare providers need to understand what makes these groups distinct so that culturally sensitive care is delivered.

BACKGROUND

In order to provide service for our nation's military commitments, there are many groups who are key to its success and support, regardless of the location (stateside or global), the function (conflicts or human-itarian efforts), or the time (war or peace). This chapter includes an examination of four diverse groups that serve or are associated with the military. Three of these groups are active within the service, the Reserve component and National Guard component, military women, and the LGBT military commu-nity. The fourth group, PMCs, provide services to the military, yet are civilians employed by agencies or businesses outside the military sector. All of these significant groups have deep military roots, have produced many important contributions, and are strategically active within our various service branch environments, although limited knowledge still exists about them (Minnick, 2014; Ursano et al., 2016).

Overall, there has been more research and observations written about service members during their Iraq/Afghanistan war deployment, and as veterans, than any other major U.S. conflict (Institute of Medicine [IOM], 2013). Yet, as with any scientific information, there is always a lag between the observations, research, analysis, and publications. Men in the military (85%) are still the majority of subjects in many Iraq and Afghanistan War studies (IOM, 2013). For this chapter the latest literature, written both during and post the Iraq/Afghanistan wars, are presented with a snapshot about each of these significant groups. The chapter highlights their presence and critical capabilities, along with their similarities and differences from the major component of men still comprising the majority of full-time military personnel. Limited information about these significant groups is reported in the lit-erature offering less support to clinicians in their effort to provide culturally sensitive, patient-centered care. Although as the composition of the military and the associated policies change, further focus about them will be important.

The Importance of Mission

For everyone in the Armed Forces, military readiness to accomplish the mission is of the utmost con-cern and in order to complete the task, one must be fit and healthy. This holistic premise becomes crucial when every military policy and regulation is created, discussed, and executed. To accomplish the prescribed readiness standards for the fighting force, the U.S. military recruits and carefully screens to seek healthy men and women. To date service branches are only finding approximately 29% that qualify for these intense service standards (U.S. Department of Defense [DoD], 2017). Immediately after joining the military, recruits complete rigorous physical training and testing. This expectation of readiness follows service members throughout their time in the military. From these rigorous expecta-tions, along with access to healthcare, some believe a sense of hardiness could be present, thus the term "healthy solider effect" has sometimes been applied to them (Conard & Armstrong, 2018).

Within this paramount "mission first" policy, military service members (MSMs) are expected to take individual responsibility for their readiness to duty by proactively seeking care when needed to maintain their health (Bruner & Woll, 2012). When the MSM does not adhere to their health readiness standards they could be creating a situation in which they become non-qualified for deployment. The latter affects the military's personnel and financial resource investment of the MSM (Baker, 2014). This readiness for duty can also affect numerous activities in combat zones including medical evacuations, as they consume significant time and mission resources. The wounded and injured are the major pri-ority. Non-urgent medical evacuations for disease or non-battle-injuries (or other examples such as pregnancy, podiatry, or dental) are deliberately attempted to be kept at a minimum so they do not neg-atively impact unit member morale due to the loss of a unit member and others having to take on more responsibilities. These standards for readiness for the first three groups described in this chapter are applied for every branch of the service, making them subject to separation from the service at any time. With PMC, their employing agencies are liable for their health concerns during any of their combat zone experiences, although some of the PMC work might be in close proximity so the military could provide some services for them, if necessary and/or possible (Swed & Crosbie, 2019).

Civilian healthcare professionals will increasingly come in contact with veterans in their work. When examining their health issues, each of these diverse groups may have comparable outcomes, although what becomes distinctive about them is the reasons, specific responses, the time of docu-mentation/detection, and/or the increasing prevalence of their healthcare concerns (Oster et al., 2017). This chapter will be assistive regardless of whether the member of this group is seeking care entirely at a Veterans Health Administration (VHA) facility or civilian health facility, or requesting services from both as many veterans are doing. In addition, the information contained in this chapter will assist clinicians in focusing their examination on both the presenting health issues of veterans, as well as being aware of future health risks unique to veterans. These crossovers for healthcare will become more frequent with the Congressional 115th Legislative Session (2018) "VA MISSION Act." (It is officially titled the John S. McCain III, Daniel K. Akaka, and Samuel R. Johnson VA Maintaining Internal Sys-tems and Strengthening Integrated Outside Networks Act.) The intent of the legislation is to provide veterans, who are currently enrolled in the VHA, increased access to timely community-based care within a 30 to 60 mile radius. In addition, it also allows veterans' opportunities to receive treatment at local civilian emergency department and urgent care centers without stipulations from participating providers. For the latter services, in most circumstances there are currently no, or minimal, co-pay per visit for the veteran.

RESERVE AND NATIONAL GUARD PERSONNEL

The foundation for our RC was the nation's early colony militia founded in 1636, yet it took almost 300 more years for the RC to be financially and administratively federalized, finally recognized for their laudable, strong, prolonged service of filling the gaps of active military personnel (Ursano et al., 2016). Following the Vietnam War, changes in the draft requirements and the move toward an all-volunteer service system prompted more attention on the RC assets to fulfill a new Armed Forces composition. Each military branch (Navy, Marine, Coast Guard, Army, and Air Force) expanded their respective Reserves, while the latter two branches also increased their National Guard personnel (Minnick, 2014). It should be noted that the words "part time" are used for RC personnel; this denotes their difference from full-time personnel that are serving on Active Duty within the military 24 hours a day, 7 days a week. When the RC component are "called up" or "activated" for deployment, they also are placed on equivalent Active Duty, just as full-time military personnel. RC personnel remain on Active Duty status until they are demobilized, then they return to part-time status. These RC changes from part-time to full-time status can occur as many times as needed throughout their military career. Within the RC, the National Guard MSM serve dual roles, being subject to their state Governor's mission demands, with possible specific deployments for humanitarian events and/or natural disaster situations, as well as fed-eralized responsibilities when deployed out of the country for wartime conflicts.

Historically, early RC mobilizations primarily supported natural disaster relief such as floods and earthquakes. Because of these types of focused missions, members of the RC, their employers, and their families typically experienced few or no long separations due to military commitments. Around the mid 1980s their major service obligations changed to war deployments and their mobilizations started to become a "probability, not a possibility" (Kelly et al., 2014, p. 347). Top operational RCs became more crucial to the military force with both an individual and/or unit readiness focus to fulfill the demand for rapid deployment around the world. The first huge test of the new Armed Forces personnel composition was Gulf War I (1991) when more than 230,000 RC men (91%) and women (9%) were swiftly activated, comprising almost 20% of the fighting force (Conard & Armstrong, 2019). They served honorably, with 70 killed in action (Minnick, 2014). The events and surrounding circumstances of Post-9/11 produced more significant military operational changes for the RC as they faced numerous, unique, and intense challenges for their services and training (Ahern et al., 2015; Angel et al., 2018). Almost a million RC men (88%) and women (12%) were activated for the Iraq/Afghanistan wars; at times comprising over 40% of the Active Duty personnel during prolonged combat operations occurring between 2001 and 2014 (Scherrer et al., 2014). As with other full-time military personnel, RC also have served multiple deployments, often for 12 months or longer, in combat situations, with little time at home between their deployments (Messecar, 2017).

To date, the military's Armed Forces comprise approximately 1.4 million full-time U.S. men (85%) and women (15%), as well as an additional 800,000 men (80%) and women (20%) in the RC (Governing, 2019). Demographically, the RC tends to be older, more educated, have higher military rank (Maung et al., 2017; Scherrer et al., 2014), and often live greater distances from military installations and/or military healthcare providers (Werber et al., 2013). Just over one quarter (26.1%) of RC members identify themselves as a racial minority, while the number of minority service members in full-time positions comprise less than one third (31.3%) of the Armed Forces (DoD, 2017). Due to directives from the Office of Management and Budget, Hispanic is not included in the minority race designation, but service members who identify their ethnicity as being Hispanic or Latino include 15.5% of full-time members and 11.5% in the RC (DoD, 2017). During the prolonged combat operations of Iraq/Afghanistan wars, over half of the RC (55%) were married with families as compared to their full-time military counterparts (39%). More RC were single parents (10%), as compared to 5% of full-time troops (Office of the Deputy Under Secretary of Defense, 2012).

Research data about RC women remain sparse. Their data often have to be extracted from small studies with few subjects, or frequently teased out from their larger RC group, that also has little written about them, when the total Armed Forces composition is examined (Obsorne et al., 2012). Yet women make up approximately 19.6% of the total RC, with 10% in the National Guard and 18% in the Reserves (DoD, 2017; Obsorne et al., 2012). This increase of Reserve women is partially due to the major presence (70%) of the military's healthcare provider cache (Maung et al., 2017). Many RC women are in the Coast Guard with the fewest in the Marines (Obsorne et al., 2012). Many "firsts" are still being revealed, both in occupations and leadership roles, for RC women. For example, in 2019 the Army selected its first RC woman infantry soldier, and the top echelon of Commanders in the Maryland National Guard are women (Rempfer, 2019).

Training, Readiness, and Expectations

All military men and women (whether full time or RC) are expected to be trained and qualified to fulfill the same mission readiness, whenever and wherever needed, although to accomplish that their training time is different (Eaton et al., 2011). Full-time military personnel train approximately 240 days annually as they build and reinforce their military skills daily (Scherrer et al., 2014). Their service time is considered full-time employment, with access to a full complement of military healthcare services. In contrast, the minimum military training expectations for the RC are 39 days annually (one weekend per month and two specific weeks during the year), hence the names "part-timers, week-end warriors, or citizen soldiers" (Hansen et al., 2018, p. e397). While in their training status, RC personnel have access to military healthcare services only for injuries that occur during training time.

When RC military units are being seriously considered for a deployment, the number of mandatory training days increases to 120 days; yet, still less than half of the days compared to their full-time military counterparts. For some military occupations, this training disparity between full-time and part-time RCs does not pose a problem. Healthcare providers are a good example as they are often employed full-time in the same role in their civilian job, yet for others it can be more difficult such as their role in combat arms (weaponry). In addition, most RC members maintain part-time or full-time civilian employment, so these RC obligations are conducted while in close communication with their employers.

MOBILIZATION

There are usually four phases associated with military mobilization as a service member leaves their duty station, although there are differences during each phase for the RC, when compared to the full-time personnel. As will be noted, both pre- and especially post-deployment phases have been the most problematic for the RC (Werber et al., 2013). Many of the problems these veterans experience arise from leaving work and their family, and the uncertainties when returning to civilian work, family, and in many cases educational pursuits.

Predeployment

Following additional training time and the completion of warning orders giving RC members a 30- to 45-day notice that some type of mobilization for deployment could be happening, RC members can then be "called-up" or "activated" for Active Duty. Reporting demands could happen as soon as within 1 to 3 days or suddenly canceled. Naturally, these swift military requirements create pending and/or immediate stress for the RC, as well as for their employers and families. If the RC actually leaves, getting all of the complex paperwork/arrangements completed expeditiously from employers, educational institutions, and financial obligations is challenging, especially when switching from civilian employment salaries to full-time military paychecks (Scherrer et al., 2014). In contrast, full-time military understand deployment arrangements are an expectation of their duty responsibilities, their family and children are supported by their military community, any educational demands put on hold, legal issues addressed on the military installation, and they experience uninterrupted military salaries.

Deployment

Besides the preparation for deployment, further challenges can include "length, and type of deployment, communication during deployment, and finally, awareness of how deployment changes the military member and the family" (Messecar, 2017, p. 269). In addition, beyond less training and preparation, the RC may or may not deploy with their unit (Scherrer et al., 2014). Instead, during the Iraq and Afghanistan Wars, often they were taken (cherry-picked) from their RC unit and sent to a combat-zone destination to fill an individual position alongside other unknown U.S. military personnel. This produced low deployment support, problematic stress-filled delayed adjustments, and/or limited camaraderie (Osborne et al., 2012; Scherrer et al., 2014). In contrast, full-time military personnel deployments were often mobilized with all or part of their unit, building group support and reinforcement.

When deployed, RC tend to "serve in roles where they are exposed to combat, rather than combat service support roles" (Agimi et al., 2019, p. 5). While in the combat zone environment, all personnel (full-time and RC) are provided healthcare by their respective medical service branch, whether they are having new, recurrent, or unresolved health issues. Most MSMs will not receive documentation of their medical visits/findings, particularly while serving in austere environments. When the records are finally available, the RCs are often already in their post-deployment phase, and historically caught in a gap of timely medical record transfers (Messecar, 2017). Upon post-deployment discharge, full-time military personnel continue to be part of the DoD system and are able to access their records. In contrast, RC members lose immediate access to the DoD healthcare system following their demobilization, so it takes them longer to obtain their medical records when they have to share them with future (VHA or civilian) providers (Randall, 2012). With slowly improving communication and collaboration between the DoD and VHA electronic medical records data systems, there is the intent for greater accessibility, seamless transition of care, less duplication, and better recovery to continue (Harris et al., 2014; U.S. Department of Veterans Affairs [VA], 2019a).

Reconstitution/Demobilization

Before all service members are released from their deployment and demobilized (readied) for home (about 7–10 days), everyone receives proactive education and screening for posttraumatic stress disorder (PTSD) concerns (Warner et al., 2011). Healthcare entitlements are also discussed, including the VA benefit process and opportunities for VHA care. Complete physicals and various interprofessional consultations with social workers and chaplains are included. Yet many are eager to return home so there is less interest in debriefing information or anything that stands in the way of going home.

Post-Deployment/Reintegration

For both full-time and RC personnel, the period of post-deployment begins with the troop's arrival at their home station and the approximate 180 days the military provides for reintegration. For all concerned, reintegration back into family, society, and life is different for every deployed service member and it requires diverse adjustments after each deployment (Scherrer et al., 2014). What became evident after Gulf War I, and even more apparent during the Iraq/Afghanistan wars, was the major reintegration problems and differences between full-time military and RC personnel (Messecar, 2017; Scherrer et al., 2014). Upon completion of their combat assignment, full-time personnel usually return to a stable, well-organized military installation centered on family/military support and resources. Their returning duty assignments are planned and phased in incrementally, while structured enough to effectively guide the service member toward further full-time on-site responsibilities as soon as possible.

In contrast, Scherrer et al. (2014) described five domains that are affected during RC reintegration including education, employment, health, legal, and family/relationship concerns. Leaving their demobilization station, RCs are flown home, often alone, with no military receiving party at their destination, creating a lack of deployment closure. This time is supposed to be an opportunity to decompress from their experiences and stress accumulated during the deployment at their place of residence, with no weekend training obligations for 90 days. However, the RC becomes quickly challenged to find their way back into life with their family, often with limited support. Given the significant emotional tensions that can occur during this delicate time of social adjustment, RC relationships with family, children, and friends can become complicated with higher levels of tension and stress both parties accumulated during the RC's deployment separation (Scherrer et al., 2014). Also, during their prolonged absence(s), the educational journey of service members could be significantly impacted. Scherrer et al. (2014) documented that 77% of their queried deployed veterans were affected when academic semester or enrollments requirements were not fulfilled. Messecar (2017) related one RC soldier's feelings of trying to "find his way," as "I came back starting … where I left off [reclaiming their family placement], while my family had moved on for a year and half … [now I am trying to find] a 'new normal'" (pp. 269–272). In addition, upon reintegration, depending on their RC obligations and unit camaraderie, they may or may not elect to continue with their part-time RC military activities, especially if they were concerned with the possibility of future deployments (Harris et al., 2014; Scherrer et al., 2014). This can produce even more separation problems and less military support.

Previously employed RC members often take little time off upon their return home because stabilizing their employment is a priority. Their employers are not pleased with extended military absences (Werber et al., 2013) and there is a common myth that RC members suffer job losses during their military absences (Kintzle et al., 2015). However, if the RC left their employment in good standing, employers are required to re-employ the RC after their deployment is completed according to the Uniformed Services Employment and Reemployment Rights Act of 1994 (PL 103-353; IOM, 2013).

With these regulations, employers are not obligated to restore them to their former position upon their return, but the job should be comparable. Employers are not required to pay RC salaries while activated, potentially creating financial hardships due to pay disruptions and differences between military and civilian salaries. During their absence, seniority, pension, and career advancement benefits should continue.

RC members (41%) who were not employed before deployment have more difficulty finding employment upon returning (IOM, 2013). Following the Iraq and Afghanistan Wars, looking for a job became more problematic for those under 30 years of age (30%) and if they suffered from service-connected disabilities and/or behavioral health issues (25%–30%; IOM, 2013; Kintzle et al., 2015; Minnick, 2014). To date, survey data documents that RC unemployment rates (including underemployment) are relatively close to their civilian counterparts for both RC women (3.5%) and men (3.9%) veterans (Bureau of Labor Statistics, 2019).

Upon reintegration, full-time military personnel may access the Outpatient Medical Clinic where military care providers quickly recognize common physical and behavioral combat-zone health concerns, and prompt treatment is prescribed. In contrast, RC personnel with service-connected health problems seem to emerge more slowly and/or are not recognized/detected as quickly following deployment (Messecar, 2017). Forty percent of RC members wait to enroll and/or even use VHA benefits, sometimes taking as much as 3 to 4 months before seeking medical treatment for their military health issues. Often this delay is due to concern about family reintegration rather than their own physical and behavioral issues (Messecar, 2017; Osborne et al., 2012; Randall, 2012). Large distances, time, and expense to receive care at the closest VHA facility further hamper this delay in treatment. RC personnel have access to VA healthcare, but report the complexities of the VA make it difficult in initiating access to healthcare services (Messecar, 2017).

In addition, a persistent myth remains within "RC units that they may lose their military career if they use the VHA; another concern is that seeking help is a sign of weakness" (Randall, 2012, p. 16). Estimates of RC using the VHA remain stable at around 45% to 57% (Harris et al., 2014; Randall, 2012); this number in 2019 has not changed (VA, 2019a). Depending on their deployment assignment (combat zone or not), RC are eligible for a 5-year VHA entitlement of care. If the RC member has a 100% combat service-connected disability, they are also granted lifetime spousal and dependent healthcare by the VHA (Messecar, 2017).

With these complexities of seeking healthcare from the VHA system, often RC members seek assistance from community care providers in civilian health facilities (Harris et al., 2014). Unfortunately, civilian providers may respond to military-related complaints with hesitancy, often without knowing what questions to ask, and any consideration of common service-related co-morbidities (Doyle & Streeter, 2016; Misra-Hebert et al., 2015; Oster et al., 2017). Even with the VA MISSION Act, some civilian clinicians are reluctant to treat veterans because they are unfamiliar with the VHA's community care program, its third-party administrator, and the bureaucratic paperwork (Kupfer et al., 2018). These encounters become challenging for the RC member, who is now without the overarching military support system and may not have reconnected well with their family (Sayer et al., 2014; Scherrer et al., 2014). This time of developing new routines during the already stress-filled reintegration process can give rise to further increases in their physical and behavioral health needs (Pflieger et al., 2018).

Health Concerns

While equally important, non-battle injuries are sometimes more problematic for RC service members when considering deployment morbidity and mortality (Eaton et al., 2011). This was reflected in the high number of RC referrals (67%) to Combat Support Hospitals during deployment where common complaints included musculoskeletal pain, depression, fatigue, as well as memory and concentration problems (Eaton et al., 2011; Finley et al., 2010). In addition, age (>30 years) and the decreased physical fitness of some RC personnel often accounted for increased non-battle injuries and risks for cardiovascular and stress-related impact, especially with long and repeated deployments (Patel et al., 2017). It has become difficult to determine whether the physical and behavioral health issues are hindering successful reintegration with the family or community, or vice versa (Koblinsky et al., 2014; Lapham et al., 2012; Sayer et al., 2014).

Highlighting the complexities of non-battle injuries, poor sleep patterns underpin many healthcare concerns. Hansen et al. (2018) reported insomnia to be a prominent disorder affecting a large number of RC combat zone military personnel, especially those with irregular sleep schedules from noise exposure, night duty patrol, limited safety equipment, and combat zone environments. Outcomes of cardiovascular disease, inflammatory responses, excess weight gain, and behavioral health issues are linked to a lack of sleep (Hansen et al., 2018).

Epidemiological findings from RC veterans who were deployed in Gulf War I are reporting "significant burden to disease," with obese conditions (BMI 29.80), reduced health functioning status, and multiple chronic conditions (Dursa et al., 2016, p. 41). This includes the unexplained vague symptoms sometimes called "Gulf War Illness" although the VHA uses the diagnostic code of "chronic multisymptom illness" (Conard & Armstrong, 2019, p. 146). Symptomology for either term includes "persistent fatigue, widespread pain, muscle aches, chronic headaches, joint pain, gastrointestinal problems, weight loss, insomnia, skin rashes, dizziness, respiratory disorders as well as neurological issues of memory concentration, mood problems, neuritis, and neuralgia" (Conard & Armstrong, 2019, p. 146).

The common behavioral health problems of recent veterans include three distinctive wounds suffered by over 45% of the Iraq and Afghanistan War veterans following their deployments to the combat zone environments. They include PTSD (4%–25%), traumatic brain injury (TBI; 19.5%–22.8%), and/or depression (5%–37%; IOM, 2013). Often these are accompanied by substance misuse and/or abuse (4.7%–39%). These behavioral health concerns may be an isolated occurrence or overlap, sometimes making the diagnosis and interventional approaches of significant co-morbid conditions difficult (El-Gabalawy et al., 2018). Behavioral health problems have been found to be five times more likely in both RC men and women, as compared to their full-time counterparts or the general public, perhaps identifying a deficit in training and TBI prevention during the Iraq and Afghanistan Wars (IOM, 2013; Scherrer et al., 2014; Ursano et al., 2018). They were especially evident if the RC member experienced low deployment preparedness, deployed without their unit, encountered perceived threats (vulnerability), and had long or multiple deployments (James et al., 2013; Ursano et al., 2016, 2018).

Self-reported PTSD symptomology noticed during deployment has been documented to be approximately 9%, but, when there are further medical examinations during post-deployment and reintegration, the numbers increase to at least 22% (Ursano et al., 2016). Agimi et al. (2019) estimate the highest number of blast events resulting in TBI rates of 20% to be found among deployed Marines and Army soldiers; although data for RC Marines and Army soldier members continue to be reviewed (Ursano et al., 2016, 2018). The combination of PTSD and depression often co-occur, especially after a mild TBI (Agimi et al., 2019). Depression is higher in RCs with a history of childhood adversity (Rudenstine et al., 2015). Tasseff and Nies (2017) noted that obese RC veterans living in rural areas, diagnosed with PTSD, TBI, and depression, are two times more likely to develop Alzheimer's disease or dementia.

Societal Concerns

Historically RC enlisted, especially Army and Marine Corp, personnel have reported an incidence of heavy weekly alcohol intake (>15 drinks for men and >7 drinks for women) before deployment (Ursano et al., 2016). Low preparedness for combat zone experiences during deployment sometimes changed alcohol patterns to daily binge drinking (>6 drinks), especially in RC enlisted men (>23%) and women (13%; Ursano et al., 2018). This rate rose even higher (up to 61%) if the RC member was not deployed with their regular unit. Behavioral health problems also occurred more frequently

(Ursano et al., 2018). If PTSD, military sexual trauma (MST), or relationship problems were present, while working in a primary male work environment, high rates of alcohol consumption were also present and troublesome for enlisted RC women (>15%; Conard & Armstrong, 2018; Osborne et al., 2012; Ursano et al., 2016). Difficulty falling asleep, nightmares, chronic pain, and trying to stay asleep were additionally reported as influencing increased alcohol consumption (Lapham et al., 2012).

Both Possis et al. (2014) and Bullman et al. (2017) compiled reviews of problematic driving behaviors in veterans (44%–45%) noting that both men and women, including RC members, engaged in more risks and incurred more motor vehicle and motorcycle accidents than the general population. These findings were documented after the Vietnam War, following Operation Enduring Freedom (OEF)/Operation Iraqi Freedom (OIF)/Operation New Dawn (OND), and in many United Kingdom veterans (Possis et al., 2014). Although more motor vehicular accidents (MVAs) usually occur six or more months after deployment; during Gulf War I 23% of non-battle deaths from MVA occurred while deployed (Bullman et al., 2017, p. 634). Several factors affected this phenomenon including deployment, behavioral health issues (especially TBI), as well as military driver training which emphasized "offensive driving, tactical awareness, and situational threats" (Goldbach & Castro, 2016). Fear, anger (78%), aggression (>28%), and thrill/sensation seeking (25%) are also cited as contributing factors (Bullman et al., 2017; Possis et al., 2014).

In any situation, suicide is tragic and there are often few answers or explanations. Deployed RC men and women have reported increased rates of suicidal thoughts, considerations, and/or plans (ideations), and non-fatal, self-directed actions with/or without injury (attempts), when compared with their full-time military counterparts (Bohnert et al., 2017; Pruitt et al., 2019). For these incidences, often drugs/alcohol (56%) are used (Pruitt et al., 2019). Since 2000, the number of actual suicides committed by MSMs has increased and now exceeds the U.S. civilian population (Pruitt et al., 2019). Deaths from suicide in never-deployed former RC members has also increased with 902 RC suicides occurring in 2016 (VA, 2018b). In those who committed suicide, 49% had behavioral health disorders, 25% had substance abuse, and 23% had adjustment disorders (Pruitt et al., 2019). Branch of service also seems to factor into veteran suicidality, as can be noted in Table 8.1.

The Army, with the largest amount of MSMs, had the highest incidence (Pruitt et al., 2019). Among National Guard members, especially the Army National Guard, the rate of suicide was also elevated when compared to the suicide rate of the U.S. adult population. Both accessibility and knowledge of firearms were noted in almost 65% of these veteran suicides (men 71% and women 41%; Pruitt et al., 2019). Most of the firearms were personally owned (94%) rather than military-issued weapons (Pruitt et al., 2019).

Before 2015, almost 64% of those who committed suicide had sought some type of healthcare but presently about that same number have not sought VHA care (VA, 2018b). Yet, nearly a quarter (23.4%) of those individuals who died by suicide reached out and communicated their thoughts or desire to take their own life in the 90 days prior to their death. This included talking, writing, or

TABLE 8.1 SUICIDES ACCORDING TO SERVICE BRANCH 2018

SERVICE BRANCH	FULL-TIME MILITARY	RESPECTIVE RESERVIST
Army	138	162
Marines	58	18
Navy	68	11
Air Force	58	3
Total	322	194

SOURCE: From Pruitt, L. D., Smolenski, D. J., Bush, N. E., Tucker, J., Issa, F., Hoyt, T. V., & Regert, M. A. (2019). Suicide in the military: Understanding rates and risk factors across the United States Armed Forces. *Military Medicine, 184*(3/4), 432–437. https://doi.org/10.1093/milmed/usy296

texting/emailing others about these thoughts (Pruitt et al., 2019). That is why healthcare providers should thoroughly assess for suicide risk in veterans with every encounter (Mallin, 2019), as reducing a veteran's risk before reaching a crisis point should be a priority, as well as supporting those veterans when they are in crisis (Department of Veterans Affairs, Veterans Health Administration, Office of Mental Health and Suicide Prevention, 2018).

For the DoD and the VA, the topic of suicide is an immense and troublesome priority with significant public health efforts in full force. At the time of publication, the VA is operating a mobile Vet Center to increase access to behavioral health services for National Guard and Reserve members. Locations can be found at the VA Directory. In addition, Vet Center staff can be reached 24-hours a day at 877-WAR-VETS (927-8387) (VA, 2018b). The President's Advisory Office of Science and Technology and the VA have formed a taskforce, known as PREVENTS (President's Roadmap to Empower Veterans, and End a National Tragedy of Suicide), to empower veterans and prevent suicides (Mallin, 2019).

Homelessness is another social problem for the RC (IOM, 2013). Veterans comprise approximately 25% of the total homeless population, with 47% serving during Vietnam, and roughly 5% serving in Iraq and Afghanistan (Guina, 2020). It is believed that almost all (89%) were honorably discharged from the military (Guina, 2020). In RC members, issues related to alcohol abuse and difficulty reintegrating after deployment place them at higher risk for homelessness and engagement in criminal acts associated with survival (IOM, 2013). Concerns for the homeless should "not be only for shelter, but also for an examination of an identification and amelioration of the risk factors such as employment, health care, social services, education, and outreach, including psychiatric and substance-use disorders" (IOM, 2013, p. 339).

MILITARY WOMEN

Recognition of Florence Nightingale's work of providing care for the military wounded in the Crimea took a long time but once it was provided, her honored contributions were remembered. Our nation's response to nurses, including women in general, serving in the military has been similar. What we know now is that historically many women who served as nurses contributed fearlessly in every one of this nation's conflicts, wars, and humanitarian efforts, although for their service they often did so without recognition and compensation. During the Revolutionary War (1775–1783), General Washington obtained Congressional approval to have one nurse provide care to every 10 wounded soldiers in military hospitals ("A History of Nurses in the Military," n.d). In the War of 1812 and the Civil War (1861–1865), when women responded to the recruitment pleas offering to provide nursing care, they had to beg to become involved, falsify their names, lie about their gender, and/or wear men's clothing ("A History of Nurses in the Military," n.d.; Ayaz, 2013). As with all of these contributions by women, during and after their care services were provided, their work became appreciated, yet they were not rendered the usual value symbols of recognition commiserate of the military organization such as a uniform and salary as the men in the military.

For this section about military women, the theme of military uniforms is incorporated to demonstrate the sluggish timeline of official integration of military women. The ability to wear the military uniform is more than a putting on a piece of clothing. It symbolizes a sense of identity, signifying that the organization that one is working for believes that the person who is wearing the uniform is a valued part of that organization. Thus, the presence of a uniform, is an important observable military sign symbolizing belonging, distinction, visibility (and/or camouflage), protection, and validation of worth for the service member (Ayaz, 2013). The journey to finally receiving military uniforms took over 125 years for women.

Over 1,500 "contract nurses" provided healthcare during the Spanish-American War (1898), yet they wore no uniforms for two reasons: first, they were private contractors and second, because there were no uniforms to issue. Fortunately, their worthy contributions of healthcare did move the U.S. War

Department (a precursor to the DoD) to establish a permanent Nurse Corps within the Army Medical Department in 1901, under the Army Reorganization Act. In that same year, Army nurses became the first women to officially enter the military (Ayaz, 2013). After their military induction, in contrast to floor length white dresses with aprons civilian nurses were still wearing, these initial military women received dresses commonly a foot off the ground and styled like the man's uniform. Later in World War I (1917–1918), nearly 25,000 women served (Ayaz, 2013). They were mostly nurses and also the first to be assigned wool utilitarian dress uniforms for their roles.

In 1920, nurses officially obtained insignia, although for a limited rank system of Second Lieutenant through Major, addressed only as "Miss," and received half the pay of their male counterparts (Ayaz, 2013). Equal pay was achieved in 1930. During World War II (1941–1945), over 350,000 women served. While nurses still comprised the most substantial women's military occupation and were issued specific white dress uniforms, for the first time women also served in the Army, Navy, and Marine Corps as administrators, secretaries, architects, pilots, and communications specialists. For some positions, women were even allowed to wear slacks (U.S. Army News, 2019). Around 7,000 women, including 1,500 nurses deployed for the Korean War (1950–1953). Men, serving as nurses, were allowed military commissions in 1955 (Ayaz, 2013).

Equality momentum was further achieved in 1959 when the U.S. Army issued solid green field uniforms for both men and women, although the design was still greatly influenced by the attire of men. This was followed by the 1967 signing of Public Law 90-130 by President Lyndon B. Johnson finally providing equal benefits, promotions, and retirement for women and men service members. This law also offered a smoother transition for women to serve in the Army RC.

Despite controversial discussions related to drafting nurses during the Vietnam War (1964–1973), over 11,000 women were "allowed" to volunteer; 80% of them were military nurses (Schwartz, 1987). Yet, their presence was under the legislated cap of women (2%; David & Woods, 1999). The passage of the Equal Rights Amendment in 1972 prompted the Pentagon to diligently review and rescind other discriminatory policies (Ganzer, 2016; Gurung et al., 2018; Jacobson & Jensen, 2011). Designers of the all-volunteer U.S. military system in 1973 started to more fully view women as a valuable group to comprise the new model of the Armed Forces; their numbers rose from 1.6% at that time to 8.5% by 1980 (Davis & Woods, 1999). By the mid-1970s, regulations included allowances for women to serve during their pregnancy but without official maternity uniforms. Pregnant women were required to revert to civilian attire, offsetting them from their uniformed colleagues. This remained until maternity uniforms were approved for wear in the late 1970s (Bemis, 2017).

During Gulf War I (1991), military women comprised 9% of the deployed force (41,000) and for the first time held wide-ranging occupations beyond the usual healthcare and logistical support (D'Aoust et al., 2017). Their specific gender attire finally began to reflect their significant occupational activities as they were issued the same universal camouflage uniforms of their service branch, as their male counterparts (Conard & Armstrong, 2018). Since Post-9/11, almost 500,000 women have served in the U.S. military in support of the Iraq and Afghanistan Wars (2001–2014).

Yet despite this integration of women in the military, there remains a meaningful lack of focus on the health/safety needs of women in uniform (Ganzer, 2016; Gurung et al., 2018; Jacobson & Jensen, 2011). Expectations remained that military uniforms, personal protective gear, and field equipment that men use would also be sufficient for women (Conard & Armstrong, 2018, 2019). This premise was still apparent with the first issue of 16-pound Interceptor Body Armor in 2003 that had been designed for men. Historically, the equipment left women without functional accommodations for differing body shape and needs of women. Not until 2018 did the DoD present body armor plates to accommodate women's breasts (Female Improved Tactical Vest), and ballistic helmets to better accommodate women's hairstyles (Sisk, 2018). Additionally, the tactics employed in Iraq and Afghanistan wars increased the exposure to blast injuries leading to TBI and musculoskeletal injuries. Thus, the lethality of the battle environments became evident in the 160 deaths of women that occurred during the OIF and OEF campaigns (Eaton et al., 2011). During this same time, over 400 combat injuries to women occurred in OIF; almost the same number of women suffered combat-related injuries in OEF (Dye et al., 2016). With women in the military serving in combat occupations, combat-related injuries are expected to increase.

The number of women serving in the military continues to increase in both the full-time (>211,000, 16.2%) and RC components (>160,000, 19.6%; DoD, 2017). Military uniforms (and physical fitness standards) continue to be part of the equality and productivity discussion for military women. Newly designed Army combat uniforms that more closely correspond to female soldier dimensions are now approved. Upon request, they can be worn by either gender (Montgomery, 2012). In addition, the new Army Physical Training testing will not have different requirements. The same minimum standards for men and women will be present for each exercise activity, eliminating segregated training (U.S. Department of Army, 2018).

Health Concerns

Increased responsibilities for military women in their service branch occupations have produced "unique readiness, deployment, and post deployment issues, not only to their biological makeup but also to their societal roles ... as they go to war and perform other duties as assigned" (Davis & Woods, 1999, p. 6/9). For full-time military personnel, constant expectations are to be ready for deployment, frequent family/loved one separation, participation in numerous field exercises, and persistent alert status. This continual pressure does affect well-being, evident since military women face many similar health issues as their counterparts. They are predisposed to numerous health, physical, and behavioral concerns; whether active duty, deployed, and/or veterans. Other health concerns are unique to women.

During Gulf War I (1991), some military women were exposed to hazardous agents and now they are part of the 25% to 33% of troops (>210,000) affected with what still is sometimes referred to as Gulf War Illness/Syndrome, a signature, or distinctive, wound of that war (Conard & Armstrong, 2019). The airborne hazards, as well as burn-pits accelerated with jet fuel (Jet Propellant 8), often burned for hours each day giving off black clouds of toxic soot and offensive fumes (Szema et al., 2017). To date, these Gulf War I men and women veterans continue to report these symptoms and have accessed care through various health facilities. The VHA has chosen to call this illness/syndrome chronic multisymptom illness (CMI), mainly because 30 years after the war there is not a clear definition, etiology, terminology, and clinical management of this Gulf War Syndrome (Conard & Armstrong, 2019). Gulf War I women are reported to have a higher CMI prevalence (8.4%) than their male counterparts (4.2%; Mohanty et al., 2019), as well as the possibility of different biomarkers of illness (Coughlin, 2016).

This hazardous agent situation with exposure to the open burn pits also occurred during the Iraq and Afghanistan Wars, when trash and feces were burned at a time when no other sanitation methods were available (VA, 2013). Unfortunately, the effects of exposure to burn pits are still emerging for both the Gulf War I, as well as the veteran population from OEF/OIF, much like the emerging health issues faced by first responders to the New York and Washington, DC Post-9/11 terror attacks. Since 2012, the VHA has been soliciting veterans to participate in a national registry used for both symptom and disease tracking among these populations (VA, 2013).

In addition, the severe environments found in Iraq and Afghanistan, coupled with close quarter working conditions, convoy operations, and the absence of toilet facilities, often resulted in women suffering from dehydration and urinary tract infections (50%). This was one of the most common health risks for deployed women (Conard & Armstrong, 2018). Troops operating in hot and humid field conditions needed to hydrate continually, although women often shunned drinking large amounts of water due to concerns about avoiding unnecessary disrobing to urinate. The female urinary diversion device (FUDD), partially designed and promoted by nurses, was first introduced to a group of women deployed in 2009 as a means for urinating while standing up. This device has been well received by women in the military and has resulted in reductions in heat injuries and urinary tract infections. Women in many of the service branches now receive a FUDD as a standard component of their military field equipment issue (Steele, 2016).

Almost 80% of women serving in Iraq and Afghanistan wars were within reproductive range of 18 to 40 years of age, so gynecological issues were an important consideration (Conard & Armstrong, 2019). Menstruation issues were compounded during long combat zone deployments in austere conditions. With some military support, alternatives for military women included consistent long-acting reversible contraceptives, not only as a method of birth control but also for menstruation cessation. Intrauterine devices and hormonal implants were other options that could provide service for an extended period without requiring user action. Unfortunately, the austere environments of Iraq and Afghanistan, the lack of education about contraceptive options, and the lack of supplies often prevented the desired compliance of the hormone implants and intrauterine device availability (Conard & Armstrong, 2018). Increased education for women service members, leadership command, and healthcare personnel was implemented, including specific content for combat medics providing gynecological care for women in the field environments (Conard & Armstrong, 2018). There also was an increased risk for candida/bacterial vaginitis, which led to the "development and implementation of a self-diagnostic kit designed by a team of nurses" (Conard & Armstrong, 2018, p. 161).

In certain situations, women who become pregnant in a combat zone may be subject to punishment under the Uniformed Code of Military Justice (Burrelli, 2013). Military policy prohibits pregnant women from serving in combat, or in overseas hazardous duty stations. Such regulations are intended to protect all concerned parties, including the unborn child from the environmental and operational stressors such as trauma, hazardous fumes, and death. During the Iraq and Afghanistan wars, an estimated 10% of deployed women became pregnant while an estimated 2% were medically evacuated due to their pregnancy (Braun et al., 2016).

The diagnosis of PTSD has become the second most commonly reported service-connected disability among all disabled veterans (30%–100%). Experiencing 18-hour workdays over weeks, or even months while remaining on alert, or survival mode, can produce a tremendous drain on the body and mind. It is also one of the factors thought to increase the prevalence of PTSD (Bruner & Woll, 2012; Stern, 2017). From the Iraq and Afghanistan wars there is further evidence that a woman's reaction to trauma and injury can be problematically different with an increased occurrence of PTSD (21%) and other behavioral health issues among veteran women (Conard & Armstrong, 2018; Williams et al., 2018). Pulverman et al. (2019) report that women who sustained childhood abuse, and then were assaulted during their military service, were over six times more likely to be diagnosed with PTSD. A significant relationship between fibromyalgia in women veterans and PTSD/depression was documented in a 2017 pilot study (D'Aoust et al., 2017). While TBI has been observed and studied frequently in military men during and following deployments, actual numbers for military women remain difficult to ascertain. In 2019, one study quantified 12.6%, or over 17,066, verified cases of TBI in women (Agimi et al., 2019). This is a long-term concern as anyone with mild TBI has a two-fold increased chance of developing dementia (Agimi et al., 2019).

Sexual assault, or repeated, threatening sexual harassment, also referred to as MST, occurring in the military setting remains a significant public health issue (Pulverman et al., 2019). Early reports of MST were first disclosed during the Vietnam War, followed by several non-war incidents, although the most frequent prevalence began to surface during the prolonged Iraq and Afghanistan Wars (Conard & Armstrong, 2018; Schwartz, 1987). Overall, more military women (20%–25%) than men (<2%) reported their sexual assault and/or harassment, yet when the total number of military men are considered, MST affects both women and men with almost the same prevalence (Kelly et al., 2014). Many believe that 80% to 90% of MST incidents are still not reported (Conard & Armstrong, 2018; IOM, 2013). Military women risk factors for MST include young ages (19 years or less when joining), enlisted ranks, and previous civilian sexual assaults (Marino et al., 2019). In 2019, several DoD Annual Reports on Sexual Assault in the Military noted an upward trend of reported MST among active duty service members. They attribute these increases to the implementation of new reporting options that are easier to complete, allow anonymity, and afford confidential support with physical examination services (Marino et al., 2019).

Any veteran who has experienced MST is entitled to free care from the VHA for both associated physical and behavioral health problems (Surís et al., 2016). On-going research continues to document that MST is linked to PTSD, depression, anxiety disorders, substance abuse, and suicide, as well as liver and chronic pulmonary disease, AIDS exposure, and weight-related problems such as obesity (Marino et al., 2019; Street et al., 2008, 2009). Women veterans have reported longer lasting and higher rates of sexual pain if they had a history of childhood sexual abuse and then were sexually assaulted in the military, when compared to their civilian counterparts (Pulverman et al., 2019). Their findings include, "those abused as children were 1.75 times more likely to have developed sexual pain, those ... assaulted during military service were 2.37 times more likely ... while ... abused as children and assaulted in the military were 4.33 times more likely to have developed sexual pain" (Pulverman et al., 2019, p. 66).

MST continues to be a troublesome concern for the DoD that prides itself on discipline and orderly conduct. Federal law protects claimants from retaliation and subversion carried out by any member of the Armed Forces (Jacobson & Jensen, 2011). Mandatory education focused on MST, and the potential consequences offenders could face, was implemented in all branches. This DoD-wide training was extended to leaders of the VHA and DoD civilian contractors (Lucas et al., 2018). In addition, the VHA has increased MST treatment access and education for their medical providers on signs, symptoms, and treatment available for all veterans suspected or known to be a MST victim (Lucas et al. 2018). As with other veteran behavioral health issues, same day Mental Health Assessment is available daily in VHA facilities, and 24/7 by telephone (Lucas et al., 2018).

Depression is common in women veterans resulting from their mobilization experiences (Sairsingh et al., 2018). Military women have cited problems when leaving family, children, and elder caregiving responsibilities before deployment. Situational factors during deployments included military women being increasingly present in combat zone environments, while working in a highly structured and male-dominated environment. Some military women have reported trying to blend in with their military counterparts, working twice as hard to please, feeling "defective," not pulling their weight, an "imposter" or compartmentalizing their experiences during their deployment time, while attempting to avoid issues like traumatic stress, military violence, and substance use (Bruner & Woll, 2012, p. 128). As veterans, their two major indicators for depressive symptomology are lack of social support and financial comfort while they are balancing work and family demands after deployments. Divorce rates are 2.5 times higher for military women than the national average (Sairsingh et al., 2018). In addition, the presence of these interpersonal stressors that have contributed to behavioral health issues often compound many of their gender specific gynecological, urological, and reproductive situations (Conard & Armstrong, 2018). Lifetime depression rates for women veterans remain high (29%) when compared to veteran men (16%), and further increased when women veterans have been abused as children and then assaulted in the military (Pulverman et al., 2019). They tend also to have increased hospitalizations for a psychiatric illness (Pulverman et al., 2019).

SPECIFIC HEALTH CONCERNS OF RESERVE COMPONENT WOMEN

In addition to the general health concerns of military women as presented, RC women have specifically reported numerous post-deployment challenges. Similar to their male counterparts, female RC members take care of themselves only after their family/home life cohesion has stabilized (Randall, 2011; Messecar, 2017; Osborne et al., 2012). Over 15% of RC women either started, or continued to smoke cigarettes heavily during deployment, due to ease of access, reduced costs, and stressful milieus (Conard & Armstrong, 2018). In one study, RC women explained their situational problems that propelled them to start/continue smoking during reintegration including complexity of their life, the loss of their military role, [personal] deployment changes, reestablishing partner connections, and being a mom again (Kelly et al., 2014). These themes from their situational problems were difficult for them as they were facing reintegrating in isolation, missing the camaraderie of those who had shared the experiences of deployment, and their families'/communities' unawareness of the deployment realities (Kelly et al., 2014).

Compared to RC men, RC women have reported higher rates of sexual harassment (>27% vs. 60%) and sexual assault (1.6% vs. >13%) (Street et al., 2008, 2009). The RC women who suffered these experiences are reporting poorer health outcomes 10 years later, when compared with those who were not involved in MST (Conard & Armstrong, 2018). Lower rank enlisted (Private or Seaman) RC women have even more unique challenges with this traumatic experience due to their junior status, work situations, lack of supportive resources, and the ability to rally prompt supportive legal/medical attention (Conard & Armstrong, 2018; Osborne et al., 2012).

Societal Concerns

Overall, suicides, a sensitive topic about the self-directed injurious behavior with intent to die, differ in the military from the civilian population in age and gender, with service members younger and often male (Pruitt et al., 2019). As the number of women in the military is increasing, so are the numbers of suicides in female veterans, especially if they were in the Army, were not involved with VHA care, and/or have experienced MST (Kimerling et al., 2016; Priuitt et al., 2019). The latter factor is a relatively new dimension perhaps not evidenced until more recently as women veterans have remained under-represented in the VHA system (Kimerling et al., 2016). When compared to their civilian counterparts, suicides are 1.8 times more likely to occur in women veterans (VA, 2018b). "In 2016, firearms were used in 41.2% of suicide deaths among women veterans compared to 32.4% of suicide deaths among non-veteran women" (Office of Mental Health and Suicide Prevention, 2019, p. 2). The lower risk for suicides among women veterans using the VHA system could be due to the incorporation of the VHA behavioral health enhancement initiatives and suicide prevention programs, as well as the wide-ranging, gender-specific women's health services for MST (Kimerling et al., 2016). Answers to the many "why" questions about military/veteran related suicides remain unanswered while the DoD and VHA continue deliberate assessments during both deployments and reintegration.

While this information is limited and difficult to obtain, women veterans unfortunately, when compared with their military counterparts (1%), are steadily becoming an increasing part of the homelessness population (IOM, 2013). As of 2018, their numbers hover around 7% and are expected to rise to 9% (40,000) by 2025 (Richman, 2018). When homeless, their children are often with them whether they are staying with family/friends, in shelters, or living outside. Risk factors are numerous including having a positive PTSD screen, MST incidences, anxiety disorders, overall fair or poor health, childhood adversity, post-military abuse, ruined relationship(s), and/or under/unemployment (Richman, 2018). Recognizing the complex situations that were, or are present, it is suggested that health providers emphasize how different resources and interventions can assist or remove some of the multiple experiences that are making it difficult to develop better housing outcomes rather than centering on the housing instability or the previous/present trauma (Richman, 2018).

Veterans Health Administration Services for Women

Congressional mandates in the mid-1980s opened VHA services for healthcare to women veterans in the late 1980s. Since then, frequent legislative hearings continue to investigate the lack of a full complement of gender services for female veterans (Conard & Armstrong, 2018; Ganzer, 2016; Jacobson & Jensen, 2011). Military women now comprise 10% or 2 million of the more than 19 million total population of veterans in the United States with demographics that are different from their military counterparts; they are younger, have a higher education level, and represent a greater percentage of minorities (Stern, 2017). They are slowly becoming more of an integral part of major military health reviews and VHA studies although the documentation of their injuries and wounds seem to have been collected at different times (IOM, 2013). For example, their physical injuries often occurred while deployed, although most of the information about their psychosocial and behavioral concerns seems to be collected after they were veterans (IOM, 2013).

Service-connected health problems common among women veterans of the Post-9/11 era are now far ranging and often severe, begging the questions of deployment exposure and/or time of detection (IOM, 2013; Street et al., 2009). Nurses should familiarize themselves with the locations of VHA facilities in their region, and the services provided at these locations. In cases where the veteran's healthcare needs cannot be met within the scope of services of the VHA, a community specialist should provide the veteran with care. This care can be coordinated and paid for by the VHA through the community care department of the VHA. Clinical case managers who are RNs that work exclusively in this line of veteran care manage community care. As a result of their service, women's disability claims filed with the Veterans Benefits Administration (VBA) in the fiscal year 2015 increased from a Pre-9/11 rate of 48% to 63%. More than half of the current women veteran population hold a service-connected disability rating from the VBA with the most common being tinnitus, resulting in a maximum 10% disability (Stern, 2017). Other frequently reported disability claims relate to hearing loss, PTSD, depression, genitourinary disease, musculoskeletal injury, and TBI (VA, 2016).

LGBT IN THE MILITARY

Collectively known with the four-letter umbrella acronym of LGBT, which "inclusively recognizes the military's range of sexual orientation and gender identity minorities," (IOM, 2011; VA, 2019d, para. 1). Everyone has a sexual orientation whether there is a "(1) relative attraction to same-sex individuals, (2) sexual activity with same-sex individuals, and/or (3) sexual identity (lesbian, gay, or bisexual)" (Meadows et al., 2018, p. 1). Each person also has a gender identity. Often the term cisgender refers to people who identify with the sex they were born with (Margolies & Brown, 2019). While civilians include Q meaning queer, as in LGBTQ, the DoD (2019d) acknowledges there are many terms associated with sexual orientation identity and sexual gender identity and prefers the veteran to use the term that best suits them. Importantly, their varied differences include race, ethnicity, age, socioeconomic level (Centers for Disease Control and Prevention [CDC], 2018), religion, culture, language, disability (physical or behavioral), sex, sexual orientation, or gender identity or expression (VHA Office of Patient Care Services & Office of Health Equity, 2014). Each subgroup is distinct with their own unique experiences and health needs (IOM, 2011; Levesque, 2015). It is difficult to determine the exact number of LGBT individuals because there is no gender-neutral language on state or national surveys or health record intake forms (Levesque, 2015). Current estimates of LGBT service members in the military are 6.1% (Meadows et al., 2018).

Historically, the *Don't Ask, Don't Tell* (DADT) policy was intended to assist the LGBT military group but instead created a communication barrier for service members to openly discuss their specific health needs regarding sexual orientation or transgender identity with their healthcare providers. They feared being discharged from the military and their military healthcare providers could not ask or discuss their situations with them (Shrader et al., 2017). The DADT exclusion also seemed to imply that understanding the health needs of this population was a low priority (Goldbach & Castro, 2016). Almost 10,000 service members left during this time, which represented a costly loss of valuable manpower as well as $22,000 to $43,000 per person for processing DADT-related discharges (Gates, 2010).

After the policy was repealed in 2011, the silence was broken, and now LGBT service members who meet readiness standards can serve openly. Currently Section 3 of the Federal Defense of Marriage Act allows military providers to care for the unique health needs of the LGBT group as well as their same-sex spouses (Campbell et al., 2017). These policies have provided an important step toward equality in the military; although the LGBT service members remain very cautious and cognizant, believing that any health disparities could affect their military readiness (Meadows et al., 2018). They are also aware that senior military and political officials could influence their military presence.

LGBT Defined

Lesbian (women) and gay (men) individuals are usually attracted to people of the same sex (Margolies & Brown, 2019). Bisexual persons may be attracted to both genders. Transgender identity refers to people experiencing a different gender from their sex at birth (Meadows et al., 2018) known as natal gender. Some may have a desire to outwardly convey the gender they desire, or connect with their gender identity (Landry, 2017). An individual assigned the male gender at birth but identifies as a woman is defined as a transfemale (male to female [MtF]; Folaron & Lovasz, 2016). Conversely, a transmale (female to male [FtM]) is assigned the female gender at birth but identifies as a male. This may include classification as heterosexual or bisexual (Margolies & Brown, 2019). Suppressing the effects of the sex assigned at birth and replacing them with those of the desired sex is the goal of hormone treatment (Hyderi et al., 2017).

LGB IN THE MILITARY

While figures remain difficult to obtain, it is believed that more than 2.2% of men in active duty military are LGB, with higher numbers in the RC (>4%; Gates, 2010). More LGB women serve in the military, with estimates as high as 43% when compared to their civilian counterparts. Gates (2010) projected that lifting the DADT restrictions would result in increases of the LGB full-time military personnel by at least 40,000 and another 9,000 in the RC, although the outcomes of these projections have been difficult to locate.

TRANSGENDER IN THE MILITARY

As of 2014, there were approximately 15,500 transgender members reported to be serving in the military (Eisenala, 2014). While some may not desire any physical changes, others are seeking gender-affirming interventions such as hormone therapy that, with careful monitoring, can begin while in the military. Not unlike other service members and veterans, the LGB community also face similar health risks including depression and anxiety, alcohol/substance abuse, tobacco use, sexually transmitted infections (STIs), obesity, eating disorders, heart disease, intimate partner violence (IPV), and MST (VA, 2019b).

Male to Female

For males transitioning to females, feminizing hormone treatments such as antiandrogens and estrogens can be administered, with the desired changes beginning in 1 month and the maximum effect taking 3 years or longer to attain (Folaron & Lovasz, 2016). The effects include breast growth, redistribution of body fat, reduction in muscle mass and body hair, sweat and body odor changes, and a decrease in erectile function, testicle size, and sperm production (Deutsch, 2019). Feminizing medications may also produce and/or increase kidney disease so signs of diabetes and high blood pressure should always be assessed (VA, 2019d).

Female to Male

For females transitioning to males the administration of exogenous testosterone is common (Folaron & Lovasz, 2016). Desired changes may be apparent in 1 month, but maximum effect may take 5 years or longer to attain (Folaron & Lovasz, 2016). The effects include development of facial and body hair, voice changes, increase in muscle mass, clitoral growth, and cessation of menses (Deutsch, 2019).

Generally, these interventions help adjust one's body to closely match an individual's desired gender identity (Levesque, 2015). Yet for either transition, close physical and laboratory monitoring are required, especially during the first year of treatment of hormone therapy (Folaron & Lovasz, 2016). This monitoring of hormone levels and assessing for adverse effects, such as screening for cancer, blood clots, edema, high blood sugar, and high blood pressure, are crucial for optimal health. These negative sequelae may also affect military readiness and deployability (Folaron & Lovascz, 2016).

Further Transgender Surgical Procedures

For the transfemale (male to female [MtF]), common surgeries include orchidectomy and vaginoplasty. Breast augmentation may be delayed for 2 to 3 years to maximize breast development from feminizing hormone treatment (Wang & Kim, 2019). Surgeries for the FtM population include hysterectomy and oophorectomy so detection of any gynecological malignancies may be difficult. Clitoral hypertrophy from hormonal treatment may be sufficient to serve as a phallus (Folaron & Lovasz, 2016), otherwise a phalloplasty could be performed. Pregnancy is still possible if FtM patients are having sex with fertile males (Hyderi et al., 2017). During each one of these gender-affirming procedures, the prostate is usually left intact to avoid incontinence and urethral stricture complications, so cancer risks remain (Metzler, 2019). Gender confirming surgical procedures are expensive so are not being performed, or paid for, by the DoD or the VHA (VA, 2018a).

Health and Societal Concerns

The military group of LGBT military personnel have faced significant, numerous, and varied challenges while serving their country, as well as when they enter veteran status (Meadows et al., 2018). In addition, many LGBT service members have faced societal stigma and discrimination due to a lack of awareness from healthcare providers, as well as insensitivity to their unique needs (VHA Office of Patient Care Services & Office of Health Equity, 2014). Now they may have increased health risks, when compared with non-LGBT members, along with unique healthcare challenges such as (a) lower health status overall, (b) lower rates of both routine and preventive care, (c) higher rates of substance abuse including smoking and alcohol, (d) higher rates of traumatic experiences, (e) higher risk for mental health conditions including anxiety and depression, (f) higher rates of sexually transmitted diseases, (g) increased occurrence of some cancers, and (h) heart disease (CDC, 2018; Office of Disease Prevention and Health Promotion, 2019; Substance Abuse and Mental Health Services Administration [SAMSA], 2012; VA, 2019c; VA, 2019d; VHA Office of Patient Care Services & Office of Health Equity, 2014). Sexually transmitted infections (STIs) such as syphilis, gonorrhea, Chlamydia, pubic lice, as well as HIV, hepatitis, human papilloma virus, and herpes, also should be assessed frequently in all military members, as well as the LGBT group.

Within the VHA and their published directives, emphasis on *Do Ask, Do Tell* confirms LGBT service members should receive equitable, respectful, and affirming clinically appropriate healthcare (VA, 2019d). They should not be discriminated against for any reason, including sex, sexual orientation, gender identity or expression, and encompasses anyone the patient broadly defines to be family (VA, 2018a). To accommodate these directives, the VHA has established a LGBT Point-of-Contact program and care coordinator to provide staff education, advocate for a welcoming environment, and assist access to appropriate clinical services for LGBT veterans (Kauth et al., 2016). Any attempts to convert or change a veteran's sexual orientation by VHA staff is prohibited (VA, 2018a). In addition, other services for the LGBT group include hormone treatment, substance use/alcohol and tobacco treatment, prevention and care of STIs, IPV reduction and treatment, heart health, including cancer screening, prevention, and treatment (VA, 2019d).

LGB VETERANS

There are approximately 1 million LGB veterans in the United States (VA, 2019b). Among both gay and lesbian veterans, body image issues are common. More than their heterosexual counterparts, depression and anxiety affects both sexes of LGB, creating more susceptibility to chronic stress from discrimination, as well as greater risk for PTSD, IPV, and MST (VA, 2019b). In 2018, Lucas et al. documented that over 30% of lesbian veterans and 15% of gay veterans experienced an assault while in the military. Increased health, relationship, employment, and legal issues can result from the higher alcohol, substance, and tobacco use that is common in the LGB population (VA, 2019b). All of these risks may contribute to suicidal thoughts and attempts (VA, 2019b).

Lesbian service members have higher rates of obesity leading to other health problems such as lung disease, lung cancer, heart disease, and high blood pressure (VA, 2019b). Lesbian and bisexual women have a propensity for breast, ovarian, cervical, and uterine cancer risk, yet are less likely to get mammograms or regular pelvic exams compared to their heterosexual counterparts (VA, 2019d). Gay and bisexual men are at greater risk for prostate, testicular, colon, and anal cancer (VA, 2019d). They are also more likely to report erectile dysfunction than their heterosexual counterparts (Campbell et al., 2017).

TRANSGENDER VETERANS

The VA (2019c) reported that there are an estimated 135,000 veterans who identify as transgender, a community significantly larger (nine times greater) in the veteran population compared to non-veterans. Suicide related event rates are more than 20 times higher than those of non-transgender veterans (Blosnich et al., 2013). Medically necessary transgender care is currently offered in VHA facilities. Gender Dysphoria, "a mental health diagnosis defined as a marked incongruence between an individual's experienced or expressed gender and their assigned gender is necessary for available care" (Levesque, 2015, p. 9). After meeting these criteria, gender transitioning hormone therapy can be started. In addition, the transgender VHA member must have the capacity to make a fully informed decision and to consent to treatment and have a medical clearance by a mental health provider or other qualified health provider (VA, 2018a). Other VHA care such as behavioral health treatments and pre-operative evaluation, along with post-operative and long-term care, can be administered in support of the specific gender-confirming surgery.

PRIVATE MILITARY CONTRACTORS

Civilians have been employed by the military ever since America's earliest wars. Commonly called PMCs, these individuals are often considered "troop multipliers" and they have continued to be used exponentially in each U.S. conflict/war, implemented to support the fighting mission while trying to decrease the number of troops (Baker, 2014; Conard & Armstrong, 2019; Swed & Crosbie, 2019). During the Vietnam War, the estimated ratio was one PMC per six MSMs and "at the height of conflicts in Iraq and Afghanistan [2005-2011], PMCs outnumbered U.S. [military members] in both [combat zone environments] with 155,826 PMC alongside 152,275 U.S. [military members]" (Dungan et al., 2013, p. xiii). Their varied PMC services ranged from specialized computer, logistics, translation, tactical combat skills, and retired military officers in advisory roles, and even general transportation, security, construction, sanitation, dietary, and/or laundry work employment. During the reduction (draw down) of troops, PMCs also provide much of the policing, prison maintenance, and military education. Tour lengths of service are "highly fluid," dependent on need and position, ranging from a few weeks to the usual 6 to 7 months assignments. It is uncommon for PMCs to remain on site as long as 1 year (Dunigan et al., 2013, p. 29).

Significant information about the PMC presence is difficult to find, rarely mentioned, and often unacknowledged (Baker, 2014; Swed & Crosbie, 2019). They are sometimes referred to as "shadow forces, operating under the radar and in the shadow of their military counterpoints" (Dunigan et al., 2013, p. 28) Some of their contractual work is under the auspices of U.S. governmental agencies with regulated employment practices, while other private PMC companies are more unregulated (Baker, 2014; Dunigan et al., 2013) and therefore "not legally obligated to share information with the public on their actions, organization, or labor force" (Swed & Crosbie, 2019, para 9).

Two limited snapshots of demographic information are available from published surveys (Dunigan et al., 2013; Swed & Crosbie, 2019). The average age of PMCs is thought to be around 40 (66%) to 50 years of age (29%; Swed & Crosbie, 2019). Many PMCs are Americans, most are men, and because previous military experience is often a prerequisite for PMC duty, countless PMCs are former or retired U.S. military officers, and/or Special Forces veterans. At the height of their contracting use, they were providing service in over 50 nations and almost 70% carried weapons in their PMC duties (Dunigan et al., 2013). Dunigan et al. (2013) reported that many PMCs felt good about their deployment preparedness, especially those with previous military experience, yet even the PMCs were surprised about their combat exposure (73%).

Increased outsourcing for widespread military support is costly. Economically, extraordinary wages paid to PMCs by their employers have resulted in even higher rates charged to the DoD, costing billions of dollars in services (Baker, 2014). Legally, it becomes difficult to distinguish PMC as civilians when they are performing similar tasks as uniformed personnel, placing both the PMCs and actual military personnel (including Commanders) in difficult situations (Baker, 2014; Swed & Crosbie, 2019). In addition, there is the concern of PMC healthcare services and costs. The Defense Base Act of 1941 requires their employing organizations to have purchased Workmen's Compensation for them so injured PMCs receive coverage for medical costs, although some PMCs (21%) arrange for higher salaries rather than include healthcare as a supportive benefit (Dunigan et al., 2013). These healthcare negotiations can rebound for the PMC as there are increased reports of denials for PMC healthcare from the Defense Base Act personnel (Swed & Crosbie, 2019). The other expense relates to human costs. PMCs experienced similar visible and invisible wounds as their military counterparts when exposed to gunfire, improvised explosive device (IED)s, burn pit fires, and handling of human remains; they also became prisoners of war and victims of kidnappings (Baker, 2014; Dunigan et al., 2013). "PMCs with the DoD contracts were up to 4.5 times more apt to be killed than their military counterparts" (Dunigan et al., 2013, p. 42). Within 18 months of 2007 to 2008, there were 455 contractors killed and 15,787 injured. By 2011 the Department of Labor recorded over 51,000 PMC injury claims and through June 2013 over 4,000 contractor deaths were reported (Baker, 2014). Additional PMC costs included "direct budgetary expenses through federal subsidies to worker compensation, insurance companies, and projected higher costs to Medicare as they age" (Baker, 2014, p. 351).

Health Concerns

As with other groups in war-zone environments PMCs have reported that their major factors associated with injuries while serving were, "deployment preparedness, combat exposure, length of deployments (>7 months), and lack of supportive resources for stress" (Dunigan et al., 2013, p. 77). Transportation PMC workers were most often affected. Subsequently, PMCs reported higher behavioral health issues related to PTSD symptomology (25%), and depression (18%) than their military counterparts did. Around 10% cited high alcohol and daily tobacco use (37%), as well as TBI (10%), and general concerns related to respiratory, back pain, and hearing problems (39%). Almost 30% still had not reported seeking healthcare at the time of the 2013 Dunigan et al. survey. The reasons for not seeking care were similar to their military counterparts including, "costs, embarrassment, demonstrating signs of weakness, as well as living in small town and rural residences, with limited amount of qualified behavioral health workers" (Dunigan et al., 2013, p. 47).

Societal Concerns

While PMCs have played important roles supporting every U.S. military conflict, their increasing physical and behavioral health issues are troublesome, perhaps offsetting the advantages of excellent salaries. Substantial risk for PMCs in war zones is always present regardless of occupation, so increased preparedness and resiliency information about combat exposure is vital; during OEF/OEF/OND this was especially significant for transportation PMCs (Dunigan et al., 2013; Swed & Crosbie, 2019). Dunigan et al. (2013) argued that the PMC group needs better resources to cope with their health problems and significant barriers when trying to access behavioral health treatments. While many have had previous military service, often the VHA will only provide supportive care for the time they served directly in the military.

IMPLICATIONS FOR NURSING EDUCATION AND PRACTICE

The military strives for a structured, uniformed, organization but within and surrounding the Armed Forces are some major subgroups discussed in this chapter. Wherever the nurse is working there could be someone who is in the service, whether on a military installation, or a RC individual who might be working in the community, attending a trade/community/university education program, or presenting to the local health facility. Any type of MSM that is now a veteran likewise can be found in churches, schools, the neighborhood, as well as all of the various types of community health facilities. Their health issues could be similar to the dominant population of the military (men), while other specific health issues relate to the distinctive groups. As before, what can become different about these groups is the reasons, specific responses, the time of documentation/detection, and/or the increasing prevalence of their healthcare concerns (Oster et al., 2017). What will be important is to reach out to them wherever they may be, as a clinician and/or educator.

Advocacy for interprofessional care for all of these important groups is essential once there is a positive response to the question, "Have you ever served in the military?" (Conard & Armstrong, 2018, 2019). Providing assistance for these specific groups should begin with an assessment and discussion about both their prior military (including combat and/or trauma) experiences and/or their recent PMC exposures, especially with any new or lingering behavioral health issues. Veterans that are experiencing a myriad of physical and mental health issues require a collaborative approach to a thorough intake assessment. With the use of an interdisciplinary team of healthcare professionals their healthcare needs can be addressed, including behavioral health, social work, pharmacy, dietary, and nursing professionals (Misra-Hebert et al., 2015; Sayer et al., 2014). The efficacy of this process increases with a clear understanding of common post-deployment health issues and available community-based veteran resources (Ganzini et al., 2013; Koblinsky et al., 2014; Williams et al., 2018).

Another advocacy question to ask is where are they receiving their healthcare? Inquire also about previous VHA enrollment. If none, contact the social worker and work closely with the VHA enrollment office in their healthcare area. In some states, county VA office personnel are staffed and trained to assist with enrollment and eligibility determinations (Oster et al., 2017). Fragmentation of care diminishes continuity and coordination, often resulting in higher use of emergency departments, increased hospitalization, duplication of tests, and increased healthcare costs. In addition, fragmented care is associated with a greater likelihood of adverse effects and medical errors. Both men and women veterans with chronic conditions and mental health diagnoses are especially vulnerable to these consequences (Angel et al., 2018). Men, for instance, often avoid or decline prostate exams and discussing sexual health concerns with women providers, as with women veterans when dealing with men examining their gynecological health concerns. These preferences may lead the veteran to seek care from other providers, and worse, failing to ask for the care that they need. Regarding the RC personnel, applicable care assessment/interventions (see Box 8.1) for their reintegration into the civilian sector will also be important.

BOX 8.1

PATIENT-CENTERED, CULTURALLY COMPETENT, AND SENSITIVE CARE FOR RC VETERANS

In order to address this population's unique healthcare needs, the following are suggested:

Educational Tools
Code of Ethics for Nurses
Military Health History Pocket card
Information on roles and responsibilities of those in the Reserves and National Guard
Introduction of military culture with Green Zone Training

Personal Assessments
Awareness of biases in performance between full- and part-time military participants
Respectfulness of veterans who have fulfilled Reserves and National Guard obligations
Understanding of RC efforts with multiple deployments and reintegrations
Knowledge of RC veteran health concerns
Expertise related to unique RC veteran societal problems, such as unemployment, homelessness, and suicides
Differences in RC veteran gender-specific health issues
Spouse, loved one, and children responses to multiple deployments and associated reintegration

Nursing Approaches
Sensitive and welcoming nature
Providing a comfortable milieu, as well as gender specific, if needed
Inquire about military occupations and their experiences
Frequently assess for signature wounds of war; for example, PTSD, TBI, and MST
Assess behavioral health issues such as depression and suicide
Explore gynecological issues for RC women
Maintain multidisciplinary care coordination among healthcare providers
Promote routine preventive screenings re: pap smear and mammograms
Assess spouse, loved one, and children responses to RC obligations

MST, military sexual trauma; PTSD, posttraumatic stress disorder; RC, Reserve component; TBI, traumatic brain injury.

As military women continue to deploy into combat areas there will be increasing amounts of both non-battle and battle injuries, as well as loss of life (Osborne et al., 2012). Capitalizing on the strength of women and their tendency to seek out healthcare providers and facilities will be important. Applicable care assessment/interventions (see Box 8.2) for military women reintegration into the civilian sector will also be important.

Within the last decade women veterans have become the fastest growing segment of the VHA, yet within that system they often experience a lack of continuity of care and inadequate gynecological care. The result is that they are likely to use two healthcare systems for their specific needs (Conard & Armstrong, 2018; Harris et al., 2014; Osborne et al., 2012). These veterans have spoken loudly and repeatedly about the importance of medical services that are exclusively for women wherever they seek care, especially within the VHA (Osborne et al., 2012; Williams et al., 2018).

Veteran reluctance to be open with their care providers about many of their physical and behavioral health issues can present challenges. Continual assessment of these signature wounds (PTSD, TBI,

BOX 8.2

PATIENT-CENTERED, CULTURALLY COMPETENT, AND SENSITIVE CARE FOR WOMEN VETERANS

In order to address this population's unique healthcare needs, the following are suggested:

Educational Tools

Code of Ethics for Nurses
Military Health History Pocket card
Center for Women Veterans Toolkit
American Academy of Nursing Expert Panel, that is, Policy Briefs: MST (Marino et al., 2019)
Introduction of military culture with Green Zone Training

Personal Assessments

Awareness of your own biases of women in the military? In combat-readiness positions?
Respectfulness of women veterans
Knowledge of women veteran health concerns
Expertise of resources and data related to many of their societal problems as veterans, such as unemployment, homelessness, and suicides

Nursing Approaches

Sensitive and welcoming nature
Providing a comfortable and hopefully gender-specific milieu
Inquire about military occupations and their experiences
Frequently assess for signature wounds of war; for example, PTSD, TBI, and MST
Assess behavioral health issues such as depression and suicide
Explore gynecological issues
Maintain multidisciplinary care coordination among healthcare providers
Promote routine preventive screenings re: pap smear and mammograms
Assess family situations re: children and caregiving for elderly

MST, military sexual trauma; PTSD, posttraumatic stress disorder; TBI, traumatic brain injury.

depression, and MST) will be important at every veteran encounter, as historically their health needs peak several decades after their deployments. This will first require the establishment of trust with the veteran before there is a likelihood for therapeutic interactions (Ganzini et al., 2013). Whether they are accessing civilian or VHA healthcare services, encouragement and support are important as they may be thinking that any assistance becomes a sign of weakness when seeking care. Emphasize thoughts of "strength, courage and compassion as they should seek the care they so selflessly earned" and remind them that when they feel better, so do others around them (Randall, 2012, p. 16). Any initiation and/ or management of their current problems can assist future healthcare needs as later there are "higher rates of cardiovascular, gastrointestinal, autoimmune, and musculoskeletal system diseases, in addition to headaches" (El-Gabalawy et al., 2018, p. 850).

As discussed, it is imperative for healthcare providers to know and understand the definitions for the LGBT community, to include questions about sexual orientation and gender identity, and to become aware of the healthcare challenges faced by LGBT veterans in their assessment for better patient outcomes. Health literature, as well as the societal response, for this group is evolving so nurses need to continue to seek the latest research for evidence-based guidelines and culturally sensitive care.

Specific topics that might benefit further examination for the LGBT veteran community could be developed into continuing education presentations for them. Applicable care assessment/interventions (see Box 8.3) for LGBT reintegration into the civilian sector will also be important.

BOX 8.3

PATIENT-CENTERED, CULTURALLY COMPETENT, AND SENSITIVE CARE FOR THE LGBT COMMUNITY

In order to address this population's unique healthcare needs, the following are suggested:

Educational Tools

Code of Ethics for Nurses
ANA Position statement: Nursing advocacy for LGBTQ+ populations

Personal Assessments

Knowledge of your own biases
Knowledge of LGBT definitions
Familiarity with the ever-changing language of LGBT individuals (Kiely, 2017)

Nursing Approaches

Sensitive and welcoming nature
Providing a comfortable milieu
Use of proper pronoun when addressing the patient/client
Awareness that name and gender may not match on health records
Routine screening based on patient's assigned sex at birth:

- prostate

- Pap smear if no hysterectomy

- mammogram if no double mastectomy

Conscious screening depending on

- hormones therapy status and/or gender affirming surgeries

- breast surgery or hysterectomy

- prostate still in place (cancer)

ANA, American Nurses Association.

PMC data and research remain sparse so creating an applicable care assessment/interventions exhibit, as has been done for the other three groups discussed in this chapter, becomes problematic for a group in which more information is still needed (Swed & Crosbie, 2019). More knowledge about their work, social situations, culture, and associated regulations/structure would be assistive to close the information gap (Baker, 2014). Certainly, PMC deployment experiences vary with their circumstances (Dunigan et al., 2013), but further information about the barriers and facilitators of safely and better lines of communication within the combat zone environments between PMCs and MSMs will be important.

Nurse educators need to include specific cultural care aspects of the military member and veteran in their curriculum. Foremost, instill that patients should be asked if they have served in the military. Awareness and acknowledgment of military exposures and experiences are vital, so helping students become comfortable and interested in the service member/veteran situations will help to ensure proper healthcare. A valuable tool for all nurses and students is the Military Health History Pocket card for Healthcare Professional Trainees and Clinicians found at (va.gov/OAA/pocketcard). This tool also includes ways to establish rapport such as asking questions in a safe and private environment, with eye contact and a supportive tone of voice. This information is important not only for seeking out military/veteran situations for the didactic portion of the student's education, but also for the clinical portion where students will be caring for veterans in hospital and community settings. Creating ways to establish interprofessional care teams for collaborative approaches, as well as instructions for completing a thorough intake assessment, will yield critical information for care.

In addition, more than 800,000 veterans are currently using their GI benefits, with some of them enrolled in nursing education programs that are using innovative curricula to guide their journey (Patterson et al., 2019). As nurse educators familiarize themselves with their students, it will be important to confirm if there are any veterans present and if they represent former MSM from any of the four distinctive groups that have been discussed in this chapter. Information about student veteran experiences enrolled in prelicensure nursing programs is emerging. While many student veterans are successful, discussing "embarking on new ventures and appreciating the implications and meaning of this education pursuit" will be meaningful for them (Patterson et al., 2019, p. 353). Other obstacles may include "financial, academic, and personal struggles such as anxiety, stress, isolation, sleep difficulties and PTSD" (Shellenbarger & Decker, 2019, p. 338). Assistance throughout the nursing program with specific advisors and Student Service support, as well as further awareness of their health issues that could impact them in the classroom or clinical setting, will be helpful (Sikes et al., 2018).

FUTURE RESEARCH PRIORITIES

Several ideas for future research include

- further examination of gender specific focus sessions regarding their behavioral health reporting and concerns, instrument development, and validation regarding use of healthcare crossovers with the VHA and civilian health facilities;
- examine types of applicable education and delivery methodologies that could better facilitate a smooth community reintegration process for RC personnel;
- outcomes evidence-based research and pilot demonstration projects will be important on topics such as
  - types of continuing identification of specific RC needs during pre-deployment and post-deployment phases to better facilitate civilian to military transitions;
  - determine the access and feasibility of Advanced Nurse Practitioners-led interprofessional collaborative practice team assessments for the RC that are experiencing healthcare disparities;
  - investigate the gender-specific impact of burn pits used to incinerate plastics, garbage, computers, and medical waste in Iraq and Afghanistan downwind from military troops throughout their deployment(s);
  - explore the injured PMCs seen in civilian health facilities to note their unmet healthcare needs, examine their deployment experiences and exposures, as well as their present health needs; and
  - targeted clinical research examining the factors contributing to MVA incidence.

CONCLUSION

This chapter provided an examination of the Reserve and National Guard component, military women, the LGBT military community, and PMCs—our diverse groups that serve or are associated with the military. While they all have some similar physical and psychosocial health needs compared with the group of men in the service that is the majority, each of these groups also have their own distinctive health issues that will require monitoring throughout their life span to ensure high quality care and optimal health outcomes. RC personnel, with pressure for similar mission readiness as their full-time counterparts, are experiencing mobilization and reintegration differences in assimilation and health concerns. Military women are experiencing increasing amounts of both non-battle and battle injuries, as well as loss of life (Osborne et al., 2012). Severe environments found in Iraq and Afghanistan produced troublesome gender-specific concerns regarding hydration, safety, behavioral health, and gynecology difficulties for women, as well as MST. The military group of LGBT individuals have faced significant, numerous, and varied challenges from healthcare providers related to a lack of awareness and insensitivity to their unique concerns. Lastly, PMCs, in their various supportive roles, still have limited known information about them. They have fewer resources to cope with their health problems and may need more supportive care than anyone thought. Nurses should be at the forefront for advocating for facilitation of patient-centered, multidisciplinary, and holistic care for all these groups.

ACKNOWLEDGMENT

The authors gratefully acknowledge the expertise of Dr. Ori Swed, Assistant Professor Department of Sociology, Texas Tech University, Lubbock, Texas, with the topic of Private Military Contractors.

REFERENCES

The complete reference list for this chapter appears in the digital version of the chapter, accessible at https://connect.springerpub.com/content/book/978-0-8261-3597-1/chapter/ch08

ENHANCING CULTURAL SENSITIVITY IN PRACTICE AND ON CAMPUS

VETERAN-CENTERED CARE IN EDUCATION AND PRACTICE: FACULTY, STUDENT, AND NURSE COMPETENCIES

LIBBA REED MCMILLAN

Let us never consider ourselves finished nurses ... we must be learning all of our lives.

Florence Nightingale

KEY TERMS

military/veteran-centered care	faculty competencies
registered nurse competencies	cultural competency
student nurse competencies	

INTRODUCTION

Due to current and past wartime realities in our nation, nurses in all practice settings are challenged to meet the need for providing competent specialized healthcare services to military service members, veterans, and their families. Providing veteran-centered care in education and clinical practice involves knowledge, expected behaviors, and application of essential competencies. As practice environments change over time, nursing faculty and clinical nurse educators are in a prime position to facilitate nurses' educational needs. Nurse educators must identify, develop, and emphasize veteran-centered competencies to modify curricular needs, ensuring relevance to clinical practice outside of nursing silos (Harada et al., 2018), and assess the military and veteran cultural competence of their students (Meyer et al., 2015). Various topics within the realm of professional competency are presented in this chapter, along with strategies educators can utilize to enhance student competency at all degree levels.

BACKGROUND

There are 18.2 million veterans in the United States, comprising 7.6% of the population; more than 9 million veterans are served each year by the U.S. Department of Veterans Affairs (VA; U.S. Department

---

The complete reference list for this chapter appears in the digital version of the chapter, accessible at https://connect.springerpub.com/content/book/978-0-8261-3597-1/chapter/ch09

of Veterans Affairs, National Center for Veterans Analysis and Statistics, 2019). An estimated 28% of these veterans receive all of their healthcare through the Veterans Health Administration, leaving 72% to seek care in civilian hospitals or in many cases using both VA and civilian providers (Wang et al., 2019). However, education about the unique needs of this population within our society has not historically been a standard inclusion in prelicensure preparation for nurses and other healthcare professionals.

Nurse educators have an ethical obligation to enhance nursing education in providing culturally sensitive care to military and veteran populations in both military and civilian settings (Cooper et al., 2016; Elliott, 2019; Elliott & Patterson, 2017; Johnson et al., 2013). The ability to possess essential knowledge, develop competent clinical skills, and master effective teaching strategies must be garnered by nursing faculty to students. Essential knowledge must also be imparted through providing relevant opportunities for professional development and continuing education to practicing RNs working in VA, military, and non- VA or civilian settings (Cooper et al., 2016; Harper et al., 2016; Johnson et al., 2013; Maiocco et al., 2019; Nedegaaed & Zwilling, 2017).

The chapter is organized into four sections related to providing competent veteran-centered care in nursing education and practice. Topics covered include (a) behaviors associated with professional competence influenced by interprofessional frameworks, competency models, and regulatory organizations; (b) unique and challenging healthcare issues practicing nurses and nursing students encounter related to military service environments, specific military conflicts, and service locations; (c) role of understanding military culture in improving patient encounters, competency and patient outcomes; and (d) future research priorities associated with competency training and/or developing nursing students and practicing nurse professionals, thus impacting veterans at national, international, and global levels.

PROFESSIONAL COMPETENCE

According to the American Nurses Association (ANA, 2015), competent nursing care is guided and informed by the scope and standards of practice regarding professional practice. Specifically, competent care comprises identifying what job tasks or functions are needed, and how to perform those identified tasks and functions to improve patient outcomes. During academic training, nursing faculty must align and acquaint students with behavioral and practice expectations to successfully complete the program of study. Additionally, faculty must provide detailed measures for evaluation of successful completion of identified tasks and behavioral expectations. Nursing faculty and administrators are pivotal in explaining the rationale to major stakeholders (public, professional organizations, accreditation bodies, peer institutions, alumni, and hospital administrators), how the behaviors are congruent with standards of professional performance, current practice, programmatic curricular outcomes, and institutional accreditation standards. Professional development in the form of on-going education should ensure standards are met and the competency upholds organizational standards and advances patient care (American Association of Colleges of Nursing [AACN], 2008a; ANA, 2015). Competencies for nursing education are identified for each degree program, whether at the undergraduate (generalist) or graduate (specialty) levels. Competencies also define curricular content of a program (Blelch, 2019), establish student expectations, and should be the primary measure of student achievement of learning objectives.

"Competency is the effective application of knowledge, skills and judgment demonstrated by an individual in daily practice or job performance" (International Council of Nurses [ICN], 2005, p. 9). According the ANA (2015), RNs are expected to perform their duties, regardless of role, population, or specialty, including adherence to standards of practice of professional performance. Each standard is accompanied by competencies for RNs, with additional competencies for graduate level prepared RNs and APRNs. These standards of practice describe proficiency levels at a competent level of nursing practice, as those that demonstrate and apply critical thinking aspects of the nursing process—assessment, diagnosis, outcomes identification, planning, implementation, and evaluation (ANA, 2015). These standards also describe competent levels of expected behavior while in the professional role appropriately aligning with academic preparation. Professional performance standards include ethics, culturally congruent practice, communication, collaboration, leadership, education, evidence-based practice and research, quality of practice, professional practice evaluation, resource utilization, and environmental health (ANA, 2015).

Competent nurses are able to master diverse challenges in specific patient situations requiring culturally centered nursing care (Darnell & Hickson, 2015; Lor et al., 2016; Torres-Alzate, 2019). The addition of Standard 8 (Cultural Congruence) to the ANA's scope and standards of professional practice, is particularly applicable to caring for the military veteran and requires demonstrated competence while practicing as an RN, undergraduate, or graduate student nurse (ANA, 2015; Bonzanto et al., 2019; Lor et al., 2016; Purnell, 2016), and continued competence to practice safely and effectively (DiLeonardi & Biel, 2012). To this end, nursing faculty are pivotal in ensuring nursing curriculum is relevant to current clinical practice, evidence-based, comprehensive, and focused on producing a graduate nurse that is competent to deliver safe and effective care (AACN, 2008b; National Academies of Sciences, Engineering, and Medicine [NASEM], 2019). This comprises understanding and executing pedagogy to teach effectively with the focus on maximizing student learning. The vision of nursing roles for nursing education includes being a generalist (associate's degree in nursing, bachelor's degree in nursing [BSN]), advanced generalist (master's level/clinical nurse leader), and advanced specialty education, the doctor of nursing practice (AACN, 2008b; ICN, 2005; National League for Nursing [NLN], 2017). Specific strategies to enhance and assess development of cultural competency, military-veteran centered competencies, APRN competencies, faculty competencies, and interprofessional collaboration competencies are included in this section.

Cultural Competency

Evolving into culturally competent nurses begins with nursing education (undergraduate and graduate) and professional development (faculty and practicing nurses). Cultural competence is recognized as continuous, dynamic, evolving, based on theories from multiple disciplines, and varied according to focus (Andrews & Boyle, 2015; Jeffreys, 2010; Papadopoulos, 2011; Purnell, 2003). Shen (2015) described cultural competence as having two sub-concepts—culture and competence. Definitions may vary depending on component focus, and the intended utility of these two subconcepts.

Cultural competence models can be theoretical or methodological in approach (Shen, 2015). Examples of cultural competence models include: The Transcultural Nursing Assessment Guide (Andrews & Boyle, 2015), the Papadopoulos Model for Developing Culturally Competent and Compassionate Healthcare Professionals (Papadopoulos, 2011), and the Cultural Competence and Confidence Model: Transcultural Self-Efficiency (Jeffreys, 2010). For practicing nurses and professional development purposes, applicable models include the Dimensional Puzzle Model of Culturally Competent Care (Schim et al., 2007). Additionally, guidelines were developed by collaborative task force members of the American Academy of Nursing that provide globally relevant examples for the caregiver and for healthcare organizations—this document is entitled "Guidelines for Implementing Culturally Competent Nursing Care" (Douglas et al., 2014). Limitations of cultural competence models are the lack of focus on patient and health outcomes and lack of measurement of the behaviors of the healthcare professional, resulting in inherent lack of validation of the culturally competent care provided (Betancourt et al., 2005; Purnell, 2016; Shen, 2015).

MILITARY CULTURAL COMPETENCY

In defining military cultural competence, cultural competence must be disentangled from military culture (Atuel & Castro, 2018). To accomplish this task, there are models helpful to the care of veterans in nursing education through providing qualitative and quantitative measures of cultural competence levels. In turn, nurse educators can examine ways these competency models can help support the abilities of healthcare providers to adequately care for military members, veterans and their family members, and inform continuing education and training in nursing school curricula as well as on-boarding of nurses in practice during orientation to healthcare facilities (Tam-Seto et al., 2020).

Nurses need to be culturally competent from a general perspective, as well as military specific, to care for service members, veterans, and their family members. There are numerous models, tools, theories, and approaches that assist with informing competency as a broader-scoped generalized concept (Purnell, 2016) and others that assist with understanding the concept of cultural competency as applied to more tailored and specific approaches regarding military and veteran-centered competencies. In response to the lack of validated models to guide healthcare interactions with military community members and families, the Military and Veteran Family Cultural Competency Model (MVF-CCM) was created as an evidence-informed resource to support the development of cultural competent healthcare curricula, continuing education opportunities, and clinical practice (Tam-Seto et al., 2020). Tam-Seto et al. (2020) posits a cultural competence model is a depiction of cultural competency outlining the personality traits required for a specific job or function. Elements contained in the MVF-CCM include internal processes of acknowledgment of the culture group of military and veteran families (awareness); internal processes of emotional acknowledgement of the healthcare realities of the culture group (caring about); specific health-related knowledge about members of the cultural group (knowledge); and culturally-informed acts used during healthcare interactions (skills). With similar findings, Shen (2015) outlined domains and dimensions in nursing and other caring professionals. Among the three identified critical dimensions are affective, cognitive, and skills/practical/behavioral dimension. Within the affective dimension is the domain of cultural sensitivity; the cognitive dimension contains awareness, knowledge, and understanding; the practical skills dimension comprises necessary skills and interaction/ encounters (Shen, 2015).

Military/Veteran-Specific Competencies

Knowledge and skills in providing competent veteran-centered care is essential to providing patient-centered healthcare to service members, veterans, and their families (Beckford & Ellis, 2013; Conard et al., 2015; Finnegan et al., 2017; Gleeson & Hernmer, 2014; Hynes & Thomas, 2016; Johnson et al., 2013; Magpantay-Monroe, 2018; McMillan et al., 2017; Moss et al., 2015; Swenty et al., 2016). Delivery of culturally sensitive care that is mindful of military culture knowledge, including chain of command structure, military norms and identity, and warrior ethos/culture, is essential (Atuel & Castro, 2018; Meyer et al., 2015). Modeling strong leadership skills (Finkleman & Kenner, 2013) and providing palliative care at the end-of–life (Brommelsiek et al., 2018) are also essential knowledge components. Faculty, student nurses, and practicing nurses need to be competent in providing care for the unique needs of the veteran patient and family members and significant others by understanding resource availability (civilian and veteran-centered organizations), training civilian care providers (Nedegaard & Zwilling, 2017), plus have a cursory understanding of historical, global, and political underpinnings of the wars in which veterans and military members have served.

Table 9.1 depicts essential knowledge and competencies gleaned from the literature of faculty, undergraduate, and graduate-level nursing students, and practicing nurses related to caring for the veteran and military member. A key concept commonly discussed by the listed authors is the representation of "military and veteran culture" as being pivotal to competency development in providing care. Other shared competencies focused on the specific health concerns experienced by the veteran, especially in combat. Among these competencies are caring for substance use disorders (SUDs), polytrauma, and mental health issues, such as suicide. Competencies related to access to healthcare, such as within a VA facility or a competent civilian medical facility, are needed to provide care once identified and to provide follow-up care.

TABLE 9.1 ESSENTIAL KNOWLEDGE AND COMPETENCIES IN CARING FOR THE VETERAN AND MILITARY MEMBER

COMPETENCY	CARLSON (2016)	CHAMPLIN ET AL. (2017)	CHAMPLIN AND KUNKEL (2017)	JOHNSON ET AL. (2013)	MCMILLAN ET AL. (2017)	MOSS ET AL. (2015)	YORK ET AL. (2016)
Military and veteran culture	X	X	X	X	X	X	X
PTSD		X	X	X	X	X	X
TBI		X	X	X	X	X	X
Depression/anxiety	X	X		X			X
Substance use disorder	X	X	X	X	X	X	X
Suicide	X	X	X	X	X	X	X
Polytrauma	X	X	X	X	X	X	X
Amputation/assistive devices/wound care		X	X	X	X	X	
Pain/chronic pain		X		X	X		
Environmental/chemical exposures		X	X	X	X	X	
MST	X	X	X	X		X	X
Homelessness	X	X	X	X		X	X
End-of-life			X			X	
Veterans Health Administration/access to healthcare	X	X	X	X	X	X	X
Caregiver assistance			X				
Care of military families	X	X	X		X		X

MST, military sexual trauma; PTSD, posttraumatic stress disorder; TBI, traumatic brain injury.

Nurse Faculty Competency

From an operational standpoint of nursing education, faculty competence development can be enhanced by identifying necessary skills needed to provide culturally competent care to veterans, identifying ways to measure cultural competency, establishing strategic priority goals, identifying viable academic practice partners, and determining resources available for training. Developing faculty competence includes activities designed to assist with personal awareness of caring for veterans and military members; articulating and understanding personal insights related to veterans and military culture. Thematic concepts for faculty competencies could include personal reflection on appreciation of veteran contributions, care and empathy for the veteran, treating veterans humanely, and personal belief of being a team player, such as embodied in military culture (Carlson, 2016). Faculty should lead efforts in understanding their own cultural competency awareness, as limited cultural awareness can undermine shared decision-making, influence perceived care treatment, and impact patient-provider relationships (Meyer, 2013).

Many academic institutions offer training and development on improving faculty cultural sensitivity, diversity, and inclusion as a generalized concept. These institutional resources can be expanded from this generalized model to inform and enhance faculty teaching skills. For example, faculty can develop understanding of veterans and military members by improving awareness of differences in culture groups, curricular bias, understanding healthcare needs, and improving communication styles with diverse patient populations. Faculty competence can be further developed by utilizing resources related to improving teaching skills, such as examining curricular content, avoiding stereotypical references to cultural groups (Betancourt et al., 2005), determining the need for special topics related to veteran care, identifying ways to integrate veteran-centered care into crowded nursing curriculum (Champlin et al., 2017; Elliott & Patterson, 2017), and effectively utilizing veteran or military clinical faculty (Olenick et al., 2015).

In terms of competency development of faculty, Carlson (2016) identified 12 multidimensional major concepts including five faculty competencies and four essential knowledge areas related to veteran-specific care. The five faculty competencies include appreciation for veteran contributions, which includes honoring veterans and recognizing their contributions—being sensitive to veterans. Another competency, care and empathy for the veteran, involves an understanding of veterans and their unique experiences. Veteran cultural competence necessitates exposure to veterans and the veteran culture and their life experiences in general. Pivotal is also being a trust builder, such as treating veterans humanely, and using nonjudgmental and sincere interactions. Lastly, faculty need to be team players, including building staff relationships and being a member of a team. This team player aspect mirrors military culture in general where there is a team-oriented approach in the military infrastructure (Carlson, 2016; Conard et al., 2016; Olenick et al., 2015).

The essential competencies faculty need to teach students to provide veteran-centered care are congruent with competencies needed to fulfill the role as a practicing RN (Moyer & Graebe, 2018). Expectations of nursing faculty include assisting and ensuring the nursing student, upon graduation, is proficient and culturally competent in performing psychomotor skills, adept at demonstrating professional communication with veteran patients, and is an active team member by contributing as a partner with families and inter-professional collaborations. Caring behaviors include acquiring a professional identity that facilitates ethical practice, with the ability to understand and provide excellent patient care which is designed, managed, and coordinated throughout patient transitions in various healthcare milieus (Truong et al., 2014).

STUDENT VETERANS AS A DIVERSE POPULATION

Faculty also need to be competent in teaching diverse student populations – which varies according to whether the student has current or prior military experience or has primarily civilian experiences.

This requires faculty commitment to intentionally learning about military culture and overcoming perceived knowledge deficits in teaching diverse student groups, including student veterans (Elliott et al., 2019; Johnson et al., 2013). Additionally, nursing faculty must be attuned to unique teaching challenges related to diverse learners, such as student veterans with prior or current combat or military experience, recognizing their unique contributions to understanding veteran healthcare needs during the student's nursing education. To achieve and develop faculty competency requires attending professional development activities aimed at improving individual cultural sensitivity (Elliott et al., 2019; Sikes et al., 2018).

Faculty teaching either military and/or veteran students or civilian students must maximize existing student knowledge and experiences while in academic settings to "real world" application. Teaching diverse student populations expands far beyond knowing student demographics, such as age, race, academic credentials, and academic degrees. Faculty are not only interfacing with students that have varied life experiences and exposure to military culture, but also teaching students personally experiencing war-related injuries resulting from assignments, deployments, and combat versus non-combat experiences (Carlson, 2016). As more veterans transition into civilian life and enter nursing education, faculty will need increased professional development to understand and support best practices in teaching and facilitating learning transfer from their military experience to nursing education (Elliott et al., 2019). Critical elements of effective teaching include supporting social status, health and well-being, and academic success. For the faculty member, a continuing educational need should also be aimed at increasing individual cultural sensitivity; student veterans possess and exhibit aspects of their military culture and value systems during their nursing education (Elliott et al., 2019).

APRN Competencies

Competency considerations for APRNs are complex and have focused on legislative policies, legal authority to practice in varied practice settings, and evaluating education and training content based on core competency attainment. In terms of graduate level nursing education, such as the APRN, there are legal barriers in many states that prohibit practicing to the full extent of education and training (Institute of Medicine [IOM], 2010). APRNs provide many services associated by the public with those of physicians, including patient assessment, prescribing and ordering medications, and evaluating diagnostic tests. In 2008, several nursing organizations developed a consensus model for standardizing the regulation of APRNs in an attempt to develop consistent regulations recognizing the competencies across state borders (IOM, 2010). The use of APRNs becomes important with providing competent care of veterans and family members, as many healthcare facilities are utilizing nurse practitioners (NPs), particularly for follow-up care, leading interprofessional collaboration efforts, and early assessment (Green & Johnson, 2015; Harada et al., 2018; Monahan et al., 2018). The achievement of competencies established by the VA Centers of Excellence in Primary Care Education with NP residency students supports improvement in most competencies needed to provide care for the veteran. However, NPs perceived a decreased ability to manage sexual trauma and traumatic brain injuries, both common conditions in the veteran population (Rugen et al., 2018a, 2018b).

In 2014, the National Organization of Nurse Practitioner Faculties (NONPF) convened a work group to identify the suggested curricular content for the NP Core Competencies. This work group consisted of members of the task force that prepared the 2011 edition of the NP Core Competencies, as well as additional representation from the NONPF Board and Curricular Leadership Committee. Core competency areas include scientific foundation, practice inquiry, technology and information literacy, policy, health delivery system, and ethics (Nurse Practitioner Core Competencies Content, 2017). The relationship of competency to NP education is particularly important in the care of veterans in acute care and community settings in performing advanced history and physical examination techniques, prioritizing differential diagnoses, recommending and interpreting laboratory data and other diagnostic studies and prescribing medications (Anthamatten et al., 2019).

York et al. (2016) identified 14 veteran-centric domains derived from a literature review, which were included in psychiatric-mental health NP curricular components and competency evaluation. Veteran-centric domains included: communication with veterans, effects of combat stress, injury/ disability related to military service, care coordination with non-VA organizations, prevention and intervention services specific to the VA, health and well-being of veteran families, mental health in a veteran context, demographics of veteran patients, service-related beliefs and values, personal values and beliefs toward veteran populations, role and gender in help-seeking veterans, unique characteristics of mental health services within the VA system, recommended evidence-based practice in VA mental health services, and quality improvement for VA mental healthcare. This holistic overview of competency domains reinforces the necessity of nurse educators, students, and practice nurses understanding personal beliefs of military culture of veterans; relating the application of these domains in navigating through established healthcare systems available to veterans in the VA and civilian sectors.

Interprofessional Collaboration Competencies

In general, BSN nursing students must be prepared to provide competent patient-centered care; work effectively in interprofessional teams; utilize evidence-based practice; be adept at quality improvement, patient safety, informatics; utilize clinical reasoning/critical thinking; provide culturally sensitive care to patients and families; exhibit professionalism; and practice across the lifespan in a complex healthcare environment (AACN, 2008; Health Professions Accreditors Collaborative, 2019). The NLN's broad framework for evidence-based practice is focused on four general program outcomes, ranging from pre-licensure to doctoral education. These four program outcomes are related to enhancing human flourishing, demonstrating sound nursing judgment, developing a professional identity, and exhibiting a spirit of inquiry (NLN, 2010). The NLN Education Competencies Model (2010) is an academic model which guides faculty involved in program design and curricular revision for all types of nursing programs. To ensure student competency, nursing faculty members must transform nursing education by providing curricular elements and frameworks conducive to meeting key stakeholder's expectations and recommendations of healthcare professionals. Mastery of content and demonstrated competence in psychomotor skills, affective and cognitive domains of performance, theory, writing ability, and synthesized knowledge must be present upon graduation and successful completion of State Boards of Nursing licensure requirements (Hayden et al., 2014).

Recognizing the need for nursing education to include information in courses related to interprofessional collaboration with other healthcare disciplines to achieve the best possible patient care outcomes (Monahan et al., 2018), many nursing curricula integrate competencies related to Quality and Safety Education for Nurses (QSEN; Altmiller, 2019; QSEN, 2014), and core competencies for Interprofessional Collaborative Practice (IPCP; Interprofessional Education Collaborative [IPEC], 2016). A document published by IPEC, which includes discussion of the core competencies, is available at the following URL: hsc.unm.edu/ipe/resources/ipec-2016-core-competencies.pdf. Also included are recommendations related to core knowledge required for demonstrating professional competency (IOM, 2010). Interprofessional education and IPCP are considered ideal environments for teaching future healthcare professionals to be competent (Altmiller, 2019; Hermann et al., 2016; Morrison-Beedy et al., 2015; Peterson et al., 2016). When practitioners and students possess competencies that provide knowledge and skills to navigate and collaborate with caregivers from other disciplines, patients and the public experience optimal care (NASEM, 2019). Future health professions educators need to either possess or develop skills in working in interprofessional teams can be collectively grouped into five main areas: leadership skills, education, health and healthcare, technology, and business (NASEM, 2019).

The interprofessional healthcare model used by the VA offers opportunities for undergraduate and graduate health profession students to collaborate with VA Interprofessional Patient Aligned Care Teams to optimize veteran health outcomes and adapt to changing healthcare systems. While in the program, students are provided with opportunities to recognize the unique health needs of veterans. Additionally, students are exposed to the complexities of VA setting academic-practice partnerships related to the role of a primary care NP in the residency program (Harper et al., 2016; Rugen et al., 2018a; Rugen et al., 2018b) and psychiatric-mental health residents (York et al., 2016), and where interprofessional practice care is modeled in clinical practice and in interprofessional clinical learning environments within the national VA systems (Felker et al., 2018; Harada et al., 2018; Harper et al., 2015, 2016; Morrison-Beedy et al., 2015; Swenty et al., 2016).

Complementary and alternative medicine (CAM) disciplines also provide similar shared competencies as those taught in nursing or other related healthcare programs. These competencies are related to patient interviewing, critical thinking, evidence-based practice, and knowledge of spiritual and cultural beliefs. Among these CAM disciplines that are widely used and effective in achieving positive health outcomes for veterans are naturopathic medicine, acupuncture and oriental medicine, massage therapy and chiropractic healthcare (Brett et al., 2013; Green & Johnson, 2015; Rosenthal et al., 2019). The joint focus offers opportunities to learn about shared beliefs and attain necessary skills for addressing cultural differences while serving as patient advocates (Brommelsiek et al., 2018; Dulay et al., 2018).

UNIQUE AND CHALLENGING VETERAN HEALTHCARE ISSUES

The proficiency of nursing educators and other healthcare professionals in teaching students and ensuring students' competent delivery of clinical skills begins with the educators being proficient in understanding the unique needs of veteran patients. Veteran-centered care should be integrated or threaded into existing curriculum from beginning through advanced levels (Champlin et al., 2017; Morrison-Beedy et al., 2015).The military should be recognized as a distinct cultural group, with members possessing typical behaviors, such as core values, worldview, and shared language (Kautzmann & Lancaster, 2018; Kuehner, 2013; Purnell, 2016), and possessing distinct educational, policy, and practice challenges (Kautzmann & Lancaster, 2018). These diverse content areas directed at caring for the unique needs of the veteran population include military sexual trauma (MST), poly-trauma, amputations, exposures to chemical and thermal stressors, traumatic brain injury (TBI), posttraumatic stress disorder (PTSD), alcohol and drug addiction, homelessness, mental health disorders, suicide, and many other healthcare concerns (Bonzanto et al., 2019; Champlin et al., 2017; Conard et al., 2016; Hynes & Thomas, 2016; Johnson et al., 2013; Kiernan et al., 2016; Marcogliese & Vandyk, 2019; Morrison-Beedy et al., 2015). Additional stressors identified by the IOM (2008) regarding Gulf War health concerns include family and marital discord, financial problems, and intimate partner violence especially affecting both men and women in their ability to transition post-deployment.

Female service members, veterans, and families also present a need for healthcare providers to understand their unique needs, educate the uninformed and unaware community-based healthcare providers on the unique needs of women's physical and behavioral health issues as different from their male counterparts (Blosnich et al., 2013; Blosnich & Silenzio, 2013; Booth et al., 2012; Brooks et al., 2016; Conrad et al., 2015; Mankowski & Everett, 2016). Lesbian and bisexual women comprise approximately 43% of the military's sexual minorities (Donaldson et al., 2019). Veterans who identify as lesbian report poorer health status than their civilian heterosexual military peers (Lehavot & Simpson, 2012), are more frequently diagnosed with depression, anxiety, and PTSD than civilian women or heterosexual female veterans (Blosnich et al., 2013; Blosnich & Silenzio, 2013), and a lifetime of reported sexual violence as compared to heterosexual women (Booth et al., 2012).

There are many healthcare concerns and challenges faced by veterans today and throughout their lifespans requiring competent and culturally sensitive care delivery, such as attentiveness to patient preferences, needs, comfort, holistic approaches, and involvement from family members and caregivers (Elliott, 2019; Ersek et al., 2015). For many veterans, advanced illness, psychological stressors, traumatic injuries, advanced psychosocial needs, and chronic pain are closely associated with military service and fragmented healthcare (Antoni et al., 2012; Golden et al., 2016; Johnson et al., 2013). Cultural competence is relevant to the care of individuals in general, to include post-deployment behavioral health problems and consideration of these gender differences in responses and needs of veterans (Adams et al., 2016; Conard et al., 2016; Darnell & Hickson, 2015; Lor et al., 2016; Morrison-Beedy et al., 2015). This care component includes training and professional development of many healthcare providers, such as undergraduate and graduate nursing students and practicing nurses that understand and demonstrate skills related to caring for veterans in acute, community, tertiary, and assisted/nursing home milieus (Acosta et al., 2014; Elliott, 2019) and understanding unique barriers to mental health-care issues experienced in community settings. Among these barriers are long waits for the initial mental health appointment, lack of awareness for available mental health services, short appointments, and provider's lack of knowledge of the military culture (Pyne et al., 2019).

The need for providing nursing care to the aging veteran population and addressing unique needs associated with aging, such as elder care, resource availability, spousal support, and care facilities has increased healthcare services for this target population. Nursing homes are increasingly providing end-of-life care particularly in patients with dementia, which is a growing public health concern (Ersek et al., 2015). Palliative care in the U.S. military system has broadened the scope of services to include improving symptom management, lowering rates of hospital admissions, decreasing lengths of stay in hospitals, and improving understanding of prognosis (Snyder, 2015). Education of healthcare providers is lacking, yet important in gaining clinical knowledge of dementia warning signs, diagnosis, and management. Fostering clinical competence and professional development of nursing and nursing students could improve patient outcomes (Adler et al., 2015).

Primary concerns noted by practicing nurses in caring for veterans include uncertainty in three main areas: delivery of routine care (identifying services needed, resources, managing PTSD while hospitalized), inexperience in how to talk with veterans (knowing what to say, unsure how to respond, not identifying with challenges faced), and the potential for lack of knowledge in handling violence while delivering care, such as veteran triggers, anger management, and safety in waking up sleeping patients (Maiocco et al., 2019). Bonzanto et al. (2019) found almost 70% of practicing nurses surveyed regarding their practice behavior, never or seldom asked veterans questions about their military service experience, or history of traumatic events, and seldom assessed for stressors related to military life or veteran status. In this same study, less than 15% of practicing RNs reported being able to teach and guide colleagues on planning healthcare for veteran patients and explaining how their personal health beliefs are influenced by military and veteran culture (Bonzanto et al., 2019). This further highlights the need for nurses to increase their capacity, receive formal training, and understand military culture influences (Bonzanto et al., 2019).

PROVIDING COMPETENT VETERAN-CENTERED ASSESSMENT

Providing competent veteran-centered care begins with the first phase of the nursing process, which includes taking a health history assessment in a safe and quiet setting. Competent nurses need to initiate applicable screening questions, establish rapport with veterans based on an understanding of military culture, and work within interprofessional teams to utilize community resources (Conard et al., 2015; Johnson et al., 2013). The goal of asking relevant questions is to adequately and empathically understand the veteran's medical problems and concerns, thus instilling trust, conveying respect to the veteran, and connecting veterans to VA benefits (Counts et al., 2015; Morgan et al., 2017). General questions include: (a) discussions of military service, specifically asking the universal assessment question of all patients "Have you ever served in the military™?"; (b) service branch; (c) specifics of job duties; (d) illnesses or injuries resulting from military service; and (e) knowledge of resources, benefits and compensation of service-connected conditions, social history, presence or risk of communicable diseases (hepatitis, sexually transmitted infections), sexual health assessments, and exposure to chemicals, living conditions, or contaminants in specific geographic areas or deployments within the past 2 years (Conard et al., 2015, 2016; Counts et al., 2015; Johnson et al., 2013). The veteran should be asked questions regarding sexual health, such as current or previous unwanted sexual experiences in the military, threatening or repeated sexual attention, comments or touching, indicating the possibility of the veteran having been victimized by MST (Mankowski & Everett, 2016).

Assessment of behavioral, emotional health, and mental health, such as PTSD, feelings of hopelessness/helplessness, lack of energy, difficulty concentrating, sleep disturbances, TBI, and thoughts of suicide or inflicting harm to oneself or others need to be addressed by healthcare professionals. The nurse should assess for the presence of drugs and alcohol, particularly those used as a coping mechanism (Conard et al., 2015, 2016; Counts et al., 2015; Johnson et al., 2013). The veteran's living situation should also be addressed, such as homelessness (Mankowski & Everett, 2016), other members living in the household, safety of the residence, concerns of losing housing, specific needs in providing self-care or of dependents and caregiver needs (Conard et al., 2017). Select resources to learn more about some of the health-related issues discussed are presented in Table 9.2.

The VA provides the public with an exhaustive amount of information to provide support and care to veterans, both in and outside the VA (https://www.publichealth.va.gov/). Additionally, they provide veterans with a multitude of innovative programs focused on health and wellness, disease prevention, and exposure monitoring to name a few. Health registry programs and evaluations for veterans gives providers information about the six VA environmental health registry programs (including two VA health surveillance programs), eligibility requirements for veteran participation, and potential benefits for both veterans and their providers when a veteran participates in a registry. Further, services for women, minorities, and those in the LGBT community have expanded in the past decade to be inclusive of all veteran groups. For more information refer to Table 9.3.

STRATEGIES TO IMPROVE COMPETENCY

To achieve the outcomes delineated in undergraduate and graduate education and to develop or refine practice-related competencies (AACN, 2008; Champlin et al., 2017; IOM, 2010), integration of learning strategies must be threaded into courses and be intentional, active, and collaborative. As faculty construct meaningful and relevant learning strategies, there must be ways to continually evaluate student learning effectiveness, assess alternative models of clinical experiences and simulated learning, consider the effect of sequencing of activities, while reducing barriers to the delivery of clinical education in developing competency (Bonzanto et al., 2019; Hansen & Bratt, 2017). There are many resources available to improve veteran-centered care competencies in the form of national and international initiatives.

In 2012, a national initiative called *Joining Forces* highlighted the need to enhance nursing education of military and veteran populations (Elliott & Patterson, 2017). The AACN partnered with the VA to enhance resources designed in particular for nursing education. As a result of this partnership, the Enhancing Veteran's Care Toolkit was developed, thus, providing key educational resources that engage faculty in curricular development related to quality care of veterans and their families. Additionally, creative learning strategies on veteran care, and a repository of resources for students, faculty, and practicing nurses caring for veterans and their families resulted (www.aacnnursing.org/Teaching-Resources/Tool-Kits/Veterans-Care). A unique VA funded 7-year program, the Veterans Affairs Nursing Academy, partnered with colleges of nursing to educate and train nurses on the unique needs of veterans and their families across hospital and community settings. Participating faculty members gained essential knowledge and teaching strategies needed to prepare baccalaureate-level nursing students to provide holistic care to veterans (Carlson, 2016; Harper et al., 2015). The key information gleaned from these partnerships could be applied to other degree programs as well.

TABLE 9.2 HEALTH-RELATED RESOURCES

RESOURCES	WEB LINK
Mental Health Resources	
The NIMH provides information on a variety of mental health topics and lists current clinical trials that allow persons to access treatment for free. Call (866) 615–6464	www.militaryonesource.mil/health-wellness/mental-health/mental-health-resources
Mental health: Posttraumatic stress disorder, depression, suicide prevention	www.va.gov/health-care/health-needs-conditions/mental-health
SUDs	www.va.gov/health-care/health-needs-conditions/substance-use-problems
Veteran suicide	www.healthaffairs.org/do/10.1377/hblog20190709.197658/full
PTSD: Caring for families and patients	www.ptsd.va.gov/apps/CRAFTPTSD
PTSD	www.ptsd.va.gov/professional/treat/essentials/index.asp
Mental health and training modules	www.mentalhealthfirstaid.org/veterans-military
Suicide prevention Department of Defense	dod.defense.gov/News/Special-Reports/0916_suicideprevention
Military sexual trauma	www.va.gov/health-care/health-needs-conditions/military-sexual-trauma
Traumatic Brain Injury Resources	
Defense and Veterans Brain Injury Center created the A Head for the Future initiative to raise awareness and lower the risk of concussion. The campaign offers information about the signs, symptoms, and treatment of brain injuries and educates service members and veterans about how to prevent them	https://dvbic.dcoe.mil/
The Defense Centers of Excellence for Psychological Health and Traumatic Brain Injury provides information and resources about psychological health, PTSD, and traumatic brain injury	https://www.usar.army.mil/DCOE-TBI/The/
Veterans Affairs Poly-trauma/TBI System of Care is an integrated network of specialized rehabilitation programs dedicated to serving veterans and service members with both combat and civilian related TBI and poly-trauma	www.polytrauma.va.gov/
DoD Clinical Recommendation (June, 2014). Management of sleep disturbances following concussion/ mild traumatic brain injury: guidance for primary care management in deployed and non-deployed settings	pueblo.gpo.gov/DVBIC/pdf/DV-4014.pdf

DoD, U.S. Department of Defense; NIMH, National Institute of Mental Health; SUD, substance use disorder; TBI, traumatic brain injury.

To accomplish the goal of refining practice-related roles and competencies as stated in the IOM (2010) report, nurses should be full partners with physicians and other healthcare professionals in redesigning healthcare in the United States. Nursing education must function as a full partner and work collaboratively with military health systems and VA professionals to improve veteran outcomes

TABLE 9.3 VA RESOURCES

RESOURCE	WEB LINK
Military Health History Pocket Card for Health Professions Trainees and Clinicians	www.va.gov/OAA/pocketcard
Academic PACT	www.va.gov/oaa/apact
Veterans Health Initiative	www.publichealth.va.gov/vethealthinitiative/index.asp
Center for Women Veterans	www.va.gov/womenvet
CMV	www.va.gov/centerforminorityveterans/partners.asp
Patient Care Service for LGBT	www.patientcare.va.gov/LGBT
Office of Rural Health for Veterans	www.ruralhealth.va.gov/index.asp
Military Exposures	www.publichealth.va.gov/exposures/index.asp
Health Registry Info	www.publichealth.va.gov/docs/exposures/healthregistryprograms.pdf#

CMV, Center for Minority Veterans; PACT, Patient Aligned Care Team; VA, U.S. Department of Veterans Affairs.

across all health settings—ranging from acute care settings to home care agencies. Nursing education faculty are pivotal in improving competencies such as leadership, health policy, system improvement, research, teamwork, and collaboration in areas where veteran care can be impacted, such as in community, public health, and geriatrics (Elliott, 2019). As further outlined by the IOM (2010) report, nurses should function as a patient advocate and work with legislators to practice to the full extent of their education and training. This practice component begins with theory and clinical experiences in nursing education programs and professional development. APRNs can address gaps in care by assisting nurse graduates in making successful transitions after graduation by developing and evaluating community settings where veterans are needing care (Champlin & Kunkel, 2017).

Interprofessional learning opportunities and creating and sustaining collaborative learning activities across academic disciplines is vital to becoming a competent student nurse, practicing nurse, being able to be both a team leader and team member and broaden perspectives from other disciplines, such as complementary and integrative health providers (Brett et al., 2013; Rosenthal et al., 2019; WHO, 2010). Examples of learning strategies include case studies (McKensie et al., 2016), simulation, story-telling, self-reflective practice, role-playing (Magpantay-Monroe, 2018), reminiscing, art therapy, and specialized programs where students have contact with veterans (Conard et al., 2016). Carlson (2016) described faculty teaching strategies as developing connections with veterans and their families, staff, and other students within a veteran community to engage the veteran and gain exposure. These teaching and student activities are particularly effective when combined together to maximize achievement of numerous competency frameworks, such as the AACN Baccalaureate Essentials (AACN, 2008a).

Using simulation exercises and case-based scenarios with disciplines other than nursing enhance interprofessional learning for undergraduate and graduate nursing students (Elliott & Patterson, 2017; Hansen & Bratt, 2017). Scenarios can be constructed with kinesiology (musculoskeletal conditions, gait training), audiology (hearing loss, tinnitus), speech pathology (communication disorders), medical schools (poly trauma, disease processes), biomedical engineering and computer technology (electronic health records, prosthetics), philosophy (ethical issues, religion), psychology (mental health issues, suicide, transitions), and healthcare administration (access to care, policy issues, leadership). Simulations can be enhanced by use of standardized patients, which are readily available in many communities and in many higher education milieus with student veteran associations, particularly with graduate level nursing students. As a starting point, simulation resources are located in Box 9.1.

BOX 9.1

SIMULATION RESOURCES AND VETERAN-SPECIFIC EXERCISES/MODULES

Magpantay-Monroe, E. R. (2016). Integration of military and veteran health in a psychiatric mental health BSN curriculum: A mindful analysis. *Nurse Education Today, 48,* 111–113. https://doi.org/10.1016/j.net.2016.009.020

McKenzie, G., Freiheit, H., Steers, D., & Noone, J. (2016). Veteran and family health: Building competency with unfolding cases. *Clinical Simulation in Nursing, 12,* 79–83. https://doi.org/10.1016/j.ecns.2015.12.011

Regan, R. V., Fay-Hillier, T., & Murphy-Parker, D. (2019). Simulation clinical experience of veteran care competence for psychiatric-mental health nurse practitioner students with standardized patients. *Issues in Mental Health Nursing, 40*(3), 223–232. https://doi.org/10.1080/01612840.2018.1543743

National League for Nursing. (n. d.). *ACEV (Unfolding case studies on Veteran related health issues).* http://www.nln.org/professional-development-programs/teaching-resources/veterans-ace-v

Graduate and undergraduate nursing students need development of their role in being a patient advocate. Development of scenarios where nursing students learn to advocate for veterans and military members include understanding of the veteran perspective, knowledge of barriers and challenges faced by veterans in receiving access to quality care, and policy implications unique to veterans. Assignments that move the student from operating in a passive professional stance toward active engagement in changing and challenging the "status quo" are pivotal to assisting students in finding their voice and developing the patient advocate role. Table 9.4 provides resources as a starting point to learn more about actualizing this goal.

Teaching assignments necessitating exposure to formal and informal leaders modeling advocacy competencies, while aimed at managing and advocating for improvements or access to veteran centered care at the local, regional, national, and international levels, provide rich advocacy opportunities. Constructing assignments where nursing students learn to advocate for veterans begins with understanding the unique organizational systems that veterans utilize (see Instructor Activities in Box 9.2). This includes collaborative work with public, private, educational, and regional VA facilities and service organizations (Conard et al., 2016; Dursa et al., 2016); VA hospitals, veteran state homes, local veteran organizations, local military bases with hospitals, and state legislators that are informing policy and actively lobbying for veteran healthcare issues. Student assignments could center on writing mock letters to policy makers, or walking a veteran-centered bill through the process toward passage.

TABLE 9.4 RESOURCES FOR PROMOTING ADVOCACY

RESOURCE	WEB LINK
American Academy of Nursing	www.aannet.org/policy-advocacy
American Nurses Association	www.nursingworld.org/practice-policy/advocacy
National League for Nursing	www.nln.org/professional-development-programs/teaching-resources/toolkits/advocacy-teaching
National Council on Aging	www.ncoa.org/public-policy-action/advocacy-toolkit
Ecology Center	www.ecocenter.org/teaching-future-nurses-advocacy

Students could include descriptions of social determinants that are challenging to veterans in rural locations and those veterans with special cognitive and physical needs.

BOX 9.2

INSTRUCTOR ACTIVITIES TO PROMOTE VETERAN-CENTERED COMPETENCY

The following instructional activities can be adapted to student level (undergraduate, graduate, or doctoral) and course objectives to facilitate development of various skills, including program development, advocacy, and interprofessional collaboration. Additional instructions on veteran-specific content and/or introduction to veteran-specific competencies may be required.

1. Choose the perspective of either (a) hospital setting, (b) academia, or (c) community clinical practice setting to debate: Would establishing accreditation standards that require veteran-centered competencies such as public health components, unique communication with veterans, health promotion topics relevant to military or veteran health histories, and veteran-centered cultural competence help facilitate interprofessional education among healthcare providers?

2. In terms of improving veteran healthcare provider competencies, design a plan for staff nurse professional development that includes specific content, such as disease management, and strategies for practicing nurses to interface with academic partners (such as preceptorship activities, and community outreach activities).

3. Of the numerous competency areas covered in this chapter, choose one competency area you feel has the greatest impact on improving veteran care. Discuss how this area impacts policy, quality, and safety considerations.

Nursing students need to experience various healthcare settings to provide cultural perspectives and reimbursement models represented in military/veteran settings as compared to civilian organizations. There are many professional nursing organization meetings conducted by VA nurses and healthcare providers that are available to civilian professionals as well as accessible to nursing students. For graduate students, there are many opportunities to develop advocacy as utilized by APRNs in both VA healthcare facilities and other facilities veterans. Graduate nurses with military and veteran status can serve as preceptors to undergraduate students in military facilities and also provide rich professional development opportunities as content experts of veteran-related issues. As advocates, an advanced practice nurse can combine research ability with clinical practice that assists with informing the public and other stakeholders of veteran problems and issues.

There are a wide range of technologies that students need to be proficient. At a minimum, the student should be familiar with the technology and computer applications geared toward improving veteran-centered health. Using a professional e-Portfolio platform to organize learning activities and showcase student work can be threaded throughout all clinical experiences where students can visualize their learning, perceptions, and clinical experiences over the course of their professional education. Technologies that support care include electronic health records, patient monitoring systems, and medication administration systems (AACN, 2008b; Bonzanto et al., 2019). Additionally, use of telemedicine opportunities and telehealth tools are critical with the increased use of telemedicine with rural veterans (NASEM, 2019). Combining electronic medical records with simulation activities concerning veteran healthcare issues are effective learning opportunities, as well as collaborations with graduate students, NPs, pharmacists, social workers, or medical students.

Role of Clinical Nurse Educators in Competency Development

There is an increased need for cultural competency training in the health professions, as well as a conclusive cultural competency framework (Bonzanto et al., 2019; Brommelsiek et al., 2018; Elliott, 2019; Truong et al., 2014). According to Elliott (2019), "it is imperative for the nursing workforce to not only assess for military veteran status but to also have some knowledge of military culture and veteran-specific healthcare issues" (p. 36). The 2003 IOM Report "Health professions education: A bridge to quality" described quality healthcare and need to focus on five core competencies identified for all healthcare professionals. Of most relevance to military/veteran care is the competency that outlines a health professional's ability to deliver patient-centered care, considering the increased diversity in the U.S. population, which includes varying cultural backgrounds, values, and expectations (IOM, 2003). Due to the complexity and magnitude placed on nursing education in preparing students to care for veterans, a need for unique resources, information, research, teaching strategies, and competency development approaches emerged. Ideally, aligning the synergy of nursing education and nursing practice focused on veteran initiatives and addressing healthcare disparities, while combined with active partnerships with academia, patients and families, and regulatory buy-in, competency in caring for veterans and their families can be maximized.

The current generation of health professional educators has a unique opportunity to shape the future of health professional education and foster an environment where future nurses can learn veteran-centered care (Jones & Breen, 2015; Keavney, 2015; Magpantay-Monroe, 2018), while cultivating a deep appreciation for their role (Jones & Breen, 2015; Keavney, 2015) and identifying underlying educational needs of the learner that contribute to professional practice gaps and design educational activities to target these gaps (Moyer & Graebe, 2018). However, functioning at a thriving competency level will require educators to think differently and adapt to moving beyond traditional silos with other health professionals (Framework for Action on Interprofessional Education and Collaborative Practice, 2010; Hansen & Bratt, 2017; National Academy of Sciences, 2019; Rosenthal et al., 2019). The key aspect of thriving in a culture change that links education and professional practice, requires education and training in newer models of collaborative practice focused on obtaining better patient outcomes (Peterson et al., 2017). Many sources address the pivotal role of nurse educators as positioned to lead efforts in providing students with the knowledge to provide veteran-centered care (Acosta et al., 2014; Bowman et al., 2011; Magpantay-Monroe, 2018; McMillan et al., 2017). A major challenge to nurse educators includes evaluating students to determine achievement of clinical competency, often considered subjective at all levels of nursing preparation.

Clinical competence providing care to veterans and military members includes the nurse's ability to observe and gather information, recognize deviations from expected patterns, prioritize data, and make sense of data. Additional components of clinical competence include maintaining a professional response demeanor, providing clear communication, executing effective interventions, and performing nursing skills correctly. Professional development of competence includes the nurse evaluating the effectiveness of nursing interventions, and self-reflection of performance improvement while practicing within a culture of safety (Hayden et al., 2014).

IMPLICATIONS FOR NURSING EDUCATION AND PRACTICE

DiLeonardi and Biel (2012) discussed the merit of establishing the definition of competence. The value of clearly defined competence definitions assists with ensuring competent practice and also provokes development of implementation strategies to move continuing competency to being operationally defined; supports decisions on continuing education, certification, and recertification requirements; and assists with evaluation of competent practice behaviors. Professional development such as assessing learner understanding, reinforcing content, or advancing knowledge to improve patient care of military veteran-centered competencies, requires leadership support and commitment. This includes evaluating nurses and other healthcare providers' understanding of veterans' unique needs, and requires resources from academia, community clinical practice settings, nurse residency programs, and local or regional veteran and civilian hospitals to meet practice gaps. Faculty should pursue these opportunities by requesting funding resources to attend local, regional, national, or international professional conferences, such as AACN, NLN, Association of Military Surgeons of the United States, Palliative Nurses Association, ANA, School Nurse Association, ICN, Sigma Theta Tau International, and QSEN. Resource support from interprofessional academic and practice leadership is critical to facilitate this development, such as paid time to attend, conference travel registration, and staff/faculty coverage of workload while in attendance. Many professional conferences offer "justification for attendance" templates that are helpful in requesting resources from decision-makers. In clinical practice settings, there are opportunities to partner with hospital or clinic training and development departments to assist with funding.

Global health understanding reinforced by nursing educators is also critical and relevant to the development of competencies necessary in providing culturally competent care of veteran and military members. Development of global health curricula to reflect the core values of nursing practice are exhibited in the foundational Nursing Global Health Competencies Framework (Torres-Alzate, 2019). Six core values shared by nurses regardless of educational level must be taught in nursing education and are congruent with competencies addressing needs of veterans. These include social justice and equity, holistic care, advocacy, health as a human right, sustainability, and collaboration (Torres-Alzate, 2019). In consideration of the health and social challenges veterans may face, such as substance abuse and homelessness, one can glean how relevant these core values are to delivery of care.

There are also clinical nurse leaders, clinical nurse specialists, regional VA or U.S. Department of Defense (DoD) experts, and faculty content experts from local academic settings that are rich resources for conducting symposia, conferences, panel discussions, and training modules. Academic or clinical academic faculty can partner with various settings to conduct needs assessments or quality assurance audits to determine specific gaps in practice, which strengthen the impact of training topics or style and format of content delivery. For example, staff-led improvement projects can impact improvements in patient outcomes, and decrease the incidence of adverse patient outcomes such as medication errors, fall injuries, sepsis, and others. Linking the need for training with cost-savings or improved patient satisfaction strengthen administration's support undergraduate and student learning gaps are often detected by practicing nurses' communication and interface with student preceptors; thus, strengthening a collaborative approach to cost-sharing of professional development resources. Home care agencies can partner with veteran state homes or area nursing homes to cost-share training resources. Additionally, there are many web-based training resources, such as videos, lunch-time webinars, and military culture on-line training modules that can be completed during non-work hours or used for continuing education credits to renew nursing licensure.

FUTURE RESEARCH PRIORITIES

Nursing education should include research regarding developing clinical competency at the student and practice level in veteran-centered care; particularly improving patient outcomes throughout the lifespan. Establishing priority areas for faculty, students, and nurses are necessary to maximize clinical and classroom resources. Cultural competence training has emerged as a strategy for improving the knowledge, skills, and attitudes of healthcare professionals. However, cultural competence training currently lacks critical evidence linking the effectiveness of achieving training objectives, such as improving patient outcomes, achieving equity across diverse ethnic groups, adherence to therapy standards, and congruence in self-care management techniques (Beach et al., 2005). Other areas lacking effectiveness data are in addressing and improving healthcare disparities (Betancourt et al., 2005). The effectiveness of evaluating continuing education on impacting veteran's healthcare needs, and preparation of non-military providers caring for veterans in civilian healthcare facilities to provide culturally competent care are currently lacking empirical data (Bonzanto et al., 2019; Counts et al., 2015; Maiocco et al., 2019; Morrison-Beedy et al., 2015). Ensuring relevance of continuing education and staff preparedness to addressing salient healthcare concerns, such as suicide, mental illness, and practice updates are needed to advance the profession (Maiocco et al., 2019).

Research should be directed toward the role of nursing education in impacting understanding the diversity of military and veteran cultures via education as increasing caregiver ability to provide culturally sensitive care (Adler et al., 2015; Darnell & Hickson, 2015; Detweiler et al., 2014; Maiocco et al., 2019). Research in diverse non-VA clinical settings is needed to support safe and caring environments to veterans and their families (Bonzanto et al., 2019). There are limited studies of the care of veterans and their families by civilian providers in non-VA health systems and exploring practicing nurses' cultural competence when caring for military veterans (Elliott, 2019). The majority of research has centered on non-VA mental health providers and nursing curricula (Beach et al., 2005; Bonzanto et al., 2019).

In terms of clinical practice, there are numerous opportunities for baccalaureate students to assist faculty with research, but this research requires access to resources, scholarships, and support for additional scholarly projects or activities. Collaborative research between academic and clinical partners can promote evidence-based practice, and may promote veteran and family-centered care by engaging staff (Gettrust et al., 2016). Future research priorities for veteran-centered care include addressing those health issues unique to military service, such as TBI, post traumatic growth (Tsai et al., 2016) poly-trauma, hazardous exposures, chronic pain, PTSD, MST, SUDs, suicide, and homelessness (Johnson et al., 2013; Morrison-Beedy et al., 2015).

Nurses, NPs, physician assistants, and primary care physicians have a pivotal role in culturally competent assessment, diagnosis, management, and evaluation of acute and chronic conditions in patients. These healthcare professionals are often the initial point of contact for the patient and family member when seeking treatment options for problematic or complex healthcare conditions, thus increasing the need for nursing research in the area of best practices in training, improving knowledge and skills, professional development competencies of faculty and advanced nursing roles. Research has also increased in addressing specific quality of life issues associated with diseases and conditions associated with military service-related health concerns. Among these are addressing disabilities, and improving overall health, symptom management, and wellbeing, tinnitus (Henry et al., 2019), sleep disorders in TBI and PTSD patients (DoD, 2014), stroke (Conard et al., 2015; Damush et al., 2014), spinal cord injuries (Hill et al., 2014), cancers, and end of life issues/palliative care. The VA (2018) cites tinnitus as the most prevalent service-connected disability for veterans receiving compensation for the past decade. In the fall of 2017, the VA Rehabilitation Research and Development Service National Center for Rehabilitative Auditory Research hosted its eighth biennial conference, titled "Translating Tinnitus Research Findings into Clinical Practice." The primary objective of the conference was to provide a forum for experts to discuss how tinnitus research findings could be implemented into clinical practice (Theodoroff & Saunders, 2019).

Another clinical practice priority area for the VA, requiring competence development, is caring for veterans with cognitive decline, such as dementia. As the number of aging veterans is growing, the risk of dementia and potentially delirium, continues to increase (Adler et al., 2015; Detweiler et al., 2014). Identifying ways to improve education via classroom activities, clinical experiences, and simulations with healthcare providers about older veteran care (Conard et al., 2016), dementia warning signs, communication within team interactions, and management is crucial to improving patient outcomes and developing cultural competence.

CONCLUSION

Nursing education is in a position to lead the profession in understanding the needs of patients, the changing needs of society, and the evolving role of other health professions in providing quality patient care. Nursing educators should be at the forefront of efforts in educating and evaluating students' clinical competence to provide safe and effective care to military members and veterans. This includes improving curricula to ensure relevance of content, creating an environment conducive to student learning, providing innovative teaching strategies and clinical opportunities, and promoteing pride in the nursing profession. Ensuring competency of graduates in undergraduate and graduate programs, as well as staff development and continuing education of practicing nurses in providing care to veterans; this is a profound responsibility and professional commitment. However, ensuring nursing students, practicing nurses, and faculty competency has many challenges due to the lack of clear objective measurement capability. Moreover, achieving faculty consensus of teaching strategies, curricular content, clinical practice site availability for veteran populations, and length of time allotted to veteran-centered content is highly subjective. Whereas faculty consensus can be achieved as to the importance of inclusion of veteran-centered content, other challenges emerge related to priorities. Among these challenges are resource availability and feasibility, faculty-student ratios, student clinical fees related to funding simulation exercises (such as standardized patient costs), and evolving accreditation criteria focused on student learning outcomes on national standardized tests and credentialing.

As nurses, nursing students, and nursing educators, learning to care for veterans is never finished; cultural competence is never finished; rather it continually develops. As more veterans seek care from non-VA facilities, and advance in age, there will be a vast need for providing culturally competent care for the veteran patient, family member, and caregivers. Nurses have the unique opportunity to impact care for those veterans and family members who have sacrificed greatly and contributed to our nation's freedom.

REFERENCES

The complete reference list for this chapter appears in the digital version of the chapter, accessible at https://connect.springerpub.com/content/book/978-0-8261-3597-1/chapter/ch09

RESOURCES

Recommended Readings

FACULTY AND STUDENT COMPETENCIES

Carlson, J. (2016). Baccalaureate nursing faculty competencies and teaching strategies to enhance the care of the veteran population: Perspective of Veteran Affairs Nursing Academy (VANA) faculty. *Journal of Professional Nursing, 32*(4), 314–323. https://doi.org/10.1016/j.profnurs.2016.01.006

Champlin, B., Linck, R., Darst, E., Foley, B., Reuer, B., & Hammill, C. (2017). Veteran-centered exemplars in a pre-licensure nursing program curriculum. *Nurse Educator, 42*(5), 255–258. https://doi.org/10.1097/nne.0000000000000395

McMillan, L. R., Crumbley, D., Freeman, J., Rhodes, M., Kane, M., & Napper, J. (2017). Caring for the veteran, military and family member nursing competencies: Strategies for integrating content into nursing school curricula. *Journal of Professional Nursing, 33*(5), 378–386. https://doi.org/10.1016/j.profnurs.2017.06.002

Moss, J. A., Moore, R. L., & Selleck, C. S. (2015). Veteran competencies for undergraduate nursing education. *Advances in Nursing Science, 38*(4), 306–316. https://doi.org/10.1097/ans.0000000000000092

Rugen, K. W., Dolansky, M. A., Dulay, M., King, S., and Harada, N. (2018). Evaluation of veterans affairs primary care nurse practitioner residency: Achievement of competencies. *Nursing Outlook, 66*(1), 25–34. https://doi.org/10.1016/j.outlook.2017.06.004

York, J., Sternke, L., Myrick, D., Lauerer, J., & Hair, C. (2016). Development of veteran-centric competency domains for psychiatric-mental health nurse practitioner residents. *Journal of Psychosocial Nursing and Mental Health Services, 54*(11), 31–36. https://doi.org/10.3928/02793695-20161024-06

CULTURAL COMPETENCY

Bonzanto, T., Swan, B., & Gaughan, J. (2019). Examining the capacity of registered nurses to deliver culturally competent health care to veterans and their families. *Journal of Nursing Care Quarterly, 34*(4) 358–363. https://doi.org/10.1097/NCQ.0000000000000401

Brommelsiek, M., Peterson, J. A., & Knopf-Amelung, S. (2018). Improving cultural competency: A patient-centered approach to interprofessional education and practice in a veterans healthcare facility. *International Journal of Higher Education, 7*(4), 157–165. https://doi.org/10.5430/ijhe.v7n4p157

Convoy, S., & Westphal, R. J. (2013). The importance of developing military cultural competence. *Journal of Emergency Nursing, 39*, 591–594. https://doi.org/10.1016/j.jen.2013.08.010

Donaldson, W., Smith, H. M., & Parrish, B. P. (2019). Serving all who served: Piloting an online tool to support cultural competency with LGBT U.S. military veterans in long-term care. *Clinical Gerontologist, 42*(2), 185–191. https://doi.org/10.1080/07317115.2018.1530323

Kautzmann, C. L., & Lancaster, R. L. (2018). Teaching culturally competent veteran nursing care in prelicensure programs. *Nursing Education Perspectives, 39*, 119–120. https://doi.org/10.1097/01.NEP.0000000000000213

Westphal, R. J., & Convoy, S. P. (2015). Military culture implications for mental health and nursing care. *The Online Journal of Issues in Nursing, 20*(1), 4. http://www.nursingworld.org/MainMenuCategories/ANA-Marketplace/ANAPeriodicals/OJIN/TableofContents/Vol-20-2015/No1-Jan-2015/Military-Culture-Implications.html

CLINICAL PRACTICE

Chargualaf, K. A. (2019). Actualizing veteran-centered nursing practice in the medical-surgical setting. *MedSurg Nursing, 28*, 8–9.

Elliott, B. (2018). Civilian nurses' knowledge, confidence, and comfort caring for military veterans: Survey results of a mixed-methods study. *Home Healthcare Now, 36*, 356–361. https://doi.org/10.1097/NHH0000000000000698

Elliott, B. (2019). Civilian nurses' experiences caring for military veterans: Qualitative data from a mixed-methods study. *Home Healthcare Now, 37*(1), 36–43. https://doi.org/10.1097/nhh.0000000000000709

Erickson-Hurt, C., McGuirk, D., & Long, C. O. (2017). Healthcare benefits for veterans: What home care clinicians need to know. *Home Healthcare Now, 35*, 248–257. https://doi.org/10.1097/NHH.0000000000000538

Gabriel, M. S., Malloy, P., Wilson, L. R., Virani, R., Jones, D. H., Luhrs, C. A., & Shreve, S. T. (2015). End-of-life nursing education consortium (ELNEC) – for veterans. *Journal of Hospice & Palliative Care Nursing, 1*, 40–47. https://doi.org/10.1097/NJH.0000000000000121

Maiocco, G., Stroupe, L. M., Rhoades, A., & Vance, B. (2019). Care of veterans in a non-veteran health administration hospital: What is the status of nursing practice after continuing education? *Journal of Clinical Nursing, 283*(4), 520–527. https://doi.org/10.1111/jocn.14641

Merkle, M. A., Tanabe, P., Sverha, J. P., & Turner, B. (2016). A quality improvement initiative for designing and implementing a military service screening tool for a community emergency department. *Journal of Emergency Nursing, 42*, 400–407. https://doi.org/10.1016/j.jen.2015.11.009

Stanton, M. (2014). Investigating veteran status in primary care assessment. *Open Journal of Nursing, 4*, 663–668. https://doi.org/10.4236/ojn.2014.49070

Vest, B. M., Kulak, J. A., & Homish, G. G. (2019). Caring for veterans in US civilian primary care: Qualitative interviews with primary care providers. *Family Practice, 36*, 343–350. https://doi.org/10.1093/fampra/cmy078

Way, D., Ersek, M., Montagnini, M., Nathan, S., Perry, S. A., Dale, H., Savage, J. L., Luhrs, C. A., Shreve, S. T., & Jones, C. A. (2019). Top ten tips palliative care providers should know about caring for veterans. *Journal of Palliative Medicine, 22*, 708–713. https://doi.org/10.1098/jpm.2019.0190

Weber, J. J., Lee, R. C., & Martsolf, D. (2019). Experiences of care in the emergency department among a sample of homeless male veterans: A qualitative study. *Journal of Emergency Nursing, 46*(1), 51–58. https://doi.org/10.1016/j.jen.2019.06.009

CURRICULAR CONSIDERATIONS AND TEACHING STRATEGIES FOR THE INTEGRATION OF VETERAN HEALTH INTO NURSING EDUCATION

KATIE A. CHARGUALAF | EDNA R. MAGPANTAY-MONROE

Caring for our veterans is the duty of a grateful nation.

Patty Murray

KEY TERMS

veteran-centered curriculum

nursing curriculum

teaching strategies

transition

veteran-specific content

veteran-health competencies

nursing education

INTRODUCTION

Veterans sustain unique injuries and health issues resulting from military service that often require ongoing care in acute and community settings. Nearly three quarters of the 19 million living veterans in the United States receive their healthcare outside of the Veterans Health Administration (VHA; McMillan et al., 2017). There is a need for healthcare providers, and nurses specifically, who are prepared to provide evidence-based, veteran-centered care. However, efforts to integrate veteran-health content in nursing curricula vary. Further, practicing nurses and nursing students report a lack of knowledge and comfort caring for veterans (Maiocco et al., 2019; Roe et al., 2019). This chapter includes a presentation of the factors influencing veterans' healthcare utilization in civilian settings, veteran-health competencies, barriers and strategies to revising curricula to achieve the *Joining Forces* goals, and teaching and learning strategies faculty may use to incorporate veteran-health content into the nursing classroom.

The complete reference list for this chapter appears in the digital version of the chapter, accessible at https://connect.springerpub.com/content/book/978-0-8261-3597-1/chapter/ch10

BACKGROUND

At the end of 2018, there were 19.6 million veterans in the United States, of which 47% were over the age of 65 years and almost 10% female (U.S. Department of Veterans Affairs [VA], 2019a). Veterans have served in one or more eras including World War II, Korea, Vietnam, Gulf War, and Operation Iraqi Freedom/Operation Enduring Freedom (collectively known as Post-9/11 or the Global War on Terrorism [GWOT]). Veteran health and health issues are directly linked to military service including work role (military occupational specialty), deployment rotations, advancements in protective gear, improved training, enhanced triage procedures, rapid evacuation of injured service members, and improved treatment modalities based on best practice (Conard et al., 2015; Cooper et al., 2016). It is important to note that service members are surviving injuries that in previous conflicts were often lethal. The results of which are veterans who often require ongoing care in acute and community settings.

Although there are more than 19 million veterans living in the United States, only 9 million are enrolled in the VHA (VA, 2019a), and even fewer receive all of their healthcare through the VHA (McMillan et al., 2017). Nearly 75% of veterans seek all or part of their healthcare needs from civilian providers or entities (McMillan et al., 2017; Rossiter et al., 2018). Some of the reasons why veterans may not use a VHA facility or provider include "geographical availability, personal preference, or even lack of awareness regarding eligibility" (Rossiter et al., 2018, p. 280). Additional reasons may include prolonged wait times, culturally insensitive care, availability of resources, and dissatisfaction (Conard et al., 2015). Provisions of the Veterans Access, Choice, and Accountability Act of 2014, and later the VA Mission Act of 2018 (U.S. Senate Committee on Veterans' Affairs, 2019) resulted in greater numbers of veterans seeking care in civilian facilities.

Strategically located in all areas of the healthcare system, nurses are in an ideal position to have a meaningful impact on the health and wellness of veterans (Conard et al., 2015). But to do so, nurses must understand military and veteran culture and fully appreciate how military service influences health and wellness. The *Joining Forces* initiative, launched in 2012 by First Lady Michelle Obama and Dr. Jill Biden, sought to bring greater attention to the needs of military service members, veterans, and their families.

BOX 10.1

JOINING FORCES PLEDGE

Educating America's future nurses to care for our nation's veterans, service members, and their families facing posttraumatic stress disorder, traumatic brain injury, depression, and other clinical issues

Enriching nursing education to ensure that current and future nurses are trained in the unique clinical challenges and best practices associated with caring for military service members, veterans, and their families

Integrating content that addresses the unique health and wellness challenges of our nation's service members, veterans, and their families into nursing curricula

Sharing teaching resources and applying best practices in the care of service members, veterans, and their families

Growing the body of knowledge leading to improvements in healthcare and wellness for our service members, veterans, and their families

Joining with others to further strengthen the supportive community of nurses, institutions, and healthcare providers dedicated to improving the health of service members, veterans, and their families

SOURCE: From https://obamawhitehouse.archives.gov/the-press-office/2012/04/11/americas-nurses-join-forces-first-lady-and-dr-biden-support-veterans-and

Nursing education organizations endorsed the initiative and schools of nursing pledged to come together to meet military and veteran needs in nursing curricula (Elliott & Patterson, 2017). However, years later, it is evident that while nursing programs consider the content important, efforts to meet the *Joining Forces* goals vary significantly (Elliott & Patterson, 2017). In nursing education, the *Joining Forces* pledge includes six goals (Box 10.1). While some schools of nursing successfully meet all, or part, of the initiative goals, most were still working toward the objective (Elliott & Patterson, 2017). Beckford and Ellis (2013) acknowledged that the ways in which nurse educators are responding to the *Joining Forces* initiatives is unclear. While faculty knowledge and comfort teaching veteran-centered content are important, barriers including an already dense curriculum and requisite time to evaluate existing curricula, frequently impacted the ability to achieve the *Joining Forces* goals (Elliott & Patterson, 2017).

The foundation for a veteran-centered nursing practice begins in undergraduate education and should continue in graduate education and ongoing professional development (Chargualaf, 2019; Roe et al., 2019). Nurse educators in the clinical setting are instrumental in updating practicing nurses about veteran health. Only when all nurses are informed about the health needs of service members, veterans, and their families will a veteran-centered nursing practice be fully achieved. Before presenting active teaching and learning strategies nurse faculty and clinical educators may use to integrate veteran-health content into the classroom or work setting, veteran-centered competencies and curricular revision are discussed.

VETERAN-CENTERED COMPETENCIES

The impetus to address veteran health in nursing education stemmed from the prolonged engagement in combat operations as part of the GWOT, rising numbers of service members returning home with chronic injuries directly linked to military service, the *Joining Forces* initiative, a preponderance of veterans who receive their healthcare outside of the VA, and a lack of civilian knowledge and training to provide veteran-centered care (McMillan et al., 2017). It became clear that healthcare professionals, and nurses in particular, needed to have a strong working knowledge of military and veteran health-related issues. This prompted nurse leaders to establish and publish veteran-health competencies which may be used to guide curricular evaluation and revision. Several publications highlight important content areas that should be included in nursing curricula (Carlson, 2016; Olenick et al., 2015). Other competencies focus on topics a practicing nurse, working in a non-VA setting, should know (Conard et al., 2015; Counts et al., 2015; Johnson et al., 2013). To date, only two formalized sets of competencies for care of the veteran are available (McMillan et al., 2017; Moss et al., 2015).

Military service members and veterans are a diverse population, abiding by a set of values, customs, norms, beliefs, and behaviors often far different than their civilian counterparts (Olenick et al., 2015). Distinct laws, codes of conduct, and military ethos including loyalty, selflessness, and teamwork by which all service members abide make the military its own culture (Coll et al., 2011; Olenick et al., 2015). For many veterans, elements of the military culture become "a permanent part of their self-identity and worldview" (Westpahl & Convoy, 2015, para. 12). As such, nurses must be educated about the military and veterans in order to develop cultural humility and provide culturally sensitive care (Tervalon & Murray-García, 1998; Yeager & Bauer-Wu, 2013). Thus, the foundation for a veteran-centered nursing practice lies in understanding military and veteran culture (Carlson, 2016; Champlin et al., 2017; McMillan et al., 2017; Moss et al., 2015; Olenick et al., 2015).

The published competencies provide a starting point for faculty interested in expanding curricular initiatives to include veteran-health concepts (McMillan et al., 2017; Moss et al., 2015). Competency is defined as "an expected level of performance that integrates knowledge, skills, abilities, and judgment" (American Nurses Association [ANA], 2015, p. 44). In alignment with the Quality and Safety Education for Nurses (QSEN) initiative, both sets of competencies outline the associated knowledge, skills, and attitudes (KSAs) needed by new graduate nurses to validate each competency. Congruence between the competency sets validates published literature, experience by nurses working with veterans, VHA

TABLE 10.1 COMPARING VETERAN-CENTERED COMPETENCIES/CONTENT AREAS ACROSS SELECT LITERATURE

COMPETENCY	MOSS ET AL. (2015)	MCMILLAN ET AL. (2017)	CARLSON (2016)	OLENICK ET AL. (2015)	VA PRIORITIES*
Military and veteran culture	X	X	X	X	
PTSD	X	X	X	X	
TBI	X	X			
Depression/anxiety				X	
Substance use disorder	X	X		X	
Suicide	X	X		X	X
Polytrauma	X	X			
Amputation/assistive devices/wound care	X	X		X	
Pain/chronic pain		X		X	
Environmental/ chemical exposures	X	X		X	
MST	X		X		X
Homelessness	X		X	X	
End of life	X				
Veterans Health Administration/ access to healthcare	X	X	X	X	X
Caregiver assistance		X			
Care of military families			X		

* VA Priorities as established by the VA FY 2018–2024 strategic plan.

FY, fiscal year; MST, military sexual trauma; PTSD, posttraumatic stress disorder; TBI, traumatic brain injury; VA, U.S. Department of Veterans Affairs.

SOURCE: U.S. Department of Veterans Affairs. (2019). *Department of Veterans Affairs FY 2018–2024 strategic plan.* https://www.va.gov/oei/docs/VA2018-2024strategicPlan.pdf

policy, and faculty expertise. Table 10.1 compares the veteran-centered competencies and content areas across nursing literature. Only those competencies explicitly stated on the competency list were noted in the table; however, in certain cases it is likely that a content area was included even though the supportive statement was written in broader terms. For example, McMillan et al. (2017) identified the influence of chronic pain in veterans with traumatic brain injury (TBI) and amputation. On the other hand, in the competencies established by Moss et al. (2015), students must be able to "recognize common problems associated with traumatic amputations" which would include pain (p. 311).

Several notable differences were found among the different competencies. Moss et al. (2015) was the only study to identify military sexual trauma (MST), although McMillan et al. (2017) highlighted the impact of polytrauma on alterations in sexual intimacy. McMillan et al. (2017) isolated advocacy of the veteran and family member(s) into a separate competency but provided only a single statement about engaging with community partners and resources. Moss et al. (2015) highlighted additional competencies likely to be addressed at a community level including homelessness. In light of the similarities and differences among the competencies and other published literature, nurse faculty should consider all of these sources to inform the integration of veteran-health content into nursing curricula.

Nurse faculty must have the knowledge to facilitate curricular redesign and successfully teach veteran-health competencies. This may be accomplished by hiring faculty who are veterans or come from a military background but more likely will entail professional development. Champlin et al. (2017) discussed a faculty development plan whereby veteran-specific disorders were presented and discussed at the beginning of regularly scheduled monthly faculty meetings. The same may be accomplished through articles reviewing veteran health issues with teaching recommendations that award contact hours (Conard et al., 2015). Accessing teaching and learning resources from reputable professional nursing organizations, such as The American Association of Colleges of Nursing (AACN) "Joining Forces: Enhancing Veterans' Care Tool Kit," is another opportunity to learn about veterans (AACN, 2019). Regardless of the method employed to learn and understand veterans and service-connected disorders, what is most important is that professional development be ongoing to ensure that content is current, relevant, and evidence-based.

NURSING CURRICULA REVISITED

Successful integration of veteran-health content requires an understanding of both change as well as the underpinning of current nursing curricula. The National League for Nursing (NLN, 2019a) defines curriculum as "the interaction among learners, teachers, and knowledge—occurring in an academic environment—that is designed to accomplish goals identified by the learners, the teachers, and the profession the learners expect to enter" (para. 6). Curricula are not just the courses a student takes, the content nurse faculty review within a course, or the experiential learning opportunities. It is the vessel by which nurse educators organize teaching and learning to prepare students for professional practice and evaluate those endeavors. Curricula should reflect best practices in instruction and healthcare delivery, incorporating research evidence with ongoing evaluation and revision to ensure continued relevance.

Several professional organizations, national reports, and detailed recommendations drive curricular development and change (Table 10.2). At a foundational level, the Essentials of Baccalaureate Education for Professional Practice (AACN, 2008) provides a framework for undergraduate education through nine curricular elements deemed fundamental for new graduate nurses. Some of the essentials incorporate recommendations outlined in the Institute of Medicine (IOM, 2000) report, *To Err Is Human: Building a Safer Health System*. The quantification of medical errors and resulting patient harm prompted nurse leaders to incorporate concepts related to safety, quality improvement, and research evidence to support best practices into nursing curricula. Soon after, a national study funded by the Robert Wood Johnson Foundation in 2005 sought to bridge the academic-practice gap in the areas of patient safety and quality. The results of the project were six quality and patient safety competencies with the requisite KSA needed to demonstrate achievement of each competency (QSEN Institute, 2019).

Later, the *Carnegie National Nursing Education Study*, led by Dr. Patricia Benner, explored learning theory, mastering a skilled practice, and developing a professional identity to uncover the strengths and weaknesses of nursing education and identify professional challenges (The Carnegie Foudation for the Advancement of Teaching, 2010). The report determined that while U.S. nursing programs are effectively helping nurses develop an ethical practice and a professional identity, they are less effective in integrating nursing, natural, and social sciences as well as technology and humanities into nursing education (The Carnegie Foundation for the Advancement of Teaching, 2010). Clinical learning experiences are especially effective when educators combine clinical and classroom teaching. To that end, the researchers recommended a radical transformation of nursing education with focuses on entry and pathways, nursing students, student experiences in education, teaching pedagogies, transition to practice, and national oversight (The Carnegie Foundation for the Advancement of Teaching, 2010). The NLN unveiled the Excellence in Nursing Model in 2006 (NLN, 2006). In it, excellence in nursing education was defined by eight core elements encompassing relevant stakeholders, resources, curricula, and pedagogy (NLN, 2006). In 2019, the NLN revised their *Hallmarks of Excellence* tool outlining

230

TABLE 10.2 UNDERPINNINGS OF CURRENT NURSING CURRICULA*

AACN	■ Essentials of BSN education (2008)
	■ Liberal education for baccalaureate generalist nursing practice
	■ Basic organizational and systems leadership for quality care and patient safety
	■ Scholarship for evidence-based practice
	■ Information management and application of patient care technology
	■ Healthcare policy, finance, and regulatory environments
	■ **Interprofessional** communication and collaboration for improving patient health outcomes
	■ Clinical prevention and **population health**
	■ Professionalism and professional values
	■ Baccalaureate generalist nursing practice
	■ Essentials of MSN education (2011)
	■ Background for Practice from Sciences and Humanities
	■ Organizational and Systems Leadership
	■ Quality Improvement and Safety
	■ Translating and Integrating Scholarship into Practice
	■ Informatics and Healthcare Technologies
	■ Health Policy and Advocacy
	■ Interprofessional Collaboration for Improving Patient and Population Health Outcomes
	■ Clinical Prevention and Population Health for Improving Health
	■ Master's-Level Nursing Practice
	■ Essentials of DNP education (2006)
	■ Scientific Underpinnings for Practice
	■ Organizational and Systems Leadership for Quality Improvement and Systems Thinking
	■ Clinical Scholarship and Analytical Methods for Evidence-Based Practice
	■ Information Systems/Technology and Patient Care Technology for the Improvement and Transformation of Healthcare
	■ Healthcare Policy for Advocacy in Health Care
	■ Interprofessional Collaboration for Improving Patient and Population Health Outcomes
	■ Clinical Prevention and Population Health for Improving the Nation's Health
	■ Advanced Nursing Practice
National League for Nursing	■ Excellence in Nursing Model (2006)
	■ Clear program standards and hallmarks that raise expectations
	■ Well-prepared faculty
	■ Qualified students
	■ Well-prepared educational administrators
	■ Evidence-based programs and teaching/evaluation methods
	■ Quality and adequate resources
	■ Student-centered, interactive, innovative programs and curricula
National League for Nursing	■ Hallmarks of Excellence (2019b)
	■ Engaged students
	■ Diverse, well-prepared faculty
	■ Culture of continuous quality improvement
	■ Innovative, **evidence-based curriculum**
	■ Innovative, evidence-based approaches to facilitate and evaluate learning
	■ Resources to support program goal attainment
	■ Commitment to pedagogical scholarship
	■ Effective institutional and professional leadership
Quality and Safety Education for Nurses	■ QSEN Competencies with KSAs (2019)
	■ **Patient-centered care**
	■ Teamwork and **collaboration**
	■ Evidence-based practice
	■ Quality improvement
	■ Safety
	■ Informatics

TABLE 10.2 (continued)

Carnegie Foundation for the Advancement of Teaching	■ Educating Nurses (2010)
	  ■ U.S. nursing programs are very effective in forming professional identity and ethical comportment
	  ■ Clinical practice assignments provide powerful learning experiences, especially in those programs where educators integrate clinical and classroom teaching
	  ■ U.S. nursing programs are not generally effective in teaching nursing science, natural sciences, social sciences, technology, and humanities
	  ■ 25 recommendations divided between six categories
	    ■ Entry and pathways
	    ■ Student population
	    ■ The student experience
	    ■ Teaching
	    ■ Entry to practice
	    ■ National oversight

American Nurses Association (2015)	■ Scope & Standards of Practice (3rd edition, 2015)
	  ■ Standard 1: Assessment
	  ■ Standard 2: Diagnosis
	  ■ Standard 3: Outcomes identification
	  ■ Standard 4: Planning
	  ■ Standard 5: Implementation
	    ■ Standard 5A: **Coordination of care**
	    ■ Standard 5B: Health teaching and health promotion
	  ■ Standard 6: Evaluation
	  ■ Standard 7: Ethics
	  ■ Standard 8: **Culturally congruent practice**
	  ■ Standard 9: **Communication**
	  ■ Standard 10: Collaboration
	  ■ Standard 11: **Leadership**
	  ■ Standard 12: **Education**
	  ■ Standard 13: Evidence-based practice and Research
	  ■ Standard 14: Quality of practice
	  ■ Standard 15: Professional practice evaluation
	  ■ Standard 16: Resource utilization
	  ■ Standard 17: **Environmental health**

IOM	■ Health Professions Education: A Bridge to Quality (2003)
	  ■ Provide **patient-centered care**
	  ■ Work in interdisciplinary teams
	  ■ Employ evidence-based practice
	  ■ Apply quality improvement
	  ■ Utilize informatics

NOTE: Keywords linked to veteran-centered health are bolded.

* Full reference and links to each organization/association are located on the reference list.

AACN, American Association of Colleges of Nursing; BSN, Bachelor of Science in Nursing; DNP, Doctor of Nursing Practice; EBP, evidence-based practice, IOM, Institute of Medicine; KSA, knowledge, skills, and attitudes; MSN, Master of Science in Nursing; NLN, National League for Nursing; QI, quality improvement; QSEN, Quality and Safety Education for Nurses.

characteristics of high performing nursing programs (NLN, 2019b). Its purpose is to guide nursing programs in their pursuit of evidence-based best practices in curriculum and teaching. Finally, *Nursing: Scope and Standards of Practice*, developed by the ANA (2015), guide professional nursing practice and inform nursing curricula.

Challenges and Barriers

Each of the curricular foundations discussed in Table 10.3 validate the inclusion of veteran health competencies in nursing curricula. And yet, undertaking a curricular revision, for any reason, is an arduous

TABLE 10.3 CURRICULAR STAKEHOLDERS

State board of nursing	Responsible to oversee the implementation of curricula to ensure teaching pedagogies, clinical learning experiences, and faculty credentials needed to sufficiently prepare new graduates for professional nursing practice
Accrediting bodies	Include NLNAC and the CCNE Responsible for evaluating outcomes such as graduation rates, first time NCLEX pass rates, job placement rates, and student feedback as a measure of program effectiveness and student satisfaction
Professional organizations	Organizations such as the IOM, AACN, NLN, and QSEN Develop frameworks and standards required for safe nursing practice, all of which directly influence curricular development and revision
Institutions of higher learning and university administrators	Nursing curricula are influenced by general education requirements outlined by the university, availability of resources such as the library or technology, financial support to hire faculty and offset programmatic costs, and assistance securing clinical practice sites
Faculty	Faculty are key stakeholders in this process (Champlin et al., 2017) because they maintain knowledge and experience in both clinical practice and nursing education. Faculty are also keenly aware of professional standards and trends impacting patient care in all settings
Students/graduates	Nursing students expect to receive a quality education that is not cost prohibitive. Nursing curricula should be flexible, timely, and accommodate the needs of adult learners
Community partners Potential employers	Collaboration with clinical nurse partners and nurse employers provide clinical learning experiences capable of meeting clinical outcomes and ensure curricula sufficiently prepares new graduates to meet current practice demands

AACN, American Association of Colleges of Nursing; CCNE, Commission on Collegiate Nursing Education; IOM, Institute of Medicine; NCLEX, National Council Licensing Exam; NLN, National League for Nursing; NLNAC, National League for Nursing Accrediting Commission; QSEN, Quality and Safety Education for Nurses

SOURCE: Shanthi, R., & Angeline, G. (2015). Curriculum development in nursing education: Where is the pathway? *IOSR Journal of Nursing and Health Science, 4,* 76–81. https://doi.org/10.9790/1959-04537681

task rife with challenges. Beischel and Davis (2014) argued that a successful revision of nursing curricula requires knowledgeable and committed change agents, faculty who recognize a need for change and are willing to do so, and a clear vision to guide the change process. Addressing and overcoming barriers to change is also necessary to facilitate an environment in which change is embraced. Common barriers impacting change in a healthcare environment include a lack of awareness and rationale for needed change, motivation, beliefs and attitudes related to change and one's ability to undertake change, and skills and resources to effectively participate in change (National Health Service, National Institute for Health and Clinical Excellence, 2007).

In nursing education, curricular revision to accommodate veteran-health content and competencies is also likely to be met with a number of challenges. The first of which is time. Curricular revision should include evaluation of program objectives, course mapping, alignment between course level learning outcomes and program objectives, and assessment strategies (Shanthi & Angeline, 2015). Faculty workload is frequently cited as a barrier to active participation in curricular evaluation and redesign (Beischel & Davis, 2014). Assigning workload credit is suggested as one method of helping nursing programs overcome this challenge. One nursing program seeking to embed QSEN competencies into an existing curriculum created a binder of QSEN-related teaching resources and challenged faculty to utilize these resources to enhance learning assignments and teaching strategies (Beischel & Davis, 2014). This idea reduces the potential workload burden on faculty and could be tailored to schools of nursing seeking to include veteran-health competencies in their curricula.

Budgetary and resource constraints also influence curricular evaluation and revision (Keating, 2015). In fact, both impact the curriculum development/revision process as well as the outcome of such an endeavor. An aging workforce, a shortage of nurse educators, decreased higher education funding, and rapidly expanding technologies to enhance teaching and learning are factors that should be acknowledged as affecting curricular change. "Assessment of current and future resources is crucial" when revising nursing curricula (Keating, 2015, p. 36).

Faculty may struggle to identify where to teach veteran-health competencies in the curriculum as well as the specific content that should be included. In many cases, nursing curricula are crowded; laden with content faculty perceive as vital to preparing new graduates for professional practice (Champlin et al., 2017). Harmer and Huffman (2012) note that technologies, changes in healthcare delivery, and content reinforcement leave faculty "overwhelmed trying to teach more content in the same amount of time" (p. 238). The struggle is compounded by a rapidly growing body of available information and resources to augment nursing education. The challenge, then, is to seek out innovative ways to embed veteran health information in an already saturated curriculum. Experiential learning opportunities such as simulation and dedicating a percentage of required clinical instructional time in a veteran health facility are proposed ways of overcoming this barrier (Cooper et al., 2016; Harmer & Huffman, 2012).

A fear of the unknown may create or foster a sense of complacency. This challenge is predicated on faculty's lack of knowledge about military and veteran culture and the health impacts of military service. Coupled with this are faculty who lack "formal preparation in curriculum development, instructional design, or performance assessment" (IOM, 2011). Hendricks (2020) argues, "Revising curricula requires faculty to possess content expertise, an understanding of how various curricular elements interact, and the ability to negotiate and manage change" (p. 156). Building a team of faculty with experience in curricular revision alongside committed faculty recognizing the need for inclusion of this content may be one solution to this barrier. Further, efforts to support faculty to step outside their comfort zone to explore relevant content areas and new student-centered teaching strategies are recommended (Baron, 2017).

Best Practices for Curricular Change or Revision

Best practices for curricular revision should be considered when working to integrate veteran health competencies. First, faculty must be committed to reexamine and update nursing curricula regularly based on "new evidence and a changing science base, changes and advances in technology, and changes in the needs of patients and the health care system" (IOM The Future of Nursing Report, 2011, Need for Updated & Adaptive Curricula section, para 1). Oermann (2019) stated that the curricular revision process "starts by recognizing the need for change" (p. 1). Relevant stakeholders (Table 10.4) should take an active part in the assessment, evaluation, and revision of curricula because each maintains a unique viewpoint of current and future trends (Hendricks, 2020). Appreciating that stakeholder knowledge and expertise related to curricular development and revision varies significantly, a task force of experienced faculty should oversee the change. Opportunities for students to share their perspectives related to the curricular change is encouraged.

No curricular revision should be undertaken without sufficient planning. Perhaps most important is ensuring the timing of the curricular change does not interfere with other initiatives requiring significant time and attention from faculty (Hendricks, 2020). Further, a successful curricular revision depends on a realistic assessment of current and future resources. This is particularly relevant as technologies influence the ways nurse educators deliver nursing education and its use expected by younger generations of students (Veltri, 2020). Nursing curricula should align with the university mission, vision, and values and also consider program characteristics (Hendricks, 2020; Oermann, 2019). Doing so ensures the learning needs of the student population are considered. Finally, curricular evaluation should follow a consistent process that assesses the strengths and weaknesses, and verifies organization of concepts and courses meet stated program outcomes (Sullivan, 2020).

CREATING OR REVISING CURRICULA TO BE VETERAN-CENTERED

To ensure culturally competent practitioners, nursing curricula should be "inclusive of all diverse populations," among them military service members, veterans, and their families (Kautzmann & Lancaster, 2018, p. 120). But military culture is vastly different from civilian society, often unfamiliar to those outside of the military. "Military culture shapes a shared set of behaviors, beliefs, and values that are learned and reinforced through the lived experience of military service" (Westpahl & Convoy, 2015, para. 10). Values including duty, honor, sacrifice, loyalty, teamwork, camaraderie, and service before self underlie the military way of life and become a part of a service member's identity. Veteran identity is defined as "the self-concept deriving from one's military experiences within a sociohistorical context" (Johnson et al., 2013, p. 27). Length of military service, era served, participation in combat operations, service-connected injuries or disabilities, and reintegration experiences all influence a veteran's identity (Johnson et al., 2013). Serving in the military maintains lifelong effects which means that regardless of the length of time since a service member left the military, positive and negative sequelae continue across the lifespan (Spiro et al., 2016). The uniqueness of the military culture, the influence of veteran identity, and varied military service experiences create a need to expand the definition of cultural competence to include service members, veterans, and their families. As such, nurses working in all care areas must understand the effect military culture has on health and wellness to ensure veterans, and their families, receive culturally congruent and patient-centered care.

Soon after pledging to *Join Forces*, schools of nursing began reporting efforts to revise curricula to be veteran-centered (Beckford & Ellis, 2013; Champlin et al., 2017; Crary, 2018; Finnegan et al., 2020; Harmer & Huffman, 2012; Jones & Breen, 2015; Magpantay-Monroe, 2017; McKenzie et al., 2016; Nye et al., 2013; Rossiter et al., 2018; Schinka & Raia, 2013; Vessey et al., 2018). York et al. (2016) recommended any veteran-directed curricular revision align with the VA's core values of compassion, commitment, excellence, professionalism, integrity, accountability, and stewardship. Three ways to develop or modify curricula to incorporate veteran competencies include (a) integrate veteran-related content across relevant courses, (b) provide opportunities to interact with veterans in the clinical setting, and (c) develop an inclusive course dedicated to the veteran population or a specific veteran competency (Rossiter et al., 2018). Veteran-centered clinical experiences are discussed elsewhere in the book; therefore, this section focuses on integration of competencies in existing curricula and an inclusive veteran health course.

Integration of Competencies Into Existing Curricula

Integration of veteran competencies does not require a complete curricular revision. "As a starting point, faculty can examine the curriculum for logical entry points for veteran-centered content, using current content with veteran examples" (Champlin et al., 2017, p. 255). In some cases, faculty may already be teaching content (e.g., posttraumatic stress disorder [PTSD]) that impacts veterans and would require only an expansion of course content to include a veteran context (Olenick et al., 2015). Curricular mapping can also help differentiate what beginning nursing students should know compared to senior nursing students or practicing nurses returning to school. For example, the competency of advocacy for the military family could be introduced in a fundamentals course when military and veteran culture is discussed. In a psychiatric/mental health course, while teaching PTSD or TBI, faculty could highlight the effect of these diagnoses on military families and then identify community resources. Finally, in a pediatrics course, the impact of frequent moves as part of any military career or long separations from a family member due to deployment could be discussed as both may cause changes in childhood behaviors and influence family dynamics.

Simulation is a popular avenue for integrating veteran-health content into existing curricula (Anthony et al., 2012; Beckford & Ellis, 2013; Harmer & Huffman, 2012; Nye et al., 2013). One benefit of using experiential learning, such as simulation, to incorporate veteran care is that sensitive topics, like MST, may be included. Further, debriefing after simulation facilitates reflection, yields opportunities for constructive feedback, and allows for emotional decompression (Harmer & Huffman, 2012). Less expensive and technologically based methods of infusing veteran healthcare content are also reported in the literature. Ideas include guest speakers who are local experts on military and veteran health (Olenick et al., 2015), unfolding case studies (McKenzie et al., 2016), and standardized patient scenarios (Peterson et al., 2018).

Several professional nursing organizations offer teaching resources that faculty may use to infuse veteran health content into an existing course. The AACN developed the *Enhancing Veterans' Care Faculty Tool Kit* for faculty (www.aacnnursing.org/Teaching-Resources/Tool-Kits/Veterans-Care). Included in the tool kit are general resources needed to understand military culture and provide culturally sensitive care, as well as educational resources such as articles, case studies, and curricular examples. The NLN dedicated a section of their online teaching resources to the care of veterans (www.nln.org/professional-development-programs/teaching-resources/veterans-ace-v). Advancing Care Excellence for Veterans (ACE.V) contains a framework for providing quality care to veterans, unfolding case studies, teaching strategies that will assist students to understand the unique health needs of the veteran population, and online professional development related to veterans for nurse faculty.

Inclusive Veteran-Health Course

Another alternative is to develop a stand-alone military and veteran-centric course. In partnership with the local VA and Veterans Affairs Nursing Academy nurse faculty, Rossiter et al. (2018) developed an elective course comprised of eight modules covering topics including military and veteran cultural competence, physical and psychological wounds of military service, the military family, women's health, and military sexual trauma. The course incorporates a variety of teaching and learning modalities that help the student to connect to veterans (interview), identify community resources for veterans (research and discussion), and understand the impacts of military service on health and wellness (view documentary; case study; Rossiter et al., 2018). Other courses are described in the literature to prepare students to effectively care for the veteran population (Keavney, 2015). While the content topics and teaching strategies are similar, efforts to reach students in other health disciplines are noted. Across publications, veteran-health courses successfully help students describe military and veteran culture, identify service-connected illness and disabilities, identify community resources, and develop a greater appreciation for veteran health needs (Crary, 2018, Keavney, 2015; Rossiter et al., 2018).

TEACHING STRATEGIES AND LEARNING ACTIVITIES FOR THE CLASSROOM

"The teaching-learning process involves the planning and implementation of experiences that are designed to lead to the achievement of student learning outcomes" (Gittings & Wittman-Price, 2017, p. 55). The process includes both the teaching strategy, the methods used by faculty to communicate knowledge and information, and learning activities, which is the engagement by students with the new information (Gittings & Wittman-Price, 2017). It is important that faculty appeal to all learning styles (Table 10.4) and vary learning activities across the three domains of learning (Table 10.5). There is no singular, best method for teaching veteran health to undergraduate and graduate nursing students. Rather, it is recommended that faculty employ a variety of teaching strategies and learning activities to ensure the KSA for each veteran-health competency is met.

Learning activities are classified as active or passive depending on the amount of learner engagement. Passive learning involves acquiring knowledge through different senses that will be recalled and used later (Scheckel, 2020). Common examples of passive learning strategies include listening to a lecture, taking notes, reading assignments, or using audiovisual media. The benefit of passive learning is that both faculty and student are comfortable with this approach to learning, faculty can communicate large volumes of information in a controlled manner, and key concepts are identified by

TABLE 10.4 LEARNING STYLES

Visual or spatial	Learners are partial to seeing and observing things, including pictures, diagrams, and written directions. These students may like to doodle, make lists, take notes, or make charts to organize information
Auditory or aural	Learners are partial to listening to a lecture rather than taking notes. Students use their own voices to reinforce new concepts by reading out loud or engage by speaking up in class. They may also reinforce their understanding by repeating the spoken words of the teacher. These learners do well in group work
Kinesthetic or tactile	Learners learn best through experiencing or doing things. They like to use their hands to touch and handle in order to understand concepts. These students might struggle to sit still and need frequent breaks when studying
Reading/ writing	Learners learn best through information displayed through text and words. They like to list their words. These students prefer PowerPoint and web-based learning

SOURCE: Cherry, G. (2019). *Which learning style do you have?* https://www.verywellmind.com/vark-learning-styles-2795156; Rolfe, A., & Cheek, B. (2012). Learning styles. *InnovAiT, 5,* 176–181. https://doi.org/10.1093/innovait/inr239

TABLE 10.5 DOMAINS OF LEARNING

Cognitive domain	The cognitive domain focuses on knowledge. Complexity of learning is presented in ascending order. Aligns with Bloom's taxonomy: remembering – understanding – applying – analyzing – evaluating – creating
Psychomotor domain	The psychomotor domain focuses on the demonstration of nursing skills in the clinical setting. Learning occurs over time with opportunities to practice and demonstrate mastery
Affective domain	The affective domain integrates the values, beliefs, and emotions of the student into the learning process. Learning should promote personal growth as an internal locus of control develops

SOURCE: Scheckel, M. (2020). Designing courses and learning experiences. In D. Billings & J. Halstead (Eds.), *Teaching in nursing: A guide for faculty* (6th ed., pp. 181–201). Elsevier.

faculty. Significant disadvantages to passive learning strategies often include insufficient time to assess understanding and clarify concepts. Active learning is widely regarded as the better learning strategy because students are actively engaged with new information (Scheckel, 2020). As a result, active learning promotes increased learning interest, motivation, understanding and retention of new information, and enhanced critical thinking abilities. However, faculty may be reluctant to pursue active learning strategies in the classroom due to a lack of knowledge related to innovative pedagogies, resistance to updating teaching strategies, and fear of the impact on teaching evaluations from students.

A collection of active learning strategies is presented in the following sections. Each active learning strategy is briefly defined followed by a presentation of how it may be used to teach veteran-specific content aligning with one or more veteran-health competencies. Learning outcomes and the domain of learning are identified for each teaching strategy and includes additional resources of information to create the content. The teaching modalities may be modified to match the needs of any course or program.

Audience/Student Response Systems

Audience response systems (ARSs) are also referred as student response systems. ARS is a two-way communication that involves use of technology where students respond to questions posed by the instructor in real time (Mareno et al., 2010). The advantages of ARSs are increased student engagement, opportunities to assess student performance (i.e., formative and summative course evaluation), opportunities to discuss/re-discuss aspects of the content that were not well understood or students can clarify concepts/ask questions, and enhanced student performance as anonymity is preserved

(Bassendowski & Petrucka, 2013; Mareno et al., 2010). The disadvantages of ARSs are the availability of an appropriate device needed for active participation, technical or connectivity issues during the class session, and use of the appropriate questions by faculty to evoke critical thinking (Mareno et al., 2010).

SAMPLE TEACHING MODALITY

Use of ARS to Understand Military Culture

Pre-work

Have students complete any or all (four total) Military Culture Course Modules. (deploymentpsych.org/military-culture-course-modules; Uniformed Services University, 2019)

Learning Outcomes

1. Demonstrate an understanding of the differences between Active Duty, Reserve, National Guard, and Veterans. (Cognitive and Affective)

2. Identify common misperceptions about caring for veterans. (Affective)

ARS, audience response system.

Many ARS programs may be freely downloaded (e.g., Poll Everywhere, Kahoot, Socrative) to any device including a smart phone or tablet. Faculty may employ this teaching modality to assess students' completion of pre-class work (e.g., assigned readings) during class to determine muddy points, or at the conclusion of the class to identify topics that require further probing and discussions. Generally, faculty must develop the questions used during this in-class learning activity although there is a sample ARS topic about homelessness found at the NLN ACE.V Teaching Strategies.

Case Study

Case studies are a teaching strategy created to direct students to a particular conclusion after an analysis of a real-life or imagined situation (Amerson, 2011). While a case study allows for application of content and fosters critical thinking and reasoning, students who lack a basic understanding of the content may struggle to engage in the analysis of the case study. Creation of case studies can address diverse backgrounds and different levels of health issues affecting veterans.

SAMPLE TEACHING MODALITY

Unfolding Case Study for Psychiatric/Mental Health Issues

Learning Outcomes

1. Identify tools and procedures to assess for suicidality and PTSD in veterans. (Cognitive and Psychomotor)

2. Differentiate assessment findings warranting immediate intervention. (Psychomotor)

3. Discuss effective communication techniques for veterans. (Psychomotor and Affective)

4. Explain the nurse's role when caring for veterans who are experiencing alterations in mental health. (Psychomotor and Affective)

5. List different veteran service organizations appropriate for the holistic care of veterans with mental health needs. (Psychomotor)

PTSD, posttraumatic stress disorder.

A 45-year-old African American male is brought to the emergency department by his wife for suicidal thoughts. He is a retired Marine and had been deployed to Iraq and Afghanistan multiple times over a 5-year period. You noticed alcohol on his breath, and he appears tearful.

QUESTIONS FOR CLASS DISCUSSION

1. What initial questions would you ask the patient?

2. What recent event(s) may have triggered this patient's suicidal thoughts?

3. What subjective and objective data might indicate that the male patient is suicidal?

As you are gathering the initial assessment information, you noticed the patient fidgeting and his wife states her husband has PTSD and also has chronic back pain from his deployment.

QUESTIONS FOR CLASS DISCUSSION

1. Discuss current treatments (pharmacology versus non- pharmacological) for this patient.

2. What is your priority plan of care for this patient?

3. What is (are) measurable and realistic goal(s) for this patient?

You are a new nursing graduate and never worked with any military patients even during your student clinical rotation.

QUESTIONS FOR CLASS DISCUSSION

1. What important military culture information would you want to ask to provide veteran-centered care?

2. How would you approach the wife during the visit?

3. What services are considered veteran-centric for this patient?

FURTHER DISCUSSIONS

Request students to create a Situation–Background–Assessment–Recommendation (SBAR) for a nurse who is relieving them for their shift. Request students create a data action response nurses note that focuses on their understanding of the applicability of veteran-centric care.

GROUP WORK

If there are nursing students who are veterans or know military culture, divide the students among the groups to share their experiences.

In addition to the sample case study presented, additional case studies are available from the AACN Teaching Resources Toolkit (www.aacnnursing.org/Teaching-Resources/Tool-Kits/Enhancing-Veterans/Educational-Resources) and the NLN ACE.V (www.nln.org/professional-development-programs/teaching-resources/veterans-ace-v/unfolding-cases). Faculty may also find the information on the We Honor Veterans website helpful in developing their own case studies (National Hospice and Palliative Care Organization, 2020).

Group Learning/Projects

Collaborative group learning and projects allows for a dialogue and exchange of information between students (Bassendowski & Petrucka, 2013). This type of active learning lends to a more interactive way of learning and teaching. A group of no more than six students can discuss a topic or issue from multiple viewpoints and clarify or develop solutions, an advantage of this active learning. The disadvantages of this strategy are the inactive involvement of individual learners, and unclear expectations of each student member to complete a defined tasked within a certain time frame (Meo, 2013). A good instructor/facilitator is required to engage all students to have equal time in providing information for any group work.

SAMPLE TEACHING MODALITY

Create a Teaching Pamphlet (or Presentation) for Any Veteran-Health Competency. Outlined by McMillan et al. (2017) or Moss et al. (2015)

Learning Outcomes

1. Define and describe unique healthcare needs of veterans. (Cognitive and Affective)

2. Identify ways to advocate for the needs of the veterans. (Cognitive and Psychomotor)

3. Create a patient and family education pamphlet on an assigned competency or disorder. (Psychomotor)

Working in a group to develop patient learning resources incorporates several skills important to professional nursing practice including retrieval and synthesis of research evidence, working in teams, patient education, and communication (public speaking). Teaching pamphlets should define the competency/health issue, identify risk factors in the veteran population, highlight signs and symptoms, outline diagnostic criteria, identify evidence-based treatment modalities and prevention strategies, and find online/community resources available to veterans. After groups present the information in class, completed teaching pamphlets may be shared with clinical and community partners. Further, course faculty could collaborate with clinical instructors to facilitate student presentations at clinical sites thus enhancing a veteran-centered practice among local practicing nurses and nurse leaders.

SAMPLE TEACHING MODALITY

Updating a List of Resources Available for Practicing Nurses to Facilitate Veteran-Centered Nursing Practice.

Learning Outcomes

1. Identify resources related to specific health issues impacting the veteran population. (Cognitive)

2. Describe how nurses could use the information to inform their nursing practice. (Psychomotor and Affective)

For this learning activity, each student group will select a health issue (e.g., PTSD, diabetes, environmental exposure) commonly encountered in the veteran population and compile an updated list of online and community resources. The list should include current research articles, professional organizations (national), and local community resources. Completed lists will be discussed in class and shared with other student groups, faculty in the school of nursing, and community clinical partners. Sharing with faculty facilitates integration of veteran-health content/competencies into other nursing courses without undue burden on faculty time and reaches a greater number of nursing students (Rossiter et al., 2018).

Concept Mapping

Concept mapping is a diagram created to organize information, analyze relationships, determine priorities, expand previous knowledge, identify less understood concepts, and examine the client from a holistic viewpoint (Schuster, 2016). This active learning strategy assists students to build critical thinking and clinical reasoning skills (Schuster, 2016). Further, concept mapping can easily be incorporated into any learning setting and scaffolding the specific elements or depth of the map may be tailored to students' knowledge and level of experience.

SAMPLE TEACHING MODALITY

TBI

Learning Outcomes

1. Describe how concept maps may be used to develop a veteran-centered nursing practice. (Cognitive and Psychomotor)

2. Create a concept map for TBI focusing on physical, cognitive, emotional, and behavioral manifestations. (Cognitive and Psychomotor)

TBI, traumatic brain injury.

Assign students to look at the Defense and Veterans Brain Injury Center (DVBIC; https://dvbic. dcoe.mil/) and Center for Deployment Psychology (deploymentpsych.org) websites, including videos, to provide a foundational knowledge about TBI prior to concept mapping. Provide students with a blank concept map. Students should identify key problems and supporting data (focusing on physical, cognitive, emotional, and behavioral manifestations), determine top priorities of care, and identify possible goals and evidence-based nursing interventions. To facilitate critical thinking and clinical reasoning faculty could ask students to draw lines to analyze relationships between data. Completed concept maps may be used to facilitate an in-class discussion allowing students to compare and contrast nursing diagnoses, goals, and nursing interventions.

Debate

Debate is a formal discussion of a particular topic that presents opposing arguments (Phillips, 2020). The advantages of a debate are it improves students' analytical skills by acknowledging the complexities of the subject matter (e.g., veteran health issues) and hones their skills in communication and teamwork (Phillips, 2020). According to Rodger and Stewart-Lord (2019), students perceived debate as a valuable teaching tool that draws on diverse viewpoints and encourages deep learning. The disadvantages of a debate are the amount of preparation time required of students to learn information and develop arguments to support assigned viewpoints, feelings of anxiety or conflict as students desire to present a well-formulated argument, and the time required to teach students the art of debate (Chen, 2014; Phillips, 2020).

SAMPLE TEACHING MODALITY

Pain Management Modalities

Learning Outcomes

Argue the advantages and disadvantages of different modalities of pain management and its effectiveness in the veteran population. (Cognitive and Affective)

Identify differences between civilian and military health teams in addressing the pain management needs of veterans. (Cognitive)

Assign students to a debate team (no greater than five or six members) addressing different modalities (e.g., pharmacologic versus non-pharmacologic) of pain management for veterans. Two teams are assigned to each modality; one team addresses the affirmative and the other the negative viewpoint. Each team should also be prepared to address the different systems of care (e.g., civilian versus military healthcare) and their role in pain management. Students may be assigned their pain management modality on the day of the debate or in advance to allow for more thoughtful debate preparation.

Following the same structure as described, assign students to a debate team addressing different laws or congressional bills impacting the health and wellness of veterans. Current legislative activities may be found online (www.congress.gov/) and entering "veteran" into the search bar will narrow results to current bills focusing on veterans.

SAMPLE TEACHING MODALITY

Veteran Advocacy

Learning Outcomes

Argue the pros and cons of the VA Mission Act of 2018 versus the Veterans Access, Choice, and Accountability Act of 2014 as improving the health and wellness of veterans. (Cognitive and Affective)

VA, U.S. Department of Veterans Affairs.

Faculty may also consider including a written component to the debate. Oros (2007) proposed several writing ideas including a group handout to accompany the debate position, an essay presenting a student's personal viewpoint on the issue, or a reflection of the learned lessons from the debate experience.

Games

Games provide content in a creative and fun way. It is an interactive activity, with rules, showcasing the player's knowledge or skill in attempting to reach a specific learning outcome (Phillips, 2020). The advantages are enhancement of critical thinking as students are more engaged with the content and support of active learning by providing immediate feedback to the students through the answers (Day-Black et al., 2015; Philips, 2020). According to Philips (2020) games help students retain newly learned information and learn from each other. On the other hand, games can be competitive, and learning can be misplaced. Other disadvantages are the time needed for faculty to create appropriate games and games may require more space to implement. Additionally, ground rules are needed to ensure a safe learning space, but faculty may not be comfortable enforcing rules.

SAMPLE TEACHING MODALITY

Military and Veteran Culture Jeopardy!

Learning Outcomes

Demonstrate an understanding of military culture. (Cognitive and Psychomotor)

Differentiate the different branches of the military and their mission/values. (Cognitive and Psychomotor)

Some examples of games are Jeopardy! or a scavenger hunt. An example scavenger hunt includes the VA Scavenger Checklist (www.aacnnursing.org/Portals/42/AcademicNursing/Tool%20Kits/Enhancing-Veterans/Student-Scavenger-Hunt-VANA.pdf). Adding a wrap-up activity, such as the muddiest point or a 1-minute paper, to the end of the game is one method faculty can use to help students identify content areas requiring clarification or a focused review.

Interview/Guest Speaker(s)

An interview is a structured meeting of people face to face. This activity allows students to gather data and understand a problem or experience from the perspective of those who lived it. The ability of the selected guest speaker to engage the students is critical to a meaningful session. The students should be trained/prompted to ask follow-up questions and record notes or thoughts during the interview. This teaching and learning modality may culminate in a number of additional activities including group discussion, reflection, journaling, or a formal written paper.

SAMPLE TEACHING MODALITY

Veterans With Disability

Learning Outcomes

1. Discuss disabilities common in the veteran population. (Cognitive and Affective)

2. Identify community resources to assist veterans with disabilities. (Psychomotor)

To facilitate an interview in the classroom setting, faculty could invite a disability coordinator from the local VA or a local non-profit organization that assists veterans with a disability. Students will apply basic information they have read or research case management strategies for veterans. Students are expected to ask questions of the guest speaker(s). Faculty may work with students to develop a list of questions ahead of the interview.

Interviews are also an ideal way for students to connect with veterans and link military service to health (Table 10.6). One interview assignment idea would include allowing students to choose a veteran to interview as part of the My Life/My Story initiative from the VA (Ringler et al., 2015). The premise of My Life/My Story is to create opportunities to get to know veterans better. The completed narratives generated from the My Life/My Story project are placed in a veteran's medical record so that practitioners may better understand them and improve patient outcomes and satisfaction.

From this interview, faculty could develop a number of follow-on assignments including a group discussion to compare and contrast health exposures during similar eras of military service, a formal paper investigating a health issue related to the veteran's military service, or students could provide a formal presentation linking military service with a noted health issue. Students could research intra-professional healthcare and community resources for the veteran they interviewed.

Journal Club

Journal clubs are defined as "organized sessions to review and discuss research articles published in scientific nursing journals to facilitate research utilization and to promote evidence-based nursing" (Häggman-Laitila et al., 2016, p. 163). The advantages of journal clubs in nursing education include increasing research awareness (Keib et al., 2017), learning the research process (Mattila et al., 2013), cultivating interest in reading nursing research (Scherzer et al., 2015), developing patterns of lifelong learning (Laaksonen, 2013), and role preparation for participation in evidence-based practice responsibilities after graduation (Keib et al., 2017). Conversely, a lack of time, interest, or research and statistical interpretation experience needed by faculty to facilitate a journal club are noted disadvantages (Häggman-Laitila et al., 2016). This teaching strategy may be used in both undergraduate and graduate nursing courses.

TABLE 10.6 VETERAN INTERVIEWS

Part 1: Initial veteran interview	Interview categories and subjects: 1. Childhood: where did they grow up, family (parents and siblings), schooling (college or vocational training), and sports, etc. 2. Military: drafted or volunteered? What branch of service, dates of service, did other family members serve in the military? Training location? Duty station(s)? Deployments? If so, where, when, and how long? Rank? Job (MOS)? And challenges when they left the military? 3. Civilian job/career? 4. Family: marriage, children 5. Hobbies: what do they like to do in their free time?

Part 2: Understanding the health impacts of military service	Using the same veteran from the first interview, students will explore the veteran's health as it relates to their military service. The questions in this interview align with the American Academy of Nursing's *Have You Ever Served* campaign:
	
	1. Were you assigned to a hostile or combat area?
	2. Did you experience enemy fire, see combat, or witness causalities?
	3. Were you wounded, injured, or hospitalized?
	4. Were you exposed to noise, chemicals, gases, demolition of munitions/ammunition, pesticides or other hazardous substances?
	5. Do you have a service-connected disability or condition?
	6. Have you ever used the VA for your healthcare? If yes, ask:
	  a. When was your last visit to the VA?
	  b. Do you have a VA primary care provider?
	7. Assess the following concerns for all veterans:
	  a. PTSD:
	    i. Have you experienced a traumatic or stressful event which you believed your life or the lives of those around you were in danger?
	    ii. Experiencing trauma-related thoughts or feelings?
	    iii. Having nightmares, vivid memories, or flashbacks?
	    iv. Feeling anxious, jittery?
	    v. Feeling a sense of panic that something bad will happen?
	    vi. Difficulty sleeping or concentrating?
	  b. Blast concussion/TBI:
	    i. During your military service did you experience heavy artillery fire, vehicle/aircraft accidents, explosions (improvised explosives, rocket propelled grenades, land mines, grenades), or fragments/bullet wounds above the shoulders?
	    ii. Did you have any of these symptoms immediately afterward? Loss of consciousness, feelings dazed or seeing stars, loss of memory about the event, or did you receive a diagnosis of concussion or head injury?

*Assignment used with permission from Dr. Julie Decker at Penn State Altoona

MOS, military occupational specialty; PTSD, posttraumatic stress disorder; TBI, traumatic brain injury; VA, Veterans Administration.

SAMPLE TEACHING MODALITY
PTSD

Learning Outcome
Compare and contrast treatment modalities for veterans with PTSD. (Cognitive)

Students are instructed to retrieve and read one research article investigating a treatment intervention for PTSD in veterans. During class, students are broken into small groups to discuss their article identifying the strengths and weaknesses of the study and treatment intervention. As a group, the treatment modalities are compared and contrasted highlighting the advantages and disadvantages for use in the veteran population.

SAMPLE TEACHING MODALITY

Pain/Chronic Pain

Learning Outcome

Describe evidence-based pharmacologic and nonpharmacologic interventions for veterans suffering from acute or chronic pain. (Cognitive)

Again, students are asked to bring a research article describing a treatment intervention for acute or chronic pain in the veteran population. Classroom discussion could include the strengths and weaknesses of the research study, the risks and benefits of each treatment intervention, and the nurse's role in implementing the treatment in different care areas. Faculty could also use a journal club to complement other teaching strategies in the classroom. For example, the retrieved articles meeting the learning outcomes could then be used alongside an unfolding case study, a simulation experience, or reflection.

Journaling/Reflection

Journaling or reflective writing is the practice of writing thoughts and impressions of situations and linking them to learning outcomes (Phillips, 2020). A guided reflection allows one to explore thoughts and feelings that are relevant to the topic. The advantages of journaling are that it encourages students to assimilate their clinical experiences with their didactic content and promotes deeper comprehension of learning and application (Phillips, 2020). Reflective writing often focuses on strengths and needs improvement of the student. The disadvantages are that students may not appreciate the full value of reflective writing and may only superficially answer the questions provided by faculty. Students may provide more factual and descriptive information instead of insightful reflection, and faculty need ample time to read and provide meaningful feedback to the students (Phillips, 2020).

SAMPLE TEACHING MODALITY

Possible Writing Prompt:

Reflect on a time when you provided care to a veteran. Discuss the following: Identify the patient's medical diagnosis. Was the diagnosis linked to military service? Describe your interactions with the patient. How were they similar or different from interactions with other patients? Describe any situations that were surprising or which you would perform differently and why. Describe any biases or stereotypes that may have impacted your nursing care. How has this experience changed these biases or stereotypes?

Learning Outcomes

1. Describe the experience of caring for a veteran. (Cognitive and Affective)
2. Identify differences in the approach to nursing care and care outcomes. (Cognitive)

Role Play

Role play is defined as acting out or performing the role of a character. According to Phillips (2020), scenarios may be scripted, spontaneous, or semi structured. The advantages of role play are that it can be a safe way to practice sensitive skills like assessing for suicide risk; allows exposure to real world situations in a safe environment; and provides additional opportunities to practice observational and decision-making skills (Phillips, 2020). The benefit of role playing is that it may be used in any teaching-learning forum including face-to-face classroom instruction or online. Role play can be uncomfortable for students who may feel they are being put on the spot. The other disadvantages of role play are that students may perceive the role play as just acting the part, and the development of scenarios and scripts may be time consuming for faculty (Phillips, 2020). This active learning strategy requires faculty to relinquish some control in the classroom which can be frustrating (Phillips, 2020).

SAMPLE TEACHING MODALITY

Screening for TBI

Learning Outcomes

1. Demonstrate proper administration of the TBI 3 question DVBIC tool. (Cognitive and Psychomotor)

2. Demonstrate empathy as a way to work with veterans with TBI. (Affective)

DVBIC, Defense and Veterans Brain Injury Center; TBI, traumatic brain injury.

In this sample teaching modality, a student volunteers to perform an assessment of a veteran with TBI using the three-question DVBIC tool. Another student volunteers to act as the veteran with a TBI. Faculty should provide general notes or a script to the student acting as the TBI patient. This is an ideal opportunity for students to practice assessing the signs and symptoms of TBI. If a veteran with TBI is available to play the part of the patient, this could be a powerful role play.

Simulation

Simulation is a teaching approach that mimics real life experience using technology or actors. When the simulation is prepared well (e.g., use of learner- and faculty-guided documents, use of reflective questions, and ample time for debriefing), the opportunity for real learning is present (Maureen et al., 2017). The use of appropriate scenarios is beneficial to help students solve problems, which may enhance critical thinking (Awad et al., 2019). Simulation can be used as an adjunct to didactic instruction especially as it helps students to synthesize didactic content to practice (Anthony et al., 2012). Standardized patients may be used in place of high-fidelity manikins. To be most effective, faculty should be trained in best practices for simulation, especially in debriefing and evaluation of course outcomes (Awad et al., 2019). The following sample teaching modality is an unfolding scenario of a veteran with psychiatric and oncological diagnoses. The holistic simulation is most appropriate for senior level undergraduate students with opportunities to apply knowledge from previous coursework. See Exhibits 10.1 (faculty document) and 10.2 (learner document) for the full simulation experience.

SAMPLE TEACHING MODALITY

Unfolding Scenario of Veteran With Psychiatric and Oncological Diagnoses (Senior Level)

Learning Outcomes

1. Apply a holistic approach to caring for patients and families with both medical-surgical and psychiatric mental health needs. (Psychomotor)

2. Synthesize the use of self through listening responses in the care of a patient and family. (Psychomotor and Affective)

3. Explore one's own biases and perceptions when rendering care to a patient and family, especially homelessness. (Affective)

4. Utilize a motivational interviewing approach to collaboratively plan care based on the client's needs. (Psychomotor and Affective)

EXHIBIT 10.1

PSYCHIATRIC AND MENTAL HEALTH NURSING COURSE SIMULATION EXPERIENCE: FACULTY DOCUMENT

Patient/Client: Leilani Mana'olana Thompson; 35 years old.
Family Member: Ekena Richards; 45 years old
NOTE: Characters names can be altered based on the diversity of the situation

Student Preparation:

1. Read the following articles:

   Johnson, B., Boubiab, L., Freundi, M., Anthony, M., Gmerek, G., & Carter, J. (2013). Enhancing veteran-centered care: A guide for nursing in non-VA settings. *American Journal of Nursing, 113*(7), 24–39

   Biggins, M., Engstron, C., Jackson, P., Sommers, E, & Thorne-Odem, S. (2013). Transforming nursing practice for veterans: Personalized, proactive and patient driven healthcare. *Nurse Leader, 11*(5), 28–32

2. Review the following web resources:

   a. Toolkit: Resources for Suicide Loss Survivors: suicidology.org/wp-content/uploads/2019/07/Resources-for-Survivors-of-Suicide.pdf

   b. National League of Nursing Resources for Veterans: www.nln.org/professional-development-programs/teaching-resources/veterans-ace-v/joining-forces/resources-for-veterans

3. Review physical assessment and care of cancer patients

4. Review mental health assessment and suicide lethality checklist

5. Review hospice care. Review the Standards of Practice for Hospice Programs 2010 (Veteran Related Programs): https://www.wehonorveterans.org/sites/default/files/public/Vet_Related_Standards_Practice.pdf

6. Review the following information from assigned text book readings (e.g., signs and symptoms, diagnostic criteria, pharmacologic and non-pharmacologic treatments, nursing interventions and management) about the following exemplars: schizophrenia, bipolar, depression, and PTSD

This simulated clinical experience (SCE) prepares the learner for the following:

NCLEX-RN Test Plan	QSEN
Safe and Effective Care Environment	Patient-Centered Care
Management of Care	Teamwork and Collaboration
Safety and Infection Control	Evidence-Based Practice
Health Promotion and Maintenance	Quality Improvement
Psychosocial Integrity	Safety
Physiological Integrity	Informatics
Basic Care and Comfort	
Pharmacological and Parenteral Therapies	
Reduction of Risk Potential	
Physiological Adaptations	

Overview of Simulation The SCE is an unfolding case. This means that each group of two students will interact with the patient at different points of care and possibly in different settings (e.g., outpatient, hospital, home hospice, and home)

Standardized patients (SPs) for the SCE will play the appropriate role. Your roles are **new graduate nurses**. *Your name is Robert (male students)/Roberta (female students).*

While two students are chosen randomly to interact with the standardized patient, all other students will be observing in the observation/debriefing room. Each set of two students will receive the scenario at a different point in time. All professional behavior expectations for simulation are required and expected. (Review the required signed documents by all participants on the learning management system as needed.)

Biographical Information: The patient is a 35-year-old female with signs and symptoms of endometrial cancer and history of bipolar disorder. Patient was in the Air Force for 4 years as a nurse. She has not worked as a nurse since her husband's death in order to take care of her child. She is preoccupied with her 17-year-old child who has schizophrenia. The diagnosis of schizophrenia was made in the past year and she has managed the diagnosis well up until this point. The patient's husband was a U.S. Army veteran who passed away last year. He participated in OIF/OEF. Cause of death was suicide. Patient's current support is her sister, Ekena. Ekena is a 45-year-old retired Lt. Col in the Marines and homeless. She frequently visits Leilani. Ekena sometimes visit with her boyfriend who was in the Marines, also homeless, with a substance abuse disorder. He primarily uses marijuana and hard liquor.

The simulation will be 3 to 4 minute vignettes and individual debriefing with the remainder of the simulation time dedicated to the debriefing of the entire group

Additions or deletions of episodes will depend on the total number of students.

Episode 1: Outpatient
Leilani goes to her doctor's office with complaints of bleeding between periods and painful intercourse (s/s of endometrial cancer). She suspects that she may have cancer and it has been confirmed by her doctor at this visit. She is showing signs of hypomania (e.g., pacing on the floor, very tangential in her thought process).
Expected Student Actions: Assessment skills, active listening.

Episode 2: Hospital
Leilani is in the hospital for preoperative testing for her total hysterectomy. Leilani is showing signs of anxiety and asks a lot of questions about the procedure.
Expected Student Actions: Assessment skills, active listening, talking to an anxious client

Episode 3: Hospital
Leilani had a total abdominal hysterectomy. She has just returned from surgery and is still feeling the effects of anesthesia (hallucinations). Her sister, Ekena, is with her.
Expected Student Actions: Dealing with hallucinations, family, and other visitors

Episode 4: Outpatient
Leilani returns to the clinic with fatigue, shortness of breath, and a cough that won't go away (lung metastases). She "knows" the cancer is back and makes statements about life not worth living. She also wants to know how her current cancer treatment will affect her bipolar meds (haldol and lithium).
Expected Student Actions: Talk to a depressed client and assess suicide lethality

Episode 5: Outpatient: Group/Family Therapy
Leilani and Ekena are in attendance at a family cancer support group led by a student nurse. Leilani focuses on her son with schizophrenia and areas of concerns such as his symptom and medication management.
Expected Student Actions: Listening skills and redirecting and knowledge about schizophrenia

Episode 6: Home
Leilani has opted not to continue treatment and to receive hospice care. Her sister is angry with her decision. *Sister leaves the room to smoke.* Leilani has ruminating thoughts of "ending it all." She talks about husband who killed himself and is asking for prescriptions to end her life.
Expected Student Actions: Talk to angry client and family, listening skills, assess suicide lethality

Episode 7: Home
Leilani is asleep and the nurses talk with Ekena who opens up about her experience in the military and being homeless. (Note: Ekena likes to swear.)
Expected Student Actions: Veteran-centered care and resources

Episode 8: Home
Leilani is actively dying, nurses stay with Ekena at her bedside.
Expected Student Actions: Care of a dying patient and family of a veteran

Episode 9: Home
Leilani passed away. Sister is showing signs of distress and anger.
Expected Student Actions: Care of family and provision of resources for a veteran, limit setting

REFERENCES

American Nurses Association. (2001). *Code of ethics for nurses with interpretive statements.* http://www.nursingworld.org/codeofethics

American Nurses Association. (2011). *Nursing: Scope and standards of practice.* http://nursingworld.org/scopeandstandardsofpractice

American Psychiatric Nurses Association. (2012). *About psychiatric mental health nursing.* http://www.apna.org/i4a/pages/index.cfm?pageid=3292

Biggins, M., Engstron, C., Jackson, P., Sommers, E, & Thorne-Odem, S. (2013, Oct). Transforming nursing practice for veterans: Personalized, proactive and patient driven healthcare. *Nurse Leader, 11*(5), 28–32.

Johnson, B., Boubiab, L., Freundi, M., Anthony, M., Gmerek, G., & Carter, J. (2013). Enhancing veteran-centered care: A guide for nursing in non-VA settings. *American Journal of Nursing, 113*(7), 24–39.

Kneisl, C. R., & Trigoboff, E. (2013). *Contemporary psychiatric-mental health nursing* (3rd ed.). Pearson Education.

National Council of State Boards of Nursing. (2019). *2019 NCLEX-RN test plan.* https://ncsbn.org/2019_RN_TestPlan-English.pdf

National League for Nursing. (2016). *Advancing care excellence for veterans.* http://www.nln.org/professional-development-programs/teaching-resources/veterans-ace-v

Quality and Safety Education for Nurses. (2011). *Quality and safety competencies.* http://www.qsen.org/competencies.php

The Joint Commission. (2012). *National patient safety goals.* http://www.jointcommission.org/standards_information/npsgs.aspx

LMS, learning management system; OEF, Operation Enduring Freedom; OIF, Operation Iraqi Freedom; PTSD, posttraumatic stress disorder; SCE, simulated clinical experience; SOB, shortness of breath; SP, standardized patient; NCLEX-RN, National Council Licensure Examination for registered nurses; QSEN, Quality and Safety Education for Nurses.

EXHIBIT 10.2

PSYCHIATRIC AND MENTAL HEALTH NURSING COURSE SIMULATION EXPERIENCE

LEARNER DOCUMENT

Patient/Client: Leilani Mana'olana Thompson 35 years old
Family Member: Ekena Richards 45 years old

Student Preparation:

1. Read the following articles:

   Johnson, B., Boubiab, L., Freundi, M., Anthony, M., Gmerek, G., & Carter, J. (2013). Enhancing veteran-centered care: A guide for nursing in non-VA settings. *American Journal of Nursing, 113*(7), 24–39

   Biggins, M., Engstron, C., Jackson, P., Sommers, E, & Thorne-Odem, S. (2013, Oct). Transforming nursing practice for veterans: Personalized, proactive and patient driven healthcare. *Nurse Leader, 11*(5), 28–32

2. Review the following web resources link related to resources:

   a. Toolkit: Resources for Suicide Loss Survivors: https://suicidology.org/wp-ontent/uploads/2019/07/Resources-for-Survivors-of-Suicide.pdf

   b. National League of Nursing Resources for Veterans: http://www.nln.org/professional-development-programs/teaching-resources/veterans-ace-v/joining-forces/resources-for-veterans

3. Review physical assessment and care of cancer patients

4. Review mental health assessment and suicide lethality checklist

5. Review hospice care. Review the Standards of Practice for Hospice Programs 2010 (Veteran Related Programs): https://www.wehonorveterans.org/sites/default/files/public/Vet_Related_Standards_Practice.pdf

6. Review the following information from class readings (e.g. signs and symptoms, diagnostic criteria, pharmacologic and non-pharmacologic treatments, nursing interventions and management) about the following exemplars: schizophrenia, bipolar, depression, and PTSD

Overview of Simulation: The simulated clinical experience (SCE) is an unfolding case. This means that each group of two students will interact with the patient at different points of care and possibly in different settings (e.g., outpatient, hospital, home hospice, and home). *SPs* for the SCE will play the appropriate role. Your roles are **new graduate nurses**

While two students are chosen randomly to interact with the standardized patient, all other students will be observing in the debriefing room. Each set of two students will receive the scenario at a different point in time. All professional behavior expectations for simulation are required and expected. (Review the required signed documents by all participants on the LMS as needed)

Biographical Information: The patient is a 35-year-old female with signs and symptoms of endometrial cancer and history of bipolar disorder. Patient was in the Air Force for 4 years as a nurse. She has not worked as a nurse since her husband's death in order to take care of her child. She is preoccupied with her 17-year-old child who has schizophrenia. The diagnosis of schizophrenia was made in the past year and has managed the diagnosis well up until this point. The patient's husband was a US Army veteran who passed away last year. He participated in OIF/OEF. Cause of death: suicide. Patient's current support is her sister, Ekena. Ekena is a 45-year-old a retired Lt. Col in the Marines and homeless. She frequently visits Leilani

The simulation will be the 3-4 minute vignettes and individual debriefing with the remainder of the simulation time dedicated to the debriefing of the entire group

REFERENCES

American Nurses Association. (2001). *Code of ethics for nurses with interpretive statements.* http://www.nursingworld.org/codeofethics

American Nurses Association. (2011). *Nursing: Scope and standards of practice.* http://nursingworld.org/scopeandstandardsofpractice

American Psychiatric Nurses Association. (2012). *About psychiatric mental health nursing.* http://www.apna.org/i4a/pages/index.cfm?pageid=3292

Biggins, M., Engstron, C., Jackson, P., Sommers, E., & Thorne-Odem, S. (2013, October). Transforming nursing practice for veterans: Personalized, proactive and patient driven healthcare. *Nurse Leader, 11*(5), 28–32.

Johnson, B., Boubiab, L., Freundi, M., Anthony, M., Gmerek, G., & Carter, J. (2013). Enhancing veteran-centered care: A guide for nursing in non-VA settings. *American Journal of Nursing, 113*(7), 24–39.

Kneisl, C. R., & Trigoboff, E. (2013). *Contemporary psychiatric-mental health nursing* (3rd ed.). Pearson Education.

National Council of State Boards of Nursing. (2019). *2019 NCLEX-RN test plan.* https://ncsbn.org/2019_RN_TestPlan-English.pdf

National League for Nursing. (2016). *Advancing care excellence for veterans.* http://www.nln.org/professional-development-programs/teaching-resources/veterans-ace-v

Quality and Safety Education for Nurses. (2011). *Quality and safety competencies.* http://www.qsen.org/competencies.php

The Joint Commission. (2012). *National patient safety goals.* http://www.jointcommission.org/standards_information/npsgs.aspx

LMS, learning management system; OEF, Operation Enduring Freedom; OIF, Operation Iraqi Freedom; PTSD, post-traumatic stress disorder; SCE, simulated clinical experience; SP, standardized patient.

Simulation is a multidimensional teaching strategy that assists students to transfer knowledge from the classroom to clinical practice. Applying communication, collaboration, assessment, clinical reasoning, and clinical judgement skills to the care of a veteran patient enhances veteran care competency and one's level of comfort interacting with veterans in the clinical setting (Regan et al., 2019).

Summary of Active Learning Strategies

The active learning strategies listed above were tailored to integrate veteran health content into undergraduate nursing curricula. However, each could easily be adapted to graduate education or clinical practice. As faculty move away from traditional, passive pedagogical instructional methods, in favor of flipped classrooms, these active learning strategies may easily be implemented (Kavanagh et al., 2017; Tagher, 2019). Additional active learning strategies faculty could use to teach veteran health content include infographics, return demonstration, storytelling, think-pair-share, and vignettes. Helping students make meaning of military and veteran culture, nurses' influence on providing culturally congruent care, and understanding the health influences of military service will result from dedicated efforts to modify existing teaching practices to include this diverse population.

Online Programs

Evidence of efforts to integrate veteran health content and competencies into online RN-Bachelor of Science in Nursing (BSN) programs is beginning to emerge in the nursing literature. Jones and

Breen (2015) described threading veteran health content across an RN-BSN program. Using a variety of active learning strategies, veteran health content was integrated into four courses; touching upon almost all of the competencies outlined by McMillan et al. (2017) and Moss et al. (2015). Keavney (2015) integrated a core course on veteran's health into a RN-BSN program at a public university. Over the eight-week course, students had the opportunity to learn about military culture, physical and psychological outcomes of military service, and understand the role of the nurse in the provision of veteran-centered care. Students from any health-related program were permitted to take the veteran health course facilitating a deeper understanding of veterans and their health through opportunities to share viewpoints and different perspectives (Keavney, 2015).

Online education is a particularly important strategy for reaching licensed, practicing nurses as little is published about the knowledge and skills of practicing nurses to meet the healthcare needs and expectations of veterans (Elliott, 2018). Like traditional undergraduate programs, existing RN-BSN courses should be examined for logical placement of veteran-health content (Keavney, 2015). Common starting points might include health assessment, pharmacology, and pathophysiology courses. Curricula could also be expanded to include a single core or elective veteran healthcare course (Keavney, 2015; Morrison-Beedy et al., 2015). The broad goal of incorporating veteran specific content educational offerings is to familiarize faculty and civilian students regarding military culture in general (Hurlbut & Revuelto, 2018). Therefore, schools of nursing are challenged to extend the "*Joining Forces*" initiative to include practicing nurses returning to school.

Graduate Level

Similar to undergraduate nursing education, Masters and Doctoral programs in the United States are working toward achieving the *Joining Forces* goals (Elliott & Patterson, 2017). Certainly, "The Essentials of Doctoral Education for Advanced Nursing Practice" (AACN, 2006) support the inclusion of veteran health content and competencies noting that "Graduate education in nursing occurs within the context of societal demands and needs as well as the interprofessional work environment" (AACN, 2006, p. 5). Evidence in the nursing literature outlining the endeavors to include veteran health in graduate education are gaining traction; although much less at the doctoral level (Caughill & Dunford, 2015; Cowan et al., 2013; Linn et al., 2015; Regan et al., 2019).

Nurse faculty recognize the need for graduate nursing students to have additional, specialized training related to veterans' healthcare aligning with their expanded role after graduation. Following a clinical rotation at a veteran-centric site, master's level nursing students participated in a focus group to assist nurse faculty in developing training for future students (Linn et al., 2015). Students in the study supported inclusion of military culture and veteran specific health issues prior to clinical placement with veterans and military families (Linn et al., 2015). In addition, hands on training can address students' self-awareness and self- management on the complexities of the care for veterans and military families. Allen et al. (2013) also recommended that graduate nursing education include healthcare policy information and implications of military service related healthcare costs.

Schools of nursing are partnering with the Veterans Health Administration (VHA) to provide opportunities to interact with veterans as part of clinical training for future nurse practitioners (Caughill & Dunford, 2015; Harper et al., 2016). Through an academic-practice partnership, psychiatric mental health nurse practitioner students complete clinical experiences at veteran serving facilities thus increasing the numbers of graduates prepared to handle complex veteran health needs (Harper et al., 2016). Nurse practitioner postgraduate training or residency programs focusing on veteran's health are also reported in the literature (Harper et al., 2016; Rugen et al., 2016). Similarly, Zapatka et al. (2014) described the success of a post-master's interprofessional fellowship program, supported by the VHA, to overcome gaps in graduate education and provide care in an outpatient primary care setting. Regan et al. (2019) also reported psychiatric nurse practitioner students' participation in a standardized patient simulation successfully enhanced veteran-care competence, improved confidence to advocate for vet-erans within the healthcare system, and assisted students to effectively manage mental health needs of veterans. While these are merely a few examples, it appears that integration of veteran health is largely directed toward mental health which is not surprising given the focus on PTSD and TBI in the *Joining Forces* initiative. Going forward, the focus of veteran health should expand beyond mental health to be more holistic.

Research in graduate education confirms challenges encountered but are beginning to be addressed by graduate nursing programs seeking to integrate veteran health content (Linn et al., 2015). These challenges include forming relationships with the VA healthcare systems, complexities of working with both physiological and behavioral health issues in the veteran population, and role differentiation of advanced practice nurses caring for veterans (Cowan et al., 2013; Linn et al., 2015; Peterson et al., 2018). Use of simulation through standardized patients and case scenarios are a safe and effective way to educate graduate nurses in a veteran-centric way (Peterson et al., 2018). Use of trained nursing faculty and clinical mentors who can serve as an advocate throughout a student's education will help overcome challenges along the way. Clear roles and meaningful, culturally sensitive training of master's prepared APRN and Doctor of Nursing Practice graduates warrants additional exploration.

Educators in the Practice Setting

Clinical educators in the practice setting also play a key role in assuring the nursing workforce is pre-pared to deliver veteran-centric care in a culturally congruent manner. Appreciating that a majority of practicing nurses do not feel prepared to care for veterans due to a lack of knowledge it is particularly important that these educators remain abreast of best practices for veteran-centered care. Further, these educators must undertake deliberate efforts to include veteran health content through ongoing educational initiatives for staff. To keep veteran-health on the forefront of nursing practice it is rec-ommended that veteran-related professional development opportunities be made available to nurses in numerous formats (e.g., online modules, annual competency assessments, and face-to-face skills sessions). To further validate veterans as a diverse population and the influence of military service and culture on the health of veterans it is recommended that annual evaluations include documentation of veteran-related professional development (Chargualaf, 2019). Any of the sample teaching modalities presented in this chapter may be modified to align with characteristics of a care setting, veteran health needs in a geographical area, or identified learning needs of staff.

IMPLICATIONS FOR NURSING EDUCATION AND PRACTICE

Veteran informed nursing practice involves providing culturally congruent and patient-centered care to veterans and their families. The fact that a majority of veterans receive their healthcare in civilian settings means that nurses, regardless of care area, will regularly encounter veterans in their profes-sional practice. Military service members and veterans are a diverse population whose health may be influenced or linked to their military service. As such, nursing education must recognize the veteran population as a unique culture worthy of inclusion in nursing curricula. Champlin et al. (2017) suggest that faculty often lack the experience or affiliation with the military limiting KSA needed to embrace integration. Therefore, nurse educators must reform nursing curriculum to assure that future nurses are knowledgeable and prepared to meet the health needs of veterans.

In academia, the willingness of administrators and faculty in the schools of nursing to incorpo-rate educational offerings and courses to create or enhance a veteran-centric curriculum is the first step. Curricular integration and educational resources should be explored to drive any needed changes (Kautzmann & Lancaster, 2018, p. 120). An assessment of students, faculty and academic-clinical partners' perceptions of the value of incorporating veteran related content in the curriculum and an understanding of military culture is a necessity. Further, self-reflection of one's knowledge, biases and attitudes about veterans allows future nurses to better their skills.

The recommendations for understanding and applying teaching strategies regarding veteran centered care to the nursing curriculum is relevant. Faculty are encouraged to begin integration of veteran health content immediately by revising existing teaching and learning activities to have a veteran focus. Deliberate efforts to scaffold veteran competencies across the curriculum by mapping courses and veteran content can take more time and requires faculty who are knowledgeable of curricular revision and military culture. A comprehensive plan for faculty professional development related to military culture and veteran health must be supported by academic administrators. Efforts to collaborate with local and national veteran organizations can support mutual interests; increased availability of teaching resources and improved veteran health outcomes.

Although nursing as a profession strives to provide evidence-based and culturally sensitive care to all patient populations; nursing education has largely failed to prepare nurses to care for veterans in ways they need and deserve. Nursing education must dedicate resources, assure an informed faculty, and deliberately include veteran health content and competencies to meet professional and community needs.

FUTURE RESEARCH PRIORITIES

There is much work to be done in regard to the classroom preparation of nursing graduates to provide care to our nation's veterans. One explanation may be largely due to a collective lack of knowledge. This includes not only lack of student knowledge, but also a lack of educator knowledge. Aside from a single descriptive study investigating efforts by schools of nursing to meet the *Joining Forces* goals, we do not know to what extent schools are incorporating veteran-specific content and the outcomes, if any, which result from this. It is from this point that future research priorities are derived.

First, a follow-up study investigating individual schools of nursing efforts to integrate veteran health content and competencies is warranted. This will help determine whether nursing education has made any progress in the years since Elliott and Patterson (2017) first published their report. Nursing faculty are encouraged to report innovative teaching and learning strategies used in both undergraduate and graduate nursing classrooms. By sharing teaching resources, faculty may feel less overwhelmed and burdened to bring veteran health into their classroom. Nursing faculty should make use of available resources and platforms to assist with curricular development (www.aacnnursing.org/Teaching-Resources/Tool-Kits/Veterans-Care). Further, empirical research that validates teaching methodologies to prepare graduates to provide veteran-centered nursing care are needed.

Efforts to validate existing veteran competencies by practicing nurses routinely caring for veterans should also be undertaken. Doing so will assure the competencies guiding nursing education align with professional practice and fully embrace the health needs of veterans. Collaborating with clinical nurse educators working inside and outside of veteran health facilities are suggested. Adding to the body of knowledge could encompass exploration of nursing students and recent graduates' perceptions of readiness to apply their learning to the military and veteran population should be undertaken. However, exploring military and veterans' perception of care provided to them by nursing students might also yield valuable information needed to meaningfully inform curricular development or revision. Finally, current and future professional development opportunities for faculty and civilian students should be explored for relevance to nursing education.

CONCLUSION

The *Joining Forces* initiative served as a catalyst for drawing attention to the health needs of veterans and efforts to integrate veteran-related health content into nursing curricula. But to date, efforts to prepare graduates to provide veteran-centered care widely vary. Veteran-centered nursing practice begins in undergraduate education and should continue through graduate education and ongoing professional development (Chargualaf, 2019; Roe et al., 2019). Efforts to examine and revise existing curricula to infuse veteran competencies are recommended. The active learning strategies and sample teaching modalities presented in this chapter serve as a starting point. Nurse faculty are called to increase their own knowledge of military and veteran culture, commit to inclusion of veteran-health content in nursing curricula, collaborate to develop teaching strategies that will prepare nurses to deliver culturally-sensitive care to veterans, and engage in research to evaluate the effectiveness of these teaching and learning strategies.

REFERENCES

The complete reference list for this chapter appears in the digital version of the chapter, accessible at https://connect.springerpub.com/content/book/978-0-8261-3597-1/chapter/ch10

RESOURCES

Recommended Readings by Content Area

VETERAN COMPETENCIES FOR NURSING EDUCATION

Carlson, J. (2016). Baccalaureate nursing faculty competencies and teaching strategies to enhance the care of the veteran population: Perspectives of veteran affairs nursing academy (VANA) faculty. *Journal of Professional Nursing, 32*, 314–323. https://doi.org/10.1016/j.profnurs.2016.01.006

McMillan, L. R., Crumbley, D., Freeman, J., Rhodes, M., Kane, M., & Napper, J. (2017). Caring for the veteran, military and family member nursing competencies: Strategies for integrating content into nursing school curricula. *Journal of Professional Nursing, 33*, 378–386. https://doi.org/10.1016/j.profnurs.2017.06.002

Moss, J., Moore, R., & Selleck, C. (2015). Veteran competencies for undergraduate nursing education. *Advances in Nursing Science, 38*, 306–316. https://doi.org/10.1097/ANS.0000000000000092

Olenick, M., Flowers, M., & Diaz, V. J. (2015). US veterans and their unique issues: Enhancing health care professional awareness. *Advances in medical education and practice, 6*, 635–639. https://doi.org/10.2147/AMEP.S89479

MILITARY AND VETERAN CULTURE

Cooper, L., Andrew S., & Fossey M. (2016). Educating nurses to care for military veterans in civilian hospitals: An integrated literature review. *Nurse Education Today, 47*, 68–73. https://doi.org/10.1016/j.nedt.2016.05.022

Counts, L., Freundl, M., & Johnson, B. (2015). Nurses providing care to military veterans in civilian hospitals. *Medical Surgical Nursing, 24*, 4–8.

Ghahramanlou-Holloway, M., Cox, D. W., Fritz, E. C., & George, B. J. (2011). An evidence-informed guide for working with military women and veterans. *Professional Psychology - Research & Practice, 42*(1), 1–7.

Johnson, B. S., Boudiab, L. D., Freundl, M., Anthony, M., Gmerek, G. B., & Carter, J. (2013). Enhancing veteran-centered care: A guide for nurses in non-VA settings. *The American Journal of Nursing, 113*(7), 24–39.

Ross, P., Ravindranath, D., Clay, M., & Lypson, M. (2015). A greater mission: Understanding military culture as a tool for serving those who have served. *Journal of Graduate Medical Education, 7*, 519–522. https://doi.org/10.4300/JGME-D-14-00568.1

Strom, T. Q., Gavian, M. E, Possis, E., Loughlin, J., Bui, T., Linardatos, E., Leskela, J., & Siegel, W. (2012). Cultural and ethical considerations when working with military personnel and veterans: A primer for VA training programs. *Training & Education in Professional Psychology, 6*(2), 67–75.

Westphal, R., & Convoy, S. (2015) Military culture implications for mental health and nursing care. *OJIN: The Online Journal of Issues in Nursing, 20*(1), Manuscript 4.

CURRICULAR CHANGE

Beckford, M., & Ellis, C. (2013). Developing nursing curriculum to facilitate the delivery of holistic care to the military veteran. *Open Journal of Nursing, 3*, 400–403. https://doi.org/10.4236/ojn.2013.35054

Cooper, L., Andrew, S., & Fossey, M. (2016) Educating nurses to care for military veterans in civilian hospitals: An integrated literature review. *Nurse Education Today, 47*, 68–73. https://doi.org/10.1016/j.nedt.2016.05.022

Elliott, B., & Patterson, B. (2017). Joining forces: The status of military and veteran health care in nursing curricula. *Journal of Professional Nursing, 33*, 145–152. https://doi.org/10.1016/j.profnurs.2016.06.006

SIMULATION

Anthony, M., Carter, J. L., Freundl, M., & Nelson, V. (2012). Using simulation to teach veteran-centered care. *Clinical Simulation in Nursing, 8*, e145–e150. https://doi.org/10.1016/j.ecns.2010.10.004

Magpantay-Monroe, E. R. (2017). Integration of military and veteran health in a psychiatric mental health BSN curriculum: A mindful analysis. *Nurse Education Today, 48*, 111–113. https://doi.org/10.1016/j.nedt.2016.09.02

GRADUATE EDUCATION

Caughill, A., & Dunford, D. (2015). A psychiatric mental health nurse practitioner program: Meeting the needs of the community and veterans as students as well as care recipients. *Issues in Mental Health Nursing, 36*, 836–839. https://doi.org/10.3109/01612840.2015.1057784

Kuehner, C. (2013). My military: A navy nurse practitioner's perspective on military culture and joining forces for veteran health. *Journal of the American Academy of Nurse Practitioners, 25*(2), 77–83.

PRACTICING NURSES

Cheney, A. M., Koenig, C. J., Miller, C. J., Zamora, K., Wright, P., Stanley, R., Payne, J., & Fortney, J. (2018). Veteran-centered barriers to VA mental healthcare services use. *BMC Health Services Research 18*, 591. https://doi.org/10.1186/s12913-018-3346-9

Currier, J. M., Stefurak, T., Carroll, T. D., & Shatto, E. H. (2017). Applying trauma-informed care to community-based mental health services for military veterans. *Best Practice in Mental Health, 13*(1), 47–64.

Elliott, B. (2018). Civilian nurses' knowledge, confidence, and comfort caring for military veterans: Survey results of a mixed-methods study. *Home Healthcare Now, 36*, 356–361.

Street, A. E., Shin, M. H., Marchany, K. E., McCaughey, V. K., Bell, M. E., & Hamilton, A. B. (2019). Veterans' perspectives on military sexual trauma-related communication with VHA providers. *Psychological Services,* 1–11. Psychological Services. Advance online publication. https://doi.org/10.1037/ser0000395

York, J., Sternke, L. M., Myrick, D. H., Lauerer, J., & Hair, C. (2016). Development of veteran-centric competency domains for psychiatric mental health nurse practitioner residents. *Journal of Psychosocial Nursing Mental Health Services, 54*, 31–36. https://doi.org/10.3928/02793695-20161024-06

VETERAN-CENTERED TEACHING STRATEGIES, LEARNING ACTIVITIES, AND RESOURCES FOR THE CLINICAL SETTING

BARBARA CHAMPLIN | RANEY LINCK

But we also remember that honoring those who've served is about more than the words we say on Veterans' Day or Memorial Day. It's about how we treat our veterans every single day of the year …

It's about serving all of you as well as you've served the United States of America.

Barack Obama

KEY TERMS

veteran-centered clinical strategies	teaching veteran-centered care
clinical care of veterans	military/veteran cultural competency

INTRODUCTION

Veterans are a population with unique healthcare needs; however, only one third are enrolled in the specialized Veterans Affairs Health Care System (VAHCS; U.S. Department of Veterans Affairs [VA], 2018a). Therefore, it is vital to determine how to meet veterans' distinctive needs in all care settings. This chapter includes an examination of veteran-centered clinical competencies for healthcare professionals and includes recommendations for educators—in both prelicensure nursing programs and staff education at healthcare facilities—to guide education material development. In addition, veteran-focused teaching strategies, learning activities, and clinical resources are provided to create new curricula and enhance existing ones. This will better prepare educators and healthcare professionals to provide culturally sensitive veteran-centered care. Suggestions for placement of possible learning activities in specific clinical courses are presented. Taken together, the veteran-centered competencies, teaching strategies, learning activities, and resources will improve care of veterans in all clinical settings.

The complete reference list for this chapter appears in the digital version of the chapter, accessible at https://connect.springerpub.com/content/book/978-0-8261-3597-1/chapter/ch11

BACKGROUND

Military service members and veterans are at risk for a number of physical and mental health issues based on the nature of their occupation, which can include training exercises or dangerous deployments. Each military service member, and their families, have a unique experience. Therefore, it is essential that nurses and healthcare providers have a basic understanding of some of the factors that influence veterans' health and well-being long-term to inform their approach in establishing rapport. These include such things as type of occupation held in the military (including branch of service—Army, Navy, Air Force, Marine Corps, or Coast Guard), number and duration of deployments, status of separation from service (e.g., medical discharge, end of time commitment, retirement), possible exposures (e.g., noise, environmental), or service-connected injuries to name a few (Elliott, 2018). The war era in which a service member served, including peacetime, is also useful to know as certain illnesses and injuries are distinctive to specific eras such as Agent Orange exposure in Vietnam Era veterans or traumatic brain injury (TBI) in Post-9/11 era veterans. Families are also impacted by the service of a parent or spouse and should be considered equally as important in the provision of care for this population.

The U.S. Census Bureau (2018) calculated there were approximately 18.2 million veterans in the United States in 2017. For the same year, the VA (2018a) reported that only 6.1 million Veterans—33% of that overall total—were enrolled in the VAHCS. With two out of three veterans receiving their care in non-VA settings, clinical competency in the care of veterans is paramount. It is estimated that 96% of veterans die outside of a VA facility (Gabriel et al., 2015), which further necessitates professional nurses, nursing faculty, and student nurses to prepare to provide quality care to veterans across their lifespan, in any and all settings. No matter the situation, military service members, veterans, and their families deserve quality, culturally-sensitive care.

Several initiatives have urged health systems to prepare nurses to effectively assess military history, general concerns of veterans, military health risks, and suicidal risk. Exemplars include the *Joining Forces* campaign led by Michelle Obama and Jill Biden (White House Archives, 2016) and the "Have You Ever Served in the Military™?" campaign by the American Academy of Nursing (AAN, 2015). The AAN (2015) has been a leader in creating tools and resources with its campaign to encourage healthcare providers to ask about and document their clients' military background. A central theme is that the healthcare needs of veterans are unique and the development of knowledge, skills, and attitudes (KSAs) to care for this population is vital. Ensuring that specific service-related questions are embedded in students' assessment tools during clinical assignments is important. This will encourage students to always inquire about veteran status and to go more in-depth in situations when their assessment reveals that a client they are caring for is a veteran. Further, inclusion of military status questions embedded in electronic health records (EHRs) would ensure all patients are properly screened across care settings so appropriate assessment, referral, and follow-up can be achieved. Box 11.1 offers examples of veteranspecific areas to assess as starting point.

In addition, the VA has invested in an Enhancing Academic Partnerships Program. Over the past decade, Veteran Affairs Nursing Academic Partnerships (VANAPs) have been established with leading nursing programs throughout the nation (U.S. Department of Veterans Affairs, 2018b). These VANAPs have contributed to the scholarship on best teaching strategies to train future nurses to provide exemplary care to veterans (Dobalian et al., 2014; Harper et al., 2015; Miltner et al., 2015). Many of the strategies presented in this chapter emerged from these partnerships, and can be adapted to educate professional nurses currently in practice.

The ability of practicing nurses to meet the healthcare needs of veterans is noteworthy and must be addressed. Empirical research and quality improvement initiatives suggest that much work is needed in the civilian sector to raise awareness and basic competency of practicing nurses (Bonzanto et al., 2019; Maiocco et al., 2019). Bonzanto et al. (2019) conducted a survey of 612 RNs that revealed the vast majority of respondents lacked the KSAs to provide culturally competent care to veterans, with only 4%

BOX 11.1

BROAD CATEGORIES OF VETERAN-SPECIFIC ASSESSMENT

VETERAN STATUS OR MILITARY SPOUSE

Branch of Service (Army, Navy, Air Force, etc.)
Role in military
Location when serving
Participation in active combat
Impact on health
Using client age or reported military conflict, identify the following utilizing the VA's Exposure Ed app:

- common exposures of the identified conflict (e.g., asbestos, burn pits, Agent Orange, blasts from bombs)

- health implications to consider regarding exposure (e.g., mesothelioma, asthma, psoriasis, PTSD, TBI, traumatic injuries). Mobile applications are discussed in more detail later in the chapter

More details and resources are available at www.haveyoueverserved.com

PTSD, posttraumatic stress disorder; TBI, traumatic brain injury; VA, U.S. Department of Veterans Affairs.

---

of nurses demonstrating the capacity to deliver culturally competent care. Maiocco et al. (2019) examined the impact of mandatory continuing education on veteran's mental health needs on the actual care nurses provided. The researchers analyzed online surveys completed by 115 hospital nurses. The majority of nurses seldom documented military history and were not aware of hospital services for veterans, despite mandatory education. Unfortunately, the study was stopped early due to concerns about violence; however, the authors concluded that a gap in care exists in the provision of veteran-centered care.

To address this gap in practice, implications and recommendations across studies includes documenting military service and care in the EHR and ongoing education (Bonzato et al., 2019; Maiocco et al., 2019). Evaluating providers' understanding of the needs of veterans, monitoring care outcomes, using VA and U.S. Department of Defense (DoD) resources (Bonzato et al., 2019), and use of veteran volunteers (Maiocco et al., 2019) have also been suggested. Clearly, nursing students and professional nurses have different learning needs; however, veteran-centered clinical competencies can serve as a springboard to developing curricula and continuing education programs to improve the care of veterans.

CLINICAL COMPETENCIES

In the United States, the American Association of Colleges of Nursing (AACN) recommends competencies and guidelines for the development of nursing curricula. They created the *AACN Essentials Series*, which defines essential competencies of graduates from nursing programs (AACN, 2020a). In addition, practice is governed by nurse practice acts and a code of ethics. Together these standards, laws, and guidelines serve as a foundation on which to design nursing curricula. Nurse leaders and faculty use this foundation to map student learning outcomes and clinical competencies in their education programs. Additional guidance comes from Quality and Safety Education for Nurses; evidence-based reports from the National Academy of Medicine, formerly known as the Institute of Medicine, and the blueprint from the North American nursing licensure exam, which is based on a practice analysis of entry-level nurses and updated every 3 years (National Council of State Boards of Nursing, 2020). Clinical competencies include the KSAs graduates should achieve by the end of the program.

The ANA (2014) defines professional role competence of nursing in the *ANA Position Statement*. Competence is described as a responsibility that is shared by individual nurses, employers, professional organizations, credentialing and regulatory agencies as well as other key stakeholders (ANA, 2014). In addition, clinical competencies are defined by AACN in many specialty areas of nursing (e.g., critical care, gerontology, palliative care, and mental health), as well as interprofessional competencies and cultural competencies (AACN, 2020b). Evaluation of clinical competence and confidence is typically assessed via the use of a clinical evaluation tool specifically designed for use at various time points in the curricula. Program outcomes, students learning outcomes, and the AACN essentials are often used to create useful evaluation tools. Once a standardized evaluation tool is created it can be individualized to a wide variety of clinical experiences. This helps to maintain consistency in the KSAs that are measured and attainment of competence and confidence of students over time.

Veteran-centered competencies that can be utilized for prelicensure level education have been developed by Moss et al. (2015) and McMillan et al. (2017). In addition, York et al. (2016) developed veteran-centered competencies specific to the domain of advanced practice psychiatric-mental health nursing. These may be of interest to readers focused on development of that specific area in their curricula. Nursing programs may elect to use the competencies of one of the cited authors or to use elements from each of these authors to develop learning experiences for their students that focus on competent nursing care of veterans. These veteran-centered competencies are examined further throughout the chapter.

Veteran-Centered Competencies

Creating opportunities in clinical settings to engage with veterans will help nursing students to develop a variety of competencies. Moss et al. (2015) and McMillan et al. (2017) developed veteran-centered competencies to guide educators in developing curricula focused on the KSAs relevant to the preparation of prelicensure nursing students to care for service members, veterans, and their families while in school and once they transition to practice. These competencies can also inform the care of current practicing nurses. Many innovative methods and strategies can be used to integrate veteran-centered content into established curricula or to develop new stand-alone content focused on veterans.

Moss et al. (2015) established *10 Veteran Competencies for Undergraduate Nursing Education* (VCUNE). The competencies include the following: (a) military and veteran culture, (b) posttraumatic stress disorder (PTSD), (c) amputation and assistive devices, (d) environmental/chemical exposures, (e) substance use disorders (SUDs), (f) military sexual trauma (MST), (g) TBI, (h) suicide, (i) homelessness, and (j) serious illness, especially at end-of life. Individual nursing programs will need to review their own curricular maps to determine placement of content mapped to particular competencies. For example, the competencies focused on PTSD, SUD, and suicide may be mapped to clinical courses focused on care of veterans in mental health settings. Other competencies such as the ones focused on amputation and assistive devices as well as TBI may be better placed in clinical courses in acute care medical-surgical clinical settings. The decisions made about placement in the curricula and the competencies used to guide clinical course development may vary from program to program, but the VCUNEs provide a strong foundation on which to build that focuses on exemplary veteran-centered care.

McMillan et al. (2017) also contributed to the growing body of knowledge regarding veteran-centered care. Based on reflective comments from students and a scheduled public forum of stakeholders interested in care of veterans, the authors developed four core competencies. The competencies included the following: (a) military culture and military specific healthcare needs, (b) physiologic nursing care for the veteran and military member, (c) mental health nursing care for the veteran and military member, and (d) nursing advocacy for the veteran and military member. The authors describe specific KSAs, and also provide resources and tool kits for each of the four areas of care. Important to highlight with this set of competencies is nursing advocacy, as it is a critical skill needed in the care provided by nurses. This is especially true considering many veterans and families lack knowledge about what resources are available to them (Elliott, 2019).

York et al. (2016) developed 14 veteran-centric competency domains to guide the practice of mental health nurse practitioners (NPs) in a VA residency program. Given the mental health needs of military service members, veterans, and in some cases their families, this work is quite relevant and timely to achieving better care for this population. The competencies include the following: (a) communication with veterans, (b) effects of combat stress, (c) injury/disability related to military service, (d) care coordination with non-VA organizations, (e) prevention and intervention services specific to the VA, (f) health and well-being of veterans' families, (g) mental health in a veteran context, (h) demographics of veteran patients, (i) service-related beliefs and values, (j) personal values and beliefs toward veteran populations, (k) role gender in help-seeking veterans, (l) unique characteristics of mental health services within the VA system, (m) recommended evidence-based practice (EBP) in VA mental health services, and (n) quality improvement for VA mental healthcare (York et al., 2016). While their work is VA centric, it can provide a foundation from which to develop NP programs to include veteran-centered elements. Further, some shared competencies can be seen across all three lists of competencies that have been presented.

Military/Veteran Cultural Competency

Military/veteran cultural competency is perhaps the most critical of all those identified as it appears to have a significant influence on the nurse-patient relationship. Lack of cultural understanding is a significant barrier to engaging this population. Veterans report it can be isolating to constantly stop and explain the most basic terms and elements of military life – "I want my [provider] to know what I'm talking about. Otherwise, there's a disconnect that's hard to get past" (Cogan, 2011, p. 4). Results of a study conducted by Nworah et al. (2018) support that veterans tend to rely heavily on self-care and self-monitoring health behaviors until seeking care is a necessary last resort. So when they do seek care, many veterans may be of the mentality of "I want them to listen. This is my body" (Nworah et al., 2018). The importance of developing a solid understanding of military and veteran culture is essential to building rapport with veterans (Westphal & Convoy, 2015).

Military service members belong to a unique culture within the larger society in the United States, which often influences who they are even after they have left the service and become a veteran. How veterans view their military service may be one of the most critical points to assess when engaging with them in any health encounter (Spiro et al., 2016). The culture within the military is very structured, governed by norms, customs, and values (Atuel & Castro, 2018). Using rank and chain of command, the hierarchical organization of the military dictates a person's place within the group, level of authority, responsibility, decision-making power, and communication flow. Through military service, individuals develop a sense of oneness or team, versus individual development (Atuel & Castro, 2018). Exemplified by Ateul and Castro (2018), "the military is part of the collective *We*, but is different from the rest of *Us*" (p. 76). This collectivist worldview translates to service members minimizing their own needs and a "suck it up" or "tough it out" attitude, which may influence health-seeking behaviors (Nworah et al., 2018).

Both student and professional nurses need to be educated on essential elements that can improve development of a therapeutic bond with veteran clients. As stated, examples include assessment of military history, discussion of general health concerns of veterans, assessment of military health risks, evaluation of suicidal risk, and so on. Developing this type of competency will be ongoing, including sessions that are integrated in multiple levels of nursing curricula and offered more than once in workplace settings. Additional support for understanding military culture is revealed in the findings of Carlson (2016), who conducted focus groups with nursing faculty to determine what faculty competencies and essential knowledge were necessary to prepare nursing students to provide holistic veteran-centered care. The author described five faculty competencies (appreciation for veteran contributions, care and empathy for veterans, veteran cultural competence, trust builder, and team player);

four essential knowledge areas (military service, military experiences, veteran experiences, and veteran affairs focus and resources); and three teaching strategies (developing connections, teaching activities, and student activities), which can serve as a guide for professional development of faculty and clinical educators.

INTEGRATION OF VETERAN COMPETENCIES INTO THE CURRICULUM

An important first step when integrating veteran-centered content into the clinical component of a course is a systematic review of current clinical experiences offered in a particular nursing program, looking for points of entry of veteran-centered experiences. This close examination should occur in both undergraduate and graduate nursing programs, and at all academic levels. In addition to placement of veteran-centered experiences and content, university and community resources and support must also be considered. Funding must be available to support this work, as well as faculty who are competent to teach and support students working with veterans. Consideration of possible clinical sites to meet student needs must be identified. Lastly, examination of facilitators who will ease integration of veteran-centered content such as faculty with military background, military-centric resources and supports on campus, and VA accessibility is vital.

Nursing programs with access to a VAHCS should strive to build clinical partnerships with the facility. Champlin et al. (2017) described clinical exemplars in a prelicensure nursing program that has an established partnership with a VAHCS. The exemplars provided include examples of curricular integration across all levels of a prelicensure program. The first clinical exemplar, a community health clinical, may be at the junior level. This community-based clinical experience could occur in a variety of community-based settings that all serve veterans. The second clinical exemplar is integrated at the senior level of the curriculum. This clinical experience could focus on care coordination in the community. Students are paired with a care coordination nurse at one of several specialty clinics serving veterans.

In situations when there is no established partnership with a VAHCS, but a facility is accessible, the first step is to build a partnership. The Health Research & Educational Trust (2016) outlines steps to initiate a new partnership. The authors suggest a strategic plan that describes partnership structures and processes, the leadership team, and roles and responsibilities. In addition, potential obstacles and challenges are discussed. The authors suggest metrics to measure success of the partnership goals as well as partner engagement. Along with evaluation of the partnership, they highlight the importance of creating a sustainability plan to ensure longevity of the partnership.

Once the partnership is established there are several ways for nursing faculty members to seize opportunities for students to provide care to veterans. For example, it may be possible for all students to complete a rotation at the facility. However, if only a subset of students can participate directly in the setting, there are ways to facilitate sharing with the larger cohort. One could consider blending post-clinical groups or seminars on campus or dedicating time in didactic class sessions to allow clinical sharing. For example, in a didactic session focused on mental health content such as PTSD, a veteran-focused film such as *Visions of Warriors* could be viewed in class. This documentary follows the lives of several veterans with a diagnosis of PTSD, as well as additional mental health diagnoses. The faculty presenter could encourage students at a veteran-centered mental health clinical site to share their relevant firsthand experiences from working with veterans.

In the next two sections, examples of veteran-centered teaching strategies in a variety of undergraduate and graduate level clinical experiences are described. Several exemplars are presented in a variety of veteran-specific clinical settings to illustrate some specific options. In addition, clinical tools and resources are embedded to provide direction for readers interested in developing veteran-centered clinical experiences. The examples presented may be used "as is" for the clinical settings as described or may be adapted for use in other clinical settings. Since nursing programs across the United States and globally vary in course offerings and sequencing, activities may need to be leveled for the academic year of students (i.e., first year, second year, etc.).

Undergraduate Programs

Opportunities for veteran-focused clinical experiences for undergraduate nursing students exist in both VA and non-VA settings. Faculty can arrange for veteran-centered clinical learning in their current settings or seek new partnerships with organizations that specifically serve veterans. There are clinical strategies and learning activities that may be used in most of the clinical courses throughout an established curricula. Several specific examples are presented to assist the reader with planning for and implementing veteran-centered clinical experiences that are a good fit within their program location. The examples, some of which are from published works, are organized by typical clinical courses within an undergraduate nursing program and can be adapted accordingly.

HEALTH ASSESSMENT

Whether Health Assessment is a stand-alone course, or integrated throughout the curricula, it is the first step in the nursing process. This is the time where nurses are able to learn about their patients, and skills evolve over time and with practice. The Veterans Health Administration has a number of free, public domain clinical resources available to facilitate this step. One is called the *Military Health History Pocket Card*, which all students should carry while at clinical sites to use as a reference (Exhibit 11.1). An easy way to incorporate this is by introducing this card as part of teaching history-taking and assessment, so that it is part of the holistic assessment from the very start. Having the card at the clinical site means this resource will be at their fingertips whenever it turns out their patient is a veteran and they need to ask more in-depth questions. The pocket card is available at www.va.gov/oaa/pocketcard.

EXHIBIT 11.1

MILITARY HEALTH HISTORY POCKET CARD

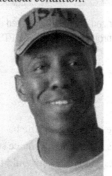

"Help me understand my medical condition."

"I had some unique experiences while serving our country, many that civilians would never have. Some of those experiences may be affecting my health, and that is why I am here at VA."

"Help me understand my medical condition, and please be patient with me. Some of my memories may be painful or difficult to discuss."

Asking the questions on this card will be helpful in understanding my medical problems and concerns.

- *Ask these questions in a safe and private place*
- *Engage with good eye contact*
- *Use a supportive tone of voice*
- *Thank veterans if they disclose stressful or traumatic experiences*
- *If you suspect someone is actively at risk for suicide, do not leave them alone*

General Questions

Would it be ok if I talked with you about your military experience?
When and where did you/do you serve and in what branch?
What type of work did you do or currently do while in the service?
Did you have **any** illnesses or injuries while in the service?

If Veterans answer "Yes" to any of the following questions, ask:
"Can you tell me more about that?"

- Did you ever become ill while you were in the service?
- Were you or a buddy wounded, injured, or hospitalized?
- Did you have a head injury with loss of consciousness, loss of memory, "seeing stars" or being temporarily disoriented?
- Did you see combat, enemy fire, or casualties?
- Were you a prisoner of war?

Compensation & Benefits

Do you have a service-connected condition?
Would you like assistance in filing for compensation for injuries or illnesses related to your service?

VA Information: 1-800-827-1000 or 844-MyVA311 (698-2311)

Living Situation

Would it be ok to talk about your living situation?
Where do you live and who do you live with? Is your housing safe?
Are you in any danger of losing your housing?
Do you need assistance in caring for yourself and/or dependents?

Unwanted Sexual Experiences in the Military

May I ask you about stressful experiences that men and women can have during military service?

1. Did you have any unwanted sexual experiences in the military? For example, threatening or repeated sexual attention, comments or touching?
2. Did you have any sexual contact against your will or when unable to say no, such as being forced, or when asleep or intoxicated?
   If Yes: I am sorry; thank you for sharing that. VA refers to this as 'military sexual trauma' or 'MST" and offers free MST-related care.
   If No: Okay, thank you. I ask all Veterans because VA offers free care related to these experiences.

 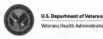 **U.S. Department of Veterans Affairs**
Veterans Health Administration

Veterans Crisis Line 1-800-273-8255 (Press 1)   APRIL 2019   Veterans Health Administration
Office of Academic Affiliations

Ask all military service members and all Veterans	Common Service-Related Exposure Concerns

Exposure Concerns

Would it be okay if I asked about some things you may have been exposed to during your service?

What... were you exposed to?

- **Chemical** (pollution, solvents, weapons, etc.)
- **Biological** (infectious diseases, weapons)
- **Psychological trauma or abuse**
- **Physical**

Blast or explosion	Radiation	Vehicular crash
Munitions or bullet wound	Shell fragment	Excessive noise
	Heat	Other injury

What... precautions were taken? *(Avoidance, PPE, Treatment)*
How... long was the exposure?
How... concerned are you about the exposure?
Where... were you exposed?
When... were you exposed?
Who... else may have been affected? Unit name, etc.

Behavior

Would it be okay if we talked about emotional responses during your service?

PTSD: Have you been concerned that you might suffer from Postraumatic Stress Disorder? Symptoms can include re-experiencing symptoms such as nightmares or unwanted thoughts, hyperarousal/being "on guard," avoiding situations that remind you of the trauma, and/or numbing of emotions.

Depression: Have you been experiencing sadness, feelings of hopelessness/helplessness, lack of energy, difficulty with concentrating, and/or poor sleep?

Risk Assessment: Have you had thoughts of harming yourself or others?

Blood Borne Viruses (Hepatitis & HIV)

- Do you have tattoos? Have you ever injected or snorted drugs, such as heroin, cocaine, or methamphetamine?
- Have you ever been tested for Hepatitis C or HIV? If not, would you like to be tested for these?

Health Risks Associated With Specific Eras

Noise Induced Hearing Loss-Ringing in the Ears	Heat Stroke/Exhaustion
Burn Pit Smoke	Hexavalent Chromium
Cold Injuries	Mustard Gas
Contaminated Water (benzene, trichloroethylene, vinyl chloride)	Nerve Agents
	Pesticides
	Radiation (Ionizing & Non-Ionizing)
Endemic Diseases	Sand, Dust, Smoke, and Particulates
Malaria Prevention: Mefloquine – Lariam	Herbicides and other dioxins like Agent Orange

Occupational Hazards: Asbestos, Industrial Solvents, Lead, Radiation, Fuels, PCBs, Noise/Vibration, Chemical Agent Resistant Coating (CARC)

Gulf War/Southwest Asia (Afghanistan, Kuwait, Iraq)

Animal Bites/Rabies	Mental Health Issues
Blunt Trauma	Multi-Drug Resistant Acinetobacter
Burn Injuries (Blast Injuries)	Oil Well Fires
Chemical or Biological Agents	Reproductive Health Issues
Chemical Munitions Demolition	Spinal Cord Injury
Combined Penetrating Injuries	Traumatic Amputation
Depleted Uranium (DU)	Traumatic Brain Injury
Dermatologic Issues	Vision Loss
Embedded Fragments (shrapnel)	

Immunizations: Anthrax, Botulinum Toxoid, Smallpox, Yellow Fever, Typhoid, Cholera, Hepatitis B, Meningitis, Whooping Cough, Polio, Tetanus

Infectious Diseases: Malaria, Brucellosis, Campylobacter jejuni, Coxiella burnetii, Mycobacterium tuberculosis, nontyphoid Salmonella, Shigella, visceral Leishmaniasis, West Nile Virus

Vietnam, Korean DMZ & Thailand

Agent Orange Exposure	Cold Injuries	Hepatitis C Risks

Cold War

Chemical Warfare Agent Experiments	Nuclear Weapons Testing or Cleanup

WWII & Korean War

Chemical Warfare Agent Experiments	Nuclear Weapons Testing or Cleanup
Cold Injuries	Biological Warfare Agents

Tell your patient about VA's
www.myhealth.va.gov
healthevet Gateway to Veteran Health Benefits and Services

Find out more about military exposures
www.publichealth.va.gov/exposures/

CARC, chemical agent resistant coating; DMZ, Demilitarized Zone; DU, depleted uranium; MST, military sexual trauma; PCB, polychlorinated biphenyls; PPE, personal protective equipment; PTSD, posttraumatic stress disorder; VA, U.S. Department of Veterans Affairs.

FOUNDATIONS OF NURSING

In a Foundations course, nursing students can be taught about the basics of military culture. Students can examine factors that may influence a person's military experience such as gender, rank, education, or war era served. Example questions for students to investigate could be: What are the major features of military culture or how does service differ for men and women? Followed by, what influence does this have on the clinical care of the veteran? This pre-work can be completed prior to clinical and discussed during post-clinical conferences to facilitate student learning on how health concerns and needs may vary between the two genders.

With this foundation of knowledge, students can then conduct an interview with a veteran patient. Depending on whether or not the student has a veteran patient sometime during the clinical portion of the course, an acquaintance or family member would be an acceptable alternative. Ideally, interviewing more than one veteran of different demographics would afford students the opportunity to compare what they heard, allowing for deeper reflection. At the Foundations level, a standard interview guide may facilitate the experience. Some basic information students may want to gather include: dates of service, discharge status (retired, medically discharged, honorable discharge, etc.), last earned rank, military occupational specialty (refers to the type of job they had), any special training or education received, number and duration of any deployments, and if they receive VA healthcare (indicates a service-connected injury/disability). Students should be encouraged to develop their own interview questions. However, faculty review is recommended to avoid use of unintended inappropriate questions such as "Have you ever shot anyone?"

A second clinical experience could be having students spend the day completing a community assessment of available military-/veteran-specific resources within a community. As a group, or maybe two to three in a group, students can then develop a resource brochure highlighting what is available. This brochure can be shared at healthcare facilities within the community or with patients they come in contact with during clinical days. As students advance in the program, this clinical experience can be expanded. Students can build on what was learned through the initial community assessment by conducting informal inquiries with key informants in the community to determine what gaps exist. Upon completion of the assessment, students can develop a health initiative focused on the veteran population. An example might include doing blood pressure screenings at the local Veterans of Foreign Wars (VFW).

MEDICAL-SURGICAL NURSING

The medical-surgical clinical setting offers many opportunities to learn about military service members, veterans, and their families. While students may learn about what disabilities are in a Foundations course, they really can start to understand how disabilities can impact a person's life during medical-surgical clinical. For military service members and veterans, this is particularly important as many suffer service-connected disabilities that are often more prevalent, and sometimes invisible, such as TBI or the long-term effects of exposure to burn pit smoke and sand particulates (Elliott, 2018; Johnson et al., 2013). These unique health risks can present an opportunity for students to not only research and learn about them, they can teach other providers on their units. One suggestion for achieving this outcome is to have students select a military/veteran-specific health issue, research the topic, and create a poster to present on a unit. Faculty can create specific guidelines to meet the course clinical objectives. These posters can be used for more than one purpose, such as learning to do peer evaluation using a standard criteria, teaching other providers within the community, or as a display on campus to increase awareness of veteran health issues. Further, this type of assignment could be threaded throughout a curricula where students conduct a literature search on a topic in their Research course and then use this same topic to highlight the clinical application using a poster presentation.

NURSING CARE OF FAMILIES

Military families face many unique stressors alongside those of a military service member. Unfortunately, these are often overlooked. Nursing Care of Families is an ideal course in which to gain clinical experience of caring for military service members, spouses, and children. As pre-work, students can explore what a military lifestyle might look like, including the impact this can have on the family unit. Frequent relocations and separations, often away from extended family supports, and deployments are among top stressors (Blue Star Families, 2018). Faculty could assign a qualitative research study by Russotti et al. (2016), which summarizes how these issues impact families with young children as explained by parents through many direct quotes. In addition, faculty could utilize the Military and Veteran Family Cultural Competency Framework developed by Tam-Seto et al. (2020) to build case studies or simulation experiences that involve a deployed parent. Interviewing a military spouse about their experiences and health concerns would also be a viable opportunity to learn.

With improvements in healthcare and evacuation from the field, service members today are surviving injuries that would have been lethal 30 years ago. This has resulted in a higher number of Post-9/11 veterans who require caregiver support (Geiling et al., 2012; Tanielan et al., 2015). While we generally associate the term "caregivers" as those who are caring for older parents, many parents and even young spouses are caring for veterans, many of whom will require care for several decades. This provides an opportunity for students to explore the needs of families on multiple levels, including the impact caring for a young veteran has on a spouse and children.

A course on caring for families is an ideal place for students to have some experiential clinical learning about patient advocacy. This could be done in several ways, with the overarching goal for students to become familiar with veteran advocacy groups and organizations. Students will be guided to select a veteran advocacy group to learn about, preferably something relatively local. Students should be guided to explore the history of the organization, what their goals are, how they are funded, what percent of their funds are used toward advocacy efforts, and how they measure the effectiveness of their work. In small groups, students can set up a time to meet with and talk to members of these groups, gaining insight into how the organization operates to assist and advocate for veterans. This can be from an organizational or personal perspective. After the visit, students will regroup and formulate their own plan/ideas to advocate for a particular concern they learned about during their experience. Students can share these experiences in future clinical conferences or through reflective journaling. If desired, clinical time could also be utilized to enhance this experience by having students develop and execute a program/project, including developing objectives and an evaluation plan, based on a selected concern. If site visits are not possible, an alternative may be to set up a panel of representatives that affords students a similar opportunity.

NURSING CARE OF THE OLDER ADULT

Military service can have both positive and negative long-term effects, some of which may be latent for decades until veterans begin to experience normative losses associated with aging (Spiro et al., 2016). End-of-life can be particularly difficult if veterans have unresolved psychosocial issues that stemmed from military service (Elliott, 2017). As stated early in the chapter, only a small percentage (about 1 in 4) of veterans die in a VA setting (Gabriel et al., 2015). This means that a large number of veterans who served during World War II, Korea, and Vietnam and are of older age, require quality, culturally sensitive care within local communities (Way et al., 2019). Students can play an integral role in caring for this population as most desire to reminisce and tell stories about their service. Community living centers and long-term care facilities are likely home to many veterans. Students attending clinical in these settings may have the opportunity to talk with veterans and be involved in planning activities with staff and families to honor their service.

Way et al. (2019) compiled a list of top 10 tips for providers who deliver palliative care to veterans. This publication is full of information useful to faculty who are interested in developing a veteran-centric clinical experience at varying levels in an academic program. Hospice experiences, or placement of students in agencies who have partnership with the VA, are ideal to gain exposure to this population. The We Honor Veterans website is an excellent resource to learn more about programs, partnerships, education, and advocacy for this population (www.wehonorveterans.org).

COMMUNITY OR PUBLIC HEALTH NURSING

Champlin and Kunkel (2017) offered an example of the implementation of a veteran-centered community health clinical experience in a prelicensure nursing program at the junior-level. In their example, a subset of students (approximately 10 per semester) participated. The experience offered opportunities in several community-based clinical settings, which included the following: (a) an adult day health program for veterans, (b) a community resource and referral center serving homeless veterans, (c) a home and community care program offering home visits to veterans, (d) a weight management program for veterans, and (e) a home telehealth program providing services to veterans unable to travel to the VAHCS. The authors described several additional learning experiences and post-clinical discussions that could broaden student learning about veteran-centered care. The students in this subset were called upon to share what they learned about veteran-centered care to their peers in seminars and in class. Champlin and Kunkel (2017) concluded that in this community health clinical experience, students met eight of 10 of the VCUNE competencies as defined by Moss et al. (2015). They cited difficulty accomplishing the two remaining competencies as they were unable to ensure all students worked with veterans with an amputation and assistive devices or who had experienced MST.

To overcome this challenge faculty can utilize Make the Connection, a free VA resource with real veterans telling their first-hand health stories (Exhibit 11.2) to augment learning and competency development. There are multiple videos of veterans sharing their personal stories of coping with amputation and MST. In fact, this resource contains a comprehensive library of videos, easily searchable by signs and symptoms, conditions, and life events. This large variety allows the instructor to easily choose videos to enhance whatever topics are being discussed in clinical that day or any areas that need to be covered. These can be streamed on the instructor's tablet or sent via a link to students' smartphones. The videos can inspire thoughtful, reflective discussions of real-life veteran situations.

EXHIBIT 11.2

MAKE THE CONNECTION VIDEOS

Make the connection: Videos from real veterans on range of symptoms and conditions

https://maketheconnection.net

Life Events & Experiences	Signs & Symptoms	Conditions	Kind of Story
☐ Coming Out to Your Healthcare Providers	☐ Alcohol or Drug Problems	☐ Adjustment Disorder	☐ My Story, My Connection
☐ Death of Family or Friends	☐ Anger and Irritability	☐ Anxiety Disorders	☐ Long Video Testimonial
☐ Family and Relationships	☐ Chronic Pain	☐ Bipolar	☐ Short Video Testimonial
☐ Financial and Legal Issues	☐ Confusion	☐ Depression	☐ Public Service Announcement
☐ Homelessness	☐ Difficulty Concentrating	☐ Effects of Military Sexual Trauma	☐ Compilation
☐ Jobs and Employment	☐ Dizziness	☐ Effects of Traumatic Brain Injury	
☐ Physical Injury	☐ Eating Problems	☐ Problems with Alcohol	
☐ Preparing for Deployment	☐ Feeling on Edge	☐ Problems with Drugs	
☐ Retirement and Aging	☐ Feelings of Hopelessness	☐ PTSD	
☐ Spirituality	☐ Flashbacks	☐ Schizophrenia	
☐ Student Veterans / Higher Education	☐ Gambling	☐ Suicide	
☐ Transitioning from Service	☐ Guilt		
	☐ Headaches		
	☐ Loss of Interest or Pleasure		
	☐ Nightmares		
	☐ Noise or Light Irritation		
	☐ Reckless Behavior		
	☐ Relationship Problems		
	☐ Social Withdrawal / Isolation		
	☐ Stress and Anxiety		
	☐ Trouble Sleeping		

PTSD, posttraumatic stress disorder.

PSYCHIATRIC/MENTAL HEALTH NURSING

Another example is to integrate veteran-centered content in an acute care mental health clinical experience. Services at a VAHCS are ideal settings for implementing veteran-centered learning opportunities focused on several VCUNE competencies, such as PTSD, SUD, TBI, and suicide. These content areas can be covered in the didactic content of a curriculum and then intentionally reinforced in the clinical setting. The likelihood is high that students in acute care mental health settings at a VAHCS will be assigned to patients who are experiencing trauma, substance misuse, TBIs, and suicidality.

Therefore, creating opportunities to present and discuss case studies based on actual clinical experiences can be readily accomplished. A modification to this is to complete a case study provided by the faculty member, which standardizes the experience for all students in the clinical group as well as in the larger cohort.

In the absence of a VA facility with mental health services, students can still learn about various mental health concerns faced by veterans through case studies, simulations, or utilizing videos (Exhibit 11.2). Further, faculty may be able to find resources or experts across campus or in the community who may be willing and able to talk to students about caring for those with mental health issues, such as faculty in Psychology or Counseling departments. In Exhibit 11.3 is a useful PTSD screening tool developed by the VA's National Center for PTSD (Prins et al., 2015). This simple tool is easy to print and can be utilized by a novice student who is assessing for PTSD with their veteran patient.

EXHIBIT 11.3

PRIMARY CARE PTSD SCREENING TOOL

Sometimes things happen to people that are unusually or especially frightening, horrible, or traumatic. For example: *a serious accident or fire, a physical or sexual assault or abuse, an earthquake or flood, a war, seeing someone be killed or seriously injured, having a loved one die through homicide or suicide.*

Have you ever experienced this kind of event? YES NO

> If no, screen total = 0. Please stop here.
> If yes, please answer the questions below.

In the past month, have you ...

1. had nightmare about the event(s) or thought about the event(s) when you did not want to?	YES	NO
2. tried hard not to think about the event(s) or went out of your way to avoid situations that reminded you of the event(s)?	YES	NO
3. been constantly on guard, watchful, or easily startled?	YES	NO
4. felt numb or detached from people, activities, or your surroundings?	YES	NO
5. felt guilty or unable to stop blaming yourself of others for the event(s) or any problems the events may have caused?	YES	NO
Total score is sum or "YES" responses in items 1-5.	**TOTAL SCORE**	

NOTE: Answering "YES" to at least 3 of the 5 questions indicates probable PTSD.

PTSD, posttraumatic stress disorder.

Students at all academic levels can participate in clinical situations that offer opportunities to work with veterans. Their knowledge base will be stronger based on the presentation of content in didactic courses. Students should be introduced to several of the assessment tools described in this chapter, as well as be well-informed regarding veteran-focused resources and supports both inside and outside the hospital setting. The intent of this section was to provide suggested activities that may be integrated into clinical experiences. Simulations, case studies, and post-clinical learning strategies are presented later in this chapter, which would be appropriate to use with students at any level.

Graduate Programs

Graduate nursing programs can benefit from the resources, mapping, and evaluation already discussed. These programs offer unique opportunities for research by PhD students or quality improvement projects conducted by Doctor of Nursing Practice (DNP) students, which could focus on veterans. The VA has an Office of Research and Development, which has identified the following topics as high priority: chronic disease management, pain management, homelessness, women's health, mental health, and prosthetics and amputation care (VA, 2017). Leaders in graduate nursing programs should invest in creating relationships with any nearby VAHCS and in initiating conversations to explicitly convey their interest in partnering on doctoral student projects.

In addition to veteran-centered DNP projects, faculty and graduate students can seek clinical placements that focus on care of veterans. For example, a graduate student interested in care of female veterans may elect to complete a women's health clinical experience focused on care of female veterans. Women are the fastest growing group within the veteran population, and every VA Medical Center has a Women Veterans Program Manager (VA, 2019a, 2019b). Contact the program manager to see what clinical opportunities might exist in women's health.

Another opportunity for graduate work is partnering with VA facilities to improve care for TBIs, which is an increasing health concern in the United States. From 2006 to 2014, the Centers for Disease Control and Prevention (CDC, 2019) reported a 54% increase in TBI-related emergency department visits as well as a 6% increase in TBI-related death rates. Nursing programs should connect with the VA Polytrauma System of Care (PSC) to explore opportunities for graduate PhD research and DNP quality improvement projects. The PSC is an integrated network of outpatient rehabilitation programs with over 150 sites to serve veterans with both combat and civilian related TBI and polytrauma (VA, 2015).

INTERPROFESSIONAL CLINICAL EXPERIENCES

Interprofessional education (IPE) and interprofessional collaborative practice challenge nursing faculty to move beyond the silo of nursing, to engage other professional education groups in interactive learning with each other (Interprofessional Education Collaborative, 2016). Using the four main competencies and sub-competencies outlined in the Interprofessional Education Collaborative (2016), rich clinical learning experiences can be created. Brommelsiek et al. (2018) reported on an 8-week IPE graduate level course on military culture, which included a practicum experience at a VA primary care clinic. Students from nursing, clinical psychology, pharmacy, and social work participated in the course. Exposure to veteran patients improved comfort and knowledge in working with this patient population (Brommelsiek et al., 2018). Further, the addition of a veteran discussion panel afforded students the opportunity to explore how culture can influence a person even after they leave military service. Such an example can be utilized as a guide to developing similar courses, both at graduate and undergraduate levels. While access to a VA clinic is helpful in establishing such clinical experiences, many communities may have veteran organizations (e.g., American Legion, VFW) that could provide a similar educational experience.

Evaluating Veteran-Centered Clinical Experiences

It is essential for nursing programs to create a curricular map documenting all the places in the curriculum where veteran-centered care is addressed in clinical, classroom, or simulation. Some programs have created a map based on the 10 VCUNE (Champlin et al., 2017). The map is a table with each competency mapped to each course with specific unit objectives created by the faculty of each course. Checking in with the faculty about these objectives each year is important. Shifting faculty assignments, clinical sites, and other changes can cause competencies to change or even be dropped. Regular curricular review helps retain the focus on exemplary veteran-centered care. Once clinical experiences have been identified or created, the next step is to find or create strategies and activities to meet the learning needs of the students and to provide quality care to veterans. In the next section of this chapter, examples of veteran-centered teaching strategies and learning activities in a variety of clinical experiences are described. Several examples are presented that may be used "as is" for the clinical settings or may be adapted.

VETERAN-CENTERED TEACHING AND LEARNING STRATEGIES FOR CLINICAL COMPETENCY DEVELOPMENT

Many nursing programs will not have access to VAHCS or other veteran-specific clinical sites. Therefore, designing alternative experiences with a focus on veterans will need to be carefully considered. As noted earlier, the majority of veterans do not receive healthcare in a VAHCS. Thus, faculty members can and should find opportunities to spotlight veteran-centered care in any clinical setting. Engaging in conversations with all clinical partners about a nursing program's intent to develop veteran-centered care competencies with students is an excellent place to start. Based on the findings of these conversations, faculty members can begin to incorporate teaching strategies in the clinical settings that focus on veterans. Several organizations beyond the VA have created high-quality resources to assist faculty and civilian healthcare providers to improve care for military service members, veterans, and their families (Box 11.2).

Johnson et al. (2013) discussed several teaching strategies for consideration when providing evidence-based care to veterans with health concerns in non-VA settings. This article provided a number of relevant resources organized by health topic, such as TBI, hazardous exposures, polytrauma, chronic pain, PTSD, MST, and SUD. This information is useful in creating assessment tools and clinical case studies, and in guiding post-clinical discussions. Furthermore, they discussed several contextual factors critical to include when caring for veterans, such as discussions of veteran identity and military culture, which can also be woven into tools, cases, and discussions (Johnson et al., 2013).

In this section, a number of teaching strategies and learning activities for the clinical setting are explored. Among these strategies are simulation and debriefing, case studies and use of guided questions, using mobile applications (referred to as "Apps"), and clinical evidence-based writing.

Simulation and Debriefing

Simulation and debriefing can be an effective strategy to teach students about veteran-centered care. Nursing faculty can easily adapt current simulation experience by making the patient a veteran. There are various types of simulation which can be utilized to enhance the clinical learning of students at all levels in a nursing program, including role play, standardized patients with actors, or use of manikins (Jefferies et al., 2016). Simulation also offers an opportunity to build interprofessional experiences into the curricula. Box 11.3 provides a list of resources for veteran-centered simulations. Keep in mind that current students and alumni who are veterans or active duty, or campus resources such as Reserve Officer Training Corps (ROTC) faculty and students, may be powerful resources. Privately talk with them beforehand to see if they have insights or stories they would like to contribute. Be sensitive to the fact that some veterans may not want to speak on these types of issues, while others will appreciate the chance to educate others about military culture and experiences. Furthermore, active duty alumni who are interested can share their wisdom and expertise from around the world due to advances in teleconferencing and smartphone video recording.

BOX 11.2

SELECT RESOURCES FOR CLINICAL TEACHING ON VETERAN-CENTERED CONCEPTS

ELNEC – FOR VETERANS
PowerPoint slides, case studies, and faculty guides available for free at www.wehonorveterans.org

ABOUT FACE: VA RESOURCES ON PTSD www.ptsd.va.gov/apps/aboutface

MORAL INJURY RESOURCES
Huffington Post: Moral Injury Project projects.huffingtonpost.com/projects/moral-injury
Also utilize this succinct article on moral injury: Guntzel, J. S. (2013). Beyond PTSD to "moral injury." *On Being.* https://onbeing.org/blog/beyond-ptsd-to-moral-injury/5069/

SERVING VETERANS: A RESOURCE GUIDE
The SAMHSA-HRSA CIHS developed this guide for primary and behavioral healthcare professionals serving veterans and their families. All of these resources and more are available from CIHS website at www.integra-tion.samhsa.gov

AMERICAN MEDICAL ASSOCIATION POPULATION CARE: VETERANS' HEALTH RE-SOURCES FOR MEDICAL PROFESSIONALS
Find resources for health issues that may affect veterans and their families, including post-traumatic stress disorder, traumatic brain injury and depression. https://www.ama-assn.org/delivering-care/population-care/veterans-healthresources-medical-professionals

APNA MILTARY AND PTSD RESOURCES
The APNA offers many general resources for caring for service members and veterans in a variety of situations, including post-deployment. They highlight VA resources for providers as well as specific resources, current research, guidelines and policies in the care of patents with PTSD. www.apna.org/i4a/pages/index.cfm?pageid=4403

EVC TOOL KIT
Developed by the AACN and the VA in 2012. It provides key educational resources to assist faculty and schools as they integrate veteran-specific content into the curricula. www.aacnnursing.org/Teaching-Resources/Tool-Kits/Veterans-Care

AACN, American Association of Colleges of Nursing; APNA, American Psychiatric Nurses Association; CIHS, Center for Integrated Health Solutions; ELNEC, End-of-Life Nursing Education Consortium; EVC, Enhancing Veterans' Care; HRSA, Health Resources and Services Administration; PTSD, posttraumatic stress disorder; SAMHSA, Substance Abuse and Mental Health Services Administration; VA, U.S. Department of Veterans Affairs.

USING MOBILE APPLICATIONS IN CLINICAL SETTINGS

The VA has its own app store and offers many apps useful to faculty and students in all settings, especially at the point of care. Most students are adept at utilizing their mobile devices, and these apps allow students access to powerful new tools. Table 11.1 highlights free apps and the VCUNE (Moss et al., 2015) competency that aligns with them.

These clinical tools could be utilized to explore a number of diseases and conditions. Box 11.4 provides a guided activity to improve understanding of veteran's unique exposures.

BOX 11.3

EXEMPLARS AND RESOURCES FOR VETERAN-CENTERED SIMULATIONS

NATIONAL LEAGUE OF NURSING: ACE.V
Excellent unfolding case study resources, available for free at www.nln.org/professional-development-programs/teaching-resources/veterans-ace-v

AACN LINKS TO VETERAN-CENTERED SIMULATIONS
Each has a different focus from mobility to physical assessment to PTSD: https://www.aacnnursing.org/Teaching-Resources/Tool-Kits/Enhancing-Veterans/Educational-Resources; https://www.aacnnursing.org/Teaching-Resources/Tool-Kits/Enhancing-Veterans/Educational-Resources

INTEGRATING WOMAN VETERAN CARE INTO SIMULATION
McKay Harmer, B., & Huffman, J. (2012). Answering the Joining Forces call: Integrating women veteran care into nursing simulations. *Nurse Educator, 37*(6), 237–241. https://doi.org/10.1097/nne.0b013e31826f2c39

EXEMPLAR OF A VETERAN-CENTERED CARE SIMULATION
Anthony, M., Carter, J., Freundl, M., Nelson, V., & Wadlington, L. (2012). Using simulation to teach veteran-centered care. *Clinical Simulation in Nursing, 8*(4), e145–e150. https://doi.org/10.1016/j.ecns.2010.10.004

EXEMPLAR OF A VETERAN-CENTERED SIMULATION USED WITH PSYCHIATRIC-MENTAL HEALTH NPs
Regan, R. V., Fay-Hillier, T., Murphy-Parker, D. (2019). Simulation clinical experience of veteran care competence for psychiatric-mental health nurse practitioner students with standardized patients. *Issues in Mental Health Nursing, 40*(3), 223–232. https://doi.org/10,1080/01612840.2018.1543743

AACN, American Association of Colleges of Nursing; ACE.V, Advancing Care Excellence for Veterans; NP, nurse practitioner; PTSD, posttraumatic stress disorder.

NOTE: Not all resources are listed in the "References" section of this chapter.

TABLE 11.1 FREE VA MOBILE APPS FOR USE IN CLASSROOM OR CLINICAL SETTING

FREE VA MOBILE APP	VETERAN COMPETENCY (MOSS ET AL., 2015)	CONTENT AREA
Exposure Ed	4. Environmental/Chemical Exposure	Medical-Surgical
Concussion Coach	7. TBI	
Psychological First Aid Mindfulness Coach PTSD Coach	2. PTSD 8. Suicide	Mental Health
Parenting to Go	*Can be used by anyone but aspects relate to:* 1. Military and Veteran Culture	OB/Pediatric
Preconception Care		
The VA App store can be accessed at mobile.va.gov/appstore		

PTSD, posttraumatic stress disorder; TBI, traumatic brain injury; VA, U.S. Department of Veterans Affairs.

Case Studies and Use of Guided Discussion Questions in Clinical

There are many veteran-centered resources available for faculty to use in the creation of veteran-centered case studies. One example is the *Enhancing Veterans' Care (EVC) Tool Kit*, developed by the AACN and the VA (2012; see Box 11.2). There are articles and case study materials in the *EVC Tool*

BOX 11.4

GUIDED ACTIVITY ON VETERAN EXPOSURES USING VA'S EXPOSURE ED APP

Ask students to look up and download the *Exposure Ed* app on their personal mobile devices (smartphone or tablet). This free VA mobile app was designed to help both VA and non-VA providers address military exposures that can cause adverse health effects. Providers can research a specific exposure, or look up all potential exposures a veteran might have experienced by date/location or by conflict.

Guide students to perform and discuss three activities in the app. First, have them look up Agent Orange – talk about the connection to type 2 diabetes mellitus and birth defects in veterans' children. Second, have them look up exposures from 1980 to 1985 and assign each student a different location from the list of options. Note how "noise" will be on every list, no matter the location. Discuss how the top service-related medical issue is hearing loss. In fact, the CDC (2011) reports veterans are 30% more likely than nonveterans to have severe hearing impairment, and over 2.7 million veterans currently receive disability benefits related to either hearing loss or tinnitus (Crouch, 2018). Finally, have students look up the Gulf War. Discuss burn pits, and then ask students to find where to sign up for a burn pit or Gulf War registry from inside the app. Once you have shown students how to use the *Exposure Ed* app, require use of the app whenever they have a veteran patient, either for assessment, assignments, and/or post-clinical discussion

CDC, Centers for Disease Control and Prevention; VA, U.S. Department of Veterans Affairs.

Kit that can be used as a springboard for developing a case study and guided question activity for post-clinical or seminar discussions. Major topics such as brain injury/TBI, clinical education, mental health and veterans, military culture, polytrauma, and PTSD are covered (AACN, 2012). The *EVC Tool Kit* is also notable for its section of resources and links for supporting student nurses who are also veterans or active duty.

Selection of an already developed case study based on a specific VCUNE competency such as PTSD can save faculty time in development. PTSD is selected as there is a higher prevalence of PTSD found within the veteran population. The lifetime prevalence of PTSD in U.S. adults is 6.8%; however, the rate is much higher in veterans, depending on conflict—from 10.1% in Gulf War veterans up to approximately 30% in Vietnam veterans (Gradus, 2019). The faculty member facilitating the discussion can select a specific article to be read before the clinical experience. One suggested publication for students to read is titled "The PTSD Tool Kit for Nurses: Assessment, Intervention, and Referral of Veterans" (Hanrahan et al., 2016 access this article by using the following link https://www.nursingworld.org/~48e191/globalassets/foundation/the_ptsd_toolkit_for_nurses__assessment.99783.pdf). The case studies embedded in the article can serve as a foundation for clinical discussions.

To build on this learning experience, faculty could use the PTSD Tool Kit and embedded case studies as a starting point, then go further by comparing this content with real world PTSD care practices that the students see in the clinical setting (whether acute care or mental health setting). The post-clinical guided questions can also be designed to meet the students' learning outcomes as designated in the course. Box 11.5 provides possible questions and activities that can be adapted based on a PTSD-focused case study selected from the Hanrahan et al. tool kit (2016), or one that is faculty developed.

Lastly, faculty can select an article or research study and develop their own case study and learning activities based on the findings of the research study or case presented. Self-selection of an article on which to base a case study can allow faculty to control the learning objectives/outcomes. The first example case study titled "Developing a Veteran-Centered Case Study Using an Evidence-Based Practice Journal Article" is guided by an EBP article and the VCUNE competencies of homelessness and MST. This case study focuses on female veterans who are experiencing homelessness. According to

BOX 11.5

POST-CLINICAL QUESTIONS AND ACTIVITIES FOR USE WITH A VETERAN-FOCUSED PTSD CASE STUDY

1. Describe the priority data based on a PTSD veteran-centered case study. Incorporate areas of assessment included in a mental status exam; that is, appearance and behavior; motor activity; speech; content of thought; flow of thought; orientation, sensorium, and memory; insight and judgment; mood and affect; and interview behavior

2. What are current care priorities for the veteran diagnosed with PTSD in the case study?

3. Develop a nursing plan of care for this veteran

   A. Identify three to four priority nursing diagnoses

   B. Identify one short-term and one long-term outcome for this client

   C. List three to four potential nursing interventions (include rationales)

   D. List examples of two to three questions to ask the veteran to determine if outcomes have been met, not met, or partially met

PTSD, posttraumatic stress disorder.

Absher (2018), the number of female veterans is increasing as is the number of female veterans who are homeless. A qualitative study conducted by Kenny and Yoder (2019) was selected for use in this example. The purpose of the study was to explore and describe the lived experience of homeless female veterans. The authors conducted phenomenological interviews and presented findings in a case study format. This article provides information that was used to create the Case Study, "Developing a Veteran-Centered Case Study Using an Evidence-Based Practice Article."

CASE STUDY

DEVELOPING A VETERAN-CENTERED CASE STUDY USING AN EVIDENCE-BASED PRACTICE JOURNAL ARTICLE

Citation: Kenny, D. J., & Yoder, L. H. (2019). A picture of the older homeless female veteran: A qualitative, case study analysis. *Archives of Psychiatric Nursing, 33,* 400–406. https://doi.org/10.1016/j.pnu.2019.05.005

Client: Sarah is an African American female veteran, age 52

Background

Sarah served in the U.S. Air Force as enlisted personnel. She participated in an active combat role when deployed during Desert Storm. Sarah is divorced and estranged from her three children. She has a family history of verbal and physical abuse as a child and experienced MST in the military. Sarah is currently using alcohol and marijuana on a daily basis and smokes a pack of cigarettes per day. The highest level of education she achieved was an associate degree in paralegal studies. Sarah is currently unemployed and residing in an urban homeless shelter for women. Her health is complicated by the following health conditions: pain, diabetes mellitus, PTSD, SUD, depression, and GAD. Sarah does not access the VAHCS and lacks awareness of healthcare benefits for veterans. She is not receiving medical assistance; she has no primary provider or clinic. She utilizes an emergency department at a nearby hospital for her healthcare needs

Current Context

Sarah regularly attends (every other week) the student/faculty led foot care clinic at the homeless shelter where she resides. The nursing student (Darryl) makes a point of providing foot care to her both times that she attends during his community health clinical rotation. During the first session, Darryl notices that Sarah is quiet, appears sad, and offers little insight into her current situation. She primarily discusses her perception that the shelter is not safe and that she wishes that she had more permanent housing. During the second session, Sarah's affect is bright, and she reports that she is feeling "better." It is during this conversation that Sarah mentions that she is interested in stopping her current substance abuse as she feels like it is not a good way to cope with her stressors and is holding her back from finding a job and housing. Darryl feels that he has developed rapport with Sarah and wants to pursue this topic with her

Guided Reflective Questions for Post-Clinical Discussion Focused on Sarah's Healthcare Priorities

1. Based on the background information provided, what are healthcare priority concerns for this Sarah? Please list five or six priority concerns. Place a star by the highest priority and explain why it is the top priority.

2. Sarah has identified a current priority. What is her priority? Is this in the priority list that you created in response to question 1? Does Sarah's priority fit with what you identified as the top priority?

3. What therapeutic communication techniques can Darryl employ to pursue Sarah's priority?

4. Identify the interprofessional team members that could play an important role in providing quality care to Sarah focused on her top priority concern. Please list five or six team members and what their role will be.

5. Use the nursing diagnosis handbook to identify three or four priority nursing diagnoses that would apply when developing a nursing plan of care of Sarah.

6. Select one nursing diagnosis and develop three or four SMART outcomes and corresponding interventions.

7. List potential health-related referrals that you would suggest to Sarah.

GAD, generalized anxiety disorder; MST, military sexual trauma; PTSD, posttraumatic stress disorder; SMART, Specific, Measurable, Attainable, Realistic, Time frame; SUD, substance use disorder; VAHCS, Veterans Affairs Health Care System.

Another case study was located in an informational article published by Wheeler and Puskar (2015). This case study presents a single 23-year-old Caucasian male veteran who is experiencing symptoms of PTSD and a blast-related TBI. The target audience for the information presented in the article is NPs. However, it can be readily adapted for use with prelicensure nursing students. Guided questions such as those presented in Case Study "Developing a Veteran-Centered Case Study Using an Evidence-Based Practice Journal Article" can be adapted for use in post-clinical discussions of this case or a new set of guided questions can be developed.

Evidence-Based Practice (EBP) Writing Activity for Clinical Use

Another teaching strategy to highlight veteran-centered care incorporates EBP, writing, and leadership. With this strategy, students search a database, write a literature summary, and lead a post-clinical discussion. The process is simple and easily adapted in a variety of clinical settings. First, ask students to select a relevant database and conduct a brief literature review targeting recent research studies with veterans. We suggest asking students to submit their articles to the faculty member in order to have them approved and to compile a complete list of the references for all students to access during the clinical experience. Following orientation and 2 to 3 weeks at the clinical setting (depending on the length of the clinical experience) to acclimate, this assignment can be introduced. One week ahead of time, require students to prepare for the following week by reading one of the student-selected veteran-centered EBP articles. The student who selected the article should do additional preparation that involves completing a brief literature summary to share with students and preparing to lead a brief discussion during post-clinical. The research article summary should include the following elements: the full citation of the reference, the purpose of the study, the method of data collection, the analysis, the findings, strengths and weaknesses, and the implications for nursing and care of the veteran.

The final element—implications for nursing—is perhaps the most important and can be emphasized by the faculty member in attendance at the post-clinical session. An additional step in the process could be to integrate this activity into more than one level of the nursing program such as the junior and senior levels. The veteran-centered research summaries could be collected and stored electronically for use as a resource as needed. The following example in Box 11.6 of an EBP research summary and guided questions for post-clinical discussion are provided to illustrate the preceding teaching strategy.

BOX 11.6

EVIDENCE-BASED PRACTICE RESEARCH SUMMARY EXAMPLE WITH GUIDED POST-CLINICAL QUESTIONS

Purpose
Cross et al. (2018) conducted a study that aimed to determine the feasibility and acceptability of rocking chair therapy as an intervention for homeless veterans experiencing mood and substance cravings. The researchers hypothesized that self-regulation (rocking) of mood and substance cravings would increase staying in SUD treatment, and would in turn, decrease recurrent homelessness

Method
Nineteen homeless veterans in SUD treatment were randomized into an intervention group ($n = 11$) and a control group ($n = 8$). The intervention group was encouraged to rock a minimum of 30 minutes a day and log the hours spent rocking. The control group was told not to sit in the rocking chairs. Participants completed an anxiety inventory and an alcohol craving questionnaire once a week for the 4 weeks of the study

Analysis
Statistical analysis was conducted to determine differences between the intervention and control groups. (Note: This brief statement is sufficient for this assignment based on the level of the undergraduate student early in the program. Statistical detail may be added as appropriate to students at a more advanced level.)

Findings
The authors found that participants used rocking (vestibular stimulation) to soothe their urge and desire to drink. They concluded that rocking has the potential to decrease risk of relapse and in turn to reduce chronic homelessness.

Strengths and Limitations
This study had three strengths: (a) purchase of the rocking chairs was a one-time, low-cost expense; (b) these rocking chairs were readily available for participants to use; (c) participants reported rocking decreased anxiety

and helped them relax. In fact, they wished that they had been able to have their own rocking chairs in their rooms. Limitations were that participants had limited access to rocking chairs due to other commitments; the rocking chairs used were not all identical; direct observation of the participants rocking was not possible; and only 10 participants completed the study.

Implications for Nursing

Nurses in acute care and community-based settings are in a position to advocate for making rocking chairs available to the clients they are working with. The purchase is relatively economical and depending on the durability the rocking chairs can be used over a relatively long period of time. In addition, nurses, in many cases, spend more time with clients than other healthcare professionals, and thus are in a prime position to encourage clients to rock as a way to self-soothe.

Guided Reflective Questions for a Post-Clinical Discussion of Evidence-Based Practice Research Summary

1. Consider the clinical setting that you are currently in. Are rocking chairs available for clients to use? If yes, are clients encouraged to use rocking as an intervention to decrease anxiety and relax?

2. If rocking chairs are not accessible to clients, what is the feasibility of changing this based on the findings of this study?

3. How would you go about suggesting the purchase of rocking chairs and how would you engage staff (including nurses) to offer rocking chair therapy as an intervention for their clients?

4. What do you imagine would be barriers to making a change to increase accessibility of rocking chairs for clients?

5. What other ways of self-soothing might nurses offer to clients?

6. What strategies can nurses use to encourage rocking as an intervention outside of the healthcare setting?

EBP, evidence-based practice; SUD, substance use disorder.

Putting It All Together and Leveling Student Experiences

The first step in creating a veteran-centered clinical experience begins with assessing the community where the nursing program is based. First, consider existing healthcare delivery systems that may already serve a higher than usual number of veterans. Faculty could meet with constituents representing the organization to propose an academic/community partnership. As an example, consider the nursing program is housed in a large university in an urban setting. There is a large homeless shelter serving men and women that is a short distance from campus. Knowing that the prevalence of veterans who are experiencing homelessness is high, faculty members seek to build a clinical partnership with the homeless shelter in close proximity to the university. Next, the faculty members and community partners could explore potential resources that can be used to guide the planning of the potential clinical experience.

Schoon et al. (2012) described the development and implementation of a foot care clinic in an urban homeless shelter. They outlined a step-by-step process that emphasizes curricular integration and faculty engagement that can serve as a guide. As noted in the article, this process will likely unfold over a period of 2 to 3 years so ample time is needed to allow for and encourage success of the project. Many of the veteran-centered examples presented in this chapter can be integrated in the early stages of establishment of the foot care clinic. They can be sustained "as is" or adapted as needed over time. The veteran-centered teaching strategies selected in this innovative example include a veteran-centered simulation and debrief exercise prior to the foot care clinic and active participation in a post-clinical conference using the article and Case Study "Developing a Veteran-Centered Case Study Using an Evidence-Based Practice Journal Article." In addition to these pre- and post-clinical exercises, faculty may consider creating reflective writing exercises focused on a variety of topics associated with veterans who are experiencing homelessness. Important to note is that students could engage with this clinical site at different levels and achieve different learning objectives throughout their course work. Repeated exposure facilitates the development of competency.

TEACHING STRATEGIES FOR NON-ACADEMIC SETTINGS

Nurses who are educators in clinical settings can modify the presented techniques and resources for their setting as well. Instead of a post-clinical conference, think about options that could be utilized during a monthly or quarterly staff meeting. One of the short videos from Make the Connection (Exhibit 11.3) could prompt a meaningful discussion. Consider developing a journal club in the unit or in the facility, or develop simulations that include a veteran patient (Chargulaf, 2019). While not an exhaustive list, Box 11.7 provides a starting point for recommended reading published since 2015 on veteran-centered care in a variety of clinical settings. The Academy of Medical-Surgical Nurses newsletter, *MedSurg Matters!*, has published some quick reference articles in their *Joining Forces* column over the past few years, which could also be a good resource for quick and easy-to-read information on various veterans' health topics. Clinical educators can also utilize the examples in Case Study "Developing a Veteran-Centered Case Study Using an Evidence-Based Practice Journal Article" to create a case study.

Educators in clinical practice are in an ideal position to work with nurses returning to school to complete bachelor's degrees or advanced practice degrees. Utilizing the content in this chapter can assist in identifying areas of opportunity on one's unit and developing quality improvement projects that focus on enhancing the care of military/veteran populations. Providing a foundation of knowledge using various methods will be needed before change can be actualized. Repeated and intentional efforts by clinical educators can be the catalyst that changes the care received. Advocating for incorporating assessment tools into the EHR and/or adding a veteran assessment to the annual nurses' skills fair are examples of how clinical educators can make an impact.

IMPLICATIONS FOR NURSING EDUCATION AND PRACTICE

Educators in both academic and practice settings must include veteran-centered content in their curricula. Nurses need to have current knowledge of the best EBPs to address the healthcare needs of veterans regardless of where they receive care. Johnson et al. (2013) suggested that education include veteran-specific assessment questions, identification of veteran-focused resources and supportive services, and access to a veteran liaison at the site, especially in non-VA settings. Nedegaard and Zwilling (2017) recommend a multi-modal approach to promoting development of military cultural competence that includes activities such as formal training, in-services, online modules, and other "field" type experiences that increase exposure to military/veteran populations.

Nursing Practice

Entry level nursing education prepares new nurses to provide care to a wide range of patients. As healthcare continues to evolve, so must nursing practice. Caring for our military and veteran population, and their families, in a culturally sensitive manner is attainable. It is not enough to simply acknowledge military service. Nurses are accountable and have a moral/ethical obligation to continue learning beyond their foundational education, in order to deliver quality healthcare to all their patients. Chargualaf (2019) suggests that nurses must first be proactive in seeking educational opportunities to

BOX 11.7

RECOMMENDED READINGS FOR EDUCATION OF PRACTICING NURSES

Conard, P. L., Allen, P., E., & Armstrong, M. L. (2015). Preparing staff to care for veterans in a way they need and deserve. *Journal of Continuing Education in Nursing, 46*, 109–118. https://doi.org/10.3928/00220124-20150220-15

Conard, P. L., & Armstrong, M. L. (2019). "Toxic wounds" of Gulf War I. *Medical Surgical Nursing, 28*, 145–151.

Conard, P. L., Armstrong, M. L., & Young, C. (2017). Unnoticed heroes caring for visible and invisible wounds of the nation's military heroes. *Medical Surgical Nursing, 26*, 365–385.

Conard, P. L., Armstrong, M. L., Young, C., Lacy, D., & Billings, L. (2016). Person-centered older military veteran care when there are consequences. *Nurse Education Today, 47*, 61–67. https://doi.org/10.1016/j.net.2016.01.014

Elliott, B. (2015). Caring for Vietnam Veterans. *Home Healthcare Now, 33*, 358–365. https://doi.org/10.1097/NHH.0000000000000261

Elliott, B. (2017). End-of-life care for WW II, Korea, and Vietnam era veterans. *Home Healthcare Now, 35*, 485–493. https://doi.org/10.1097/NHH.0000000000000607

Elliott, B. (2018). Civilian nurses' knowledge, confidence, and comfort caring for military veterans: Survey results of a mixed-methods study. *Home Healthcare Now, 36*, 356–361. https://doi.org/10.1097/NHH0000000000000698

Elliott, B. (2019). Civilian nurses' experiences caring for military veterans: Qualitative data from a mixed-methods study. *Home Healthcare Now, 37*, 36–43. https://doi.org/10.1097/NHH.0000000000000709

Klippel, C., & Sullivan, G. (2018). Older adults as caregivers for veterans with PTSD. *Journal of the American Society on Aging, 42*, 41–46.

Lee, H., Holden, B. E., Adams, P., & Mason, D. (2017). Coping strategies of older American Korean War veterans: A mixed research study. *Activities, Adaptation, & Aging, 41*, 220–238. https://doi.org/10.1080/01924788.2017.1310582

Olenick, M., Flowers, M., & Diaz, V. (2015). U.S. veterans and their unique issues: Enhancing health care professional awareness. *Advances in Medical Education and Practice, 6*, 635–639. https://doi.org/10.2147/AMEP.S89479

Way, D., Ersek, M., Montagnini, M., Nathan, S., Perry, S. A., Dale, H., …Jones, C. A. (2019). Top ten tips palliative care providers should know about caring for veterans. *Journal of Palliative Medicine, 22*, 708–713. https://doi.org/10.1098/jpm.2019.0190

Weber, J. J., Lee, R. C., & Martsolf, D. (2019). Experiences of care in the emergency department among a sample of homeless male veterans: A qualitative study. *Journal of Emergency Nursing, 46*(1), 51–58. https//doi.org/10.1016/j.jen.2019.06.009

Westphal, R. J., & Convoy, S. P. (2015). Military culture implications for mental health nursing care. *Online Journal of Nursing Issues, 20*(1). http://www.nursingworld.org/MainMenuCategories/ANAMarketplace/ANAPeriodicals/OJIN/TableofContents/Vol-20-2015/No1-Jan-2015/Military-Culture-Implications.html

Young, C., Conard, P. L., Armstrong, M. L., & Lacy, D. (2018). Older military veterans care: Many still believe they are forgotten. *Journal of Holistic Nursing, 36*, 291–300. https://doi.org/10.1177/0898010117713582

NOTE: Not all readings are listed in the References section of this chapter.

learn about military/veteran health issues, thus acknowledging the unique needs of this population and committing to improve one's knowledge and skills. Nurses in practice are encouraged to examine policies and procedures in their facilities for the identification of military/veteran status, and to advocate for change where needed. Learning about the effects of military service on individuals and families is a good starting point for those already in practice. While civilian nurses are not expected to be experts in military/veteran healthcare, having knowledge about resources available to veterans through the VA and within surrounding communities where they work, may be the one action that shows the patients that the nurse cares about who they are.

Nursing Education

Carlson (2016) identified five holistic themes required of nurse educators to be effective in this area, including appreciation of veteran contributions, veteran cultural competence, care and empathy for the veteran, as well as being a trust builder and team player. Careful self-reflection on one's own potential biases and blind spots is an essential part of this process. Further, as veterans enter nursing education as students, having this foundational knowledge may enhance faculty's ability to effectively engage and support these students.

Naturally, there may be challenges in educational and practice settings as educators enhance existing curricula or create new curricula focused on the care needs of veterans. There are several important steps in the process. First, it is critical that organizational leadership buys into the importance of the need to include veteran-centered content in the curriculum. Second, funds and time must be allocated for faculty to create content as well as to build clinical partnerships. Third, attention needs to be paid to the sustainability of the veteran-centered content with the curriculum into the future. Faculty champions can play an important role in creating and developing the curriculum, and in advocating for the implementation of veteran-centered content in academia and practice.

FUTURE RESEARCH PRIORITIES

There is much work to be done in regard to the clinical aspect of caring for veterans due to the lack of knowledge. Assessing patient military status has become a recommended practice. Future research should be conducted on what is done with this information and how it impacts patient outcomes. We also need to conduct research with nursing programs about use of veteran-centered clinical competencies and veteran-specific content (including clinical elements) and the outcomes, if any, that result. One research priority is to link how students are taught veterans' healthcare and patient outcomes, whether in direct clinical care or simulation.

It is important to understand that the veteran population itself is changing—more women; more veterans surviving polytrauma and living with TBI; differences in culture among veterans from World War II, Korea, Vietnam, Afghanistan, and the Gulf Wars. This creates opportunities and challenges in providing care. Further research may lead to reevaluating or expanding the veteran-centered competencies framework in light of the changing demographics of veterans. Determining best practices in veteran-centered care is never a "one and done" project; instead, this work must be continuously evolving and improving.

CONCLUSION

As of 2016, 7% of U.S. adults were veterans (Bialik, 2017). It can be all too easy to lose sight of the needs of a minority population. But the words of President Obama that started this chapter inspire us as nurses to remember that "honoring those who've served is about ... how we treat our veterans every single day of the year ... serving all of you as well as you've served the United States of America"

(U.S. Department of Defense, 2010). As nurses, we are in a position to lead change in educating future nurses to care for this population.

The clinical teaching strategies and resources presented in this chapter offer ways to begin or to build on veteran-centered healthcare in nursing programs. While not exhaustive, they are intended to serve as stepping-stones and a foundation upon which to build clinical experiences that focus on the provision of high-quality care to veterans. The nursing profession must be intentional and committed in integrating the VCUNE competencies to ensure these unique healthcare needs are thoroughly addressed and that veterans are always well served.

REFERENCES

The complete reference list for this chapter appears in the digital version of the chapter, accessible at https://connect.springerpub.com/content/book/978-0-8261-3597-1/chapter/ch11

STUDENT VETERANS IN HIGHER EDUCATION

KATIE A. CHARGUALAF | BRENDA ELLIOTT | BARBARA PATTERSON

Action is the fundamental key to success.

Pablo Picasso

KEY TERMS

student veteran	military
nontraditional student	nurse faculty
higher education	military friendly institution
baccalaureate nursing education	veteran friendly
transition	Post-9/11 GI Bill

INTRODUCTION

To facilitate their transition back into civilian life, many military service members enter into higher education in hopes of improving employment and economic opportunities. Student veterans bring a wealth of knowledge, skills, and experiences to the college classroom which can positively impact faculty teaching practices and peer learning experiences. However, faculty frequently report feeling unprepared to teach student veterans due to a lack of understanding about military culture, an appreciation of the challenges and facilitators faced by student veterans in higher education, and an unfamiliarity with available resources targeted to the student veteran population (Cox, 2019). This chapter provides a brief history of veteran education benefits, summarizes the experiences of veterans in higher education, examines the transition from the military to higher education, and highlights resources and recommendations for improving student veteran success in higher education.

BACKGROUND

Education benefits afforded by the GI Bill mean that increasing numbers of veterans are seeking college degrees (Dyar, 2016; Jones, 2017). The first GI Bill, entitled "The Serviceman's Readjustment Act of 1944," was signed into law following World War II for the purpose of supporting the transition back

---

The complete reference list for this chapter appears in the digital version of the chapter, accessible at https://connect.springerpub.com/content/book/978-0-8261-3597-1/chapter/ch12

into civilian society (Coll & Weiss, 2015; Vacchi & Berger, 2014). Entitlements included unemployment benefits, business loans, low interest home loans, and education benefits (Coll & Weiss, 2015). Almost half of WWII veterans (7.8 million) completed courses in an education or training program (U.S. Department of Veterans Affairs [VA], 2013). Iterations of the GI Bill emerged following the Korean and Vietnam Wars. Significant changes in benefits, social unrest, and rising tuition costs created challenges for veterans seeking a post-secondary education (Coll & Weiss, 2015; Jones, 2017). The Montgomery GI Bill (MGIB, 1984) was the first to provide benefits to those serving in the National Guard and Reserve components, although education benefits remained largely unchanged from previous versions of the GI Bill (Coll & Weiss, 2015; Jones, 2017). The Post-9/11 GI Bill, effective since August 2009, allows active duty and honorably discharged veterans, and their dependents, access to substantial education benefits. Depending on length of active duty service, the Post-9/11 GI Bill covers 36 months of benefits including full tuition and fees for students attending public (in-state) colleges and universities, up to $18,000 annually to students attending private or foreign schools, an annual stipend for books and supplies, and a monthly housing allowance for qualifying students (VA, 2019). From 2009 to 2016, the Veterans Benefits Administration (VBA) allocated $65 billion to fund the Post-9/11 GI Bill (Congressional Budget Office [CBO], 2019).

As drawdowns from the wars in Iraq and Afghanistan continue, it is estimated that by 2020, more than 5 million service members will leave the military (Ang & Molina, 2014). However, several barriers have been identified as influencing veterans' access to higher education. Prolonged periods away from an academic setting may result in a lack of knowledge about academia or access to assistance navigating the college admission process (Coll & Weiss, 2015). Veterans from "economically disadvantaged groups" may encounter additional challenges being a first-generation college student, identify as a racial or ethnic minority, or qualify as low income (Coll & Weiss, 2015, p. 7). Recommendations for supporting veterans' access and transition to college have included mentoring programs, targeted recruitment efforts, assistance accessing GI Bill education benefits, and campus support of veterans in transition (McBain et al., 2012). Although only a small percentage of the U.S. population (7% in 2016) serve in the military, there remains an influx of veterans pursuing post-secondary degrees (Bialik, 2017). As such, college and university faculty, staff, and administrators must be prepared to meet their needs.

Several terms are used to describe persons who serve or have previously served in the military and are now college students. There are no universally accepted criteria defining who is and is not a veteran (Vacchi & Berger, 2014). Some veterans believe a lack of combat experience precludes receiving veteran entitlements, including education benefits (Vacchi & Berger, 2014). According to Vacchi and Berger (2014), those currently on active duty would not be considered veterans as they are still serving. Barry (2015) added that service members in the National Guard and Reserve component would also not qualify as a veteran because they, too, are still serving. Defining characteristics of veterans, held by different entities such as higher education or the federal government, only contribute to this confusion (Vacchi & Berger, 2014). Frequently, in the higher education and nursing education literature this population of students incur the title *student veterans* (Jenner, 2017; Naphan & Elliott, 2015; Patterson et al., 2019a). Vacchi (2012) defined student veterans as "any student who is a current or former member of the active-duty military, the National Guard, or Reserves regardless of deployment status, combat experience, legal veteran status, or GI Bill use" (p. 17). Barry (2015) advocated applying the term student service members/ veterans to describe "military personnel—active, inactive, or retired-participating in higher education" (p. 415). In this chapter, *student veteran* is used to identify students currently serving or students who maintain any previous military service who may or may not receive service-related education benefits.

WHO ARE STUDENT VETERANS?

Veterans are a diverse population of students comprising all racial, ethnic, and socioeconomic backgrounds (Vacchi & Berger, 2014). According to the American Council on Education (ACE, 2014), approximately 63% of student veterans are White, 17% Black, 14% Hispanic, 6% are multicultural, and 6% are foreign-born citizens. By 2045, the numbers of Hispanic, Black, and Asian veterans are expected to increase (Bialik, 2017). Veterans are often compared to other non-traditional college students due to age proximity, full or part time employment, and family commitments. Student veterans average 25 years of age when they begin taking college courses having been away from the educational environment for approximately five years (ACE, 2014; Student Veterans of America [SVA], 2017). Almost half of student veterans are married (45%) and have children (46%; SVA, 2017). Excluding those participating in work study programs, between 42% and 46% of student veterans are employed full or part time while enrolled in college (ACE, 2014; SVA, 2017). Finally, results of the National Veteran Education Success Tracker project revealed that 51% of student veterans report a service-related disability contributing to stress while in school (Altman, 2017; SVA, 2017).

Military and veteran enrollments significantly increased from 2009 to 2012 although data vary widely across reporting sources (ACE, 2014). The ACE (2014) reported that a majority of veterans apply for and receive financial assistance although not all utilize veterans' education benefits. As of 2016, more than 1.6 million veterans accessed their Post-9/11 GI Bill education benefits (CBO, 2019). A study conducted by SVA (2017) determined that 70% of Post-9/11 veterans used their GI Bill to fund all or part of their college education. Typically, student veterans pursue degrees far different than their military specialization with the top three areas of study being business (27%), science/technology/engineering/math (14%), or healthcare (10%) fields (SVA, 2017). A commonly held myth holds that student veterans do not perform well and have lower completion rates. However, student veterans maintain a higher GPA (3.35 vs. 2.94) than their civilian peers nationally (SVA, 2017). Between 2002 and 2010, more than half (51.7%) of student veterans receiving service-related education benefits successfully fulfilled requirements for a certificate or college degree (Ang & Molina, 2014). Since 2009, the attrition rate among student veterans dropped as 72% successfully completed a certificate or degree (approximately 340,000 veterans; SVA, 2017).

Unlike traditional students, veterans acknowledge going to college was not always the plan or goal, but a choice afforded by a service-related benefit (Gregg et al., 2016). As a result, student veterans often attend colleges close to home (Jones, 2017) with a majority taking classes at 2-year public institutions (38%; ACE, 2014). This is not surprising given that tuition costs are lower in community colleges as compared to 4-year universities and Post-9/11 education benefits are stratified according to tuition rates at state (public) institutions.

Several risk factors impacting degree attainment for student veterans have been identified. These risks included delayed college enrollment, no high school diploma, taking classes part time, having dependents or being a single parent, financial independence, and working full time (Ang & Molina, 2014). In their study, Ang and Molina (2014) concluded that more than 40% of student veterans had four or more of these risk factors. Therefore, it is imperative that nurse educators have a working knowledge of military and veteran culture, understand the challenges and facilitators faced by student veterans, participate in professional development to enhance their teaching practice, and gain a familiarity with veterans' resources on campus and in the community. This chapter serves as a starting point for such professional development. The various sections of the chapter include transitioning from the military to higher education, an overview of student veterans in higher education, veterans in nursing education, recommendations for supporting student veterans at the individual and institutional levels, and implications for nursing education.

TRANSITIONING FROM THE MILITARY TO HIGHER EDUCATION

Moving out of military service into the civilian world or academia involves multiple, simultaneous transitions. Naphan and Elliott (2015) asserted the first transition involves becoming a veteran. Becoming a veteran entails leaving a previous role that contributed significantly to personal identity and replacing it with a new one, a process known as role exit (Naphan & Elliott, 2015). The process encompasses not only learning a new role but also determining the values, norms, and expectations of the previous role that are no longer useful (Elliott et al., 2017; Naphan & Elliott, 2015). This can prove particularly challenging for veterans because military values are deeply embedded in a service member's identity and worldview which may be difficult to shed (Elliott et al., 2017; Naphan & Elliott, 2015). "The experience of serving in the military transforms individual's civilian identities, values, and norms to reflect military identities, values, and norms" (Coll & Weiss, 2015, p. 11). Influencing this transition is a widening cultural gap between the military and civilian society in the United States (McCormick et al., 2019). Transition involves integrating the explicit (roles, rituals, symbols) and implicit (ideals, discipline, etiquette) elements of military culture into a civilian context (Chargualaf, 2016; McCormick et al., 2019). Jones (2017) cautioned that acculturation to academia should not seek to undo or remove the "character traits" acquired and embraced while serving but rather to remove the sense of "otherness" resulting from military service (p. 118).

The transition from the military to higher education has been described as complex and challenging due to stark differences between military culture and the campus environment (Jones, 2017; Patterson et al., 2019a). Although each branch of the military maintains a core set of values, their purpose is the same; to define and regulate role expectations, conduct, and authority over all aspects of service members' lives (Coll & Weiss, 2015). The military spends considerable time and energy building and enforcing a collectivist value system in its members. Uniformity, conformity, cohesion, teamwork, order, and discipline underpin the military way of life (Elliott et al., 2017; McCormack et al., 2019). A focus on mission readiness guides day-to-day activities and functions as the goal by which all are working toward (McCormick et al., 2019). The "hierarchical, authoritarian structure" is defined by military rank and a chain of command facilitating communication, training, education, role expectations, and promotion (McCormick et al., 2019, p. 287).

Military training facilitates the progressive inculcation of military/warrior ethos. Military ethos serves as a set of guiding principles by which all who serve follow. In the Army, for example, warrior ethos includes mission above self, never accepting defeat, never quitting, and never leaving a fallen comrade (U.S. Army, 2011). Over time, these values become enmeshed in the personal and professional identities of service members (Dyar & Brown, 2019). Service members live, work, and train together, building camaraderie and becoming trusted sources of support. This takes on a new dimension when service members deploy. There is an unwritten understanding that each has the other's back and is willing to lay down their life to protect each other, if needed. At all times, it is imperative that service members do their best, act with integrity, communicate clearly and effectively, and demonstrate strong leadership.

Higher education, on the other hand, is more nebulous. Although veterans are required to complete counseling before leaving the military, often they do not receive comprehensive information about higher education (Jones, 2017). Students are expected to function independently until such time they seek clarification or assistance (Gibbs et al., 2019). Advancement depends on individual gain; for example, getting accepted into a program of study or making good grades. In higher education, students are encouraged to formulate opinions, think independently, and challenge the status quo. "Attitudes toward hierarchy, questioning authority, civil discourse, and even punctuality and time" vastly oppose traditional military values and customs which may result in a state of dissonance or culture shock for student veterans (Jenner, 2017, p. 35). While some student veterans appreciate the freedom to make choices about their education and personal lives, others report the lack of structure as daunting (Gregg et al., 2016; Jones, 2017; Naphan & Elliott, 2015). For student veterans, attending classes and working toward degree completion became a job, their new mission (Gregg et al., 2016; Naphan & Elliott, 2015).

The literature is replete with references describing the challenges student veterans encounter as they leave the military and transition to higher education (Dyar, 2019; Griffin & Gilbert, 2015; Jenner, 2017). Across disciplines, these challenges remain consistent. Further, the obstacles endured by student veterans during transition are identified as a significant barrier to degree attainment (Jenner, 2017; Morse & Molina, 2017). The transitional issues commonly reported by student veterans may be grouped by interpersonal, financial, social, physical and psychological ailments, work and family demands, and administrative challenges. Each is described in the following section.

Interpersonal Challenges

Interpersonal challenges surface as student veterans perceive they are unprepared for higher education. For some, there is a demoralizing realization that despite previous military and life accomplishments entering higher education required starting over (Naphan & Elliott, 2015). Time lost to military service seemed to perpetuate academic adjustment struggles (Ackerman et al., 2009). Student veterans voiced a need to relearn study skills to be successful (Ackerman et al., 2009; DiRamio et al., 2008). Surprising for some is the experience of role reversal; that is, no longer being the teacher or expert (Gregg et al., 2016). Student veterans described difficulty going from being a role model to being in the background (Gregg et al., 2016).

Elements of student veterans' self-identity, cultivated during military service, contributed to additional interpersonal challenges. In the military, service members routinely participate in physical fitness and training to ensure they are mentally and physically prepared to meet mission requirements. Being unprepared or ineffective can have devastating consequences. As a result, some student veterans may not ask questions or request help (Dyar & Brown, 2019; Elliott et al., 2019; Lighthall, 2012). Nursing faculty have noted that student veterans were reluctant to seek academic help (Elliott et al., 2019). Perhaps this is due to a desire to avoid appearing weak in front of peers or faculty. Naphan and Elliott (2015) observed that engagement was a transferrable skill that facilitated success for student veterans. Efforts to enhance engagement could help avoid untoward outcomes resulting from a disinclination to seek academic assistance. Getting to know student veterans, timely communication, promoting campus learning resources, and structured group learning activities are suggested methods for assisting these students to fit in and achieve academic success (ACE, 2018; Schellenbarger & Decker, 2019; Sportsman & Thomas, 2015).

Financial Challenges

Student veterans frequently receive assistance to pay for their college education. For those receiving the Post-9/11 GI Bill education benefit, challenges resulting from a lack of knowledge about the process for establishing education benefits, communication with the VA, and timely tuition payments and disbursements for living expenses have been reported (Allen et al., 2014; Coll & Weiss, 2015; Dyar, 2016). Military transition programs largely fail to clearly articulate the scope of education benefits, how to access such entitlements, and overcoming frequently reported challenges (Jones, 2017). Student veterans are left to decipher the process alone, depending on campus officials to provide the guidance needed. As stated by Naphan and Elliott (2015), student veterans had to learn to "disentangle communication for pertinent information" (p. 41).

Student veterans report frustration when dedicated veterans' assistance is lacking on campus (Jones, 2017). Although many colleges and universities have established a veterans' services office there remains antiquated administrative processes and bureaucratic red tape that make common tasks in higher education, such as financial aid and class registration, more challenging for student veterans. The lack of institutional support can leave student veterans feeling lost (Naphan & Elliott, 2015). Student veterans desire a veterans' support office that serves as a one-stop shop for all veteran related needs that is staffed by employees who are familiar with military and veteran culture, GI Bill benefits, campus resources for veterans, and who can guide the student through an otherwise unfamiliar culture of higher education (Dyar, 2019; Griffin & Gilbert, 2015; Jones, 2017). It is crucial that student veterans receive support to bridge the military and higher education gap during the transition period. Recommendations for embedding student veteran liaisons into individual programs or schools have been proposed. One recurring suggestion is to include liaisons, or advisors, capable of mentoring veterans on a one to one basis to reduce stress, frustration, and ultimately attrition (DiRamio et al., 2008; Morrison-Beedy & Rossiter, 2018; Norman et al., 2015; Schellenbarger & Decker, 2019; Sportsman & Thomas, 2015).

Socialization Challenges

Student veterans are uniquely different from other nontraditional students, and certainly traditional students, creating social challenges as they transition to higher education. As older students, veterans bring significant life experience to the student role. To date, more than 2 million U.S. service members deployed to Iraq and Afghanistan in support of military operations (Sportsman & Thomas, 2015). More than half of these men and women deployed two or more times (Sportsman & Thomas, 2015). Military service instills a level of maturity, discipline, and work ethic not observed in non-military connected students (Cox, 2019). In the literature, student veterans describe traditional students as kids (Jones, 2017; Naphan & Elliott, 2015), whiny (Kato et al., 2016), ignorant (Kato et al., 2016), disrespect-ful (Jones, 2017), and out of touch with reality (Graf et al., 2015). What traditional students viewed as an issue was often deemed trivial by student veterans (Graf et al., 2015; Kato et al., 2016). Behaviors including packing up before class ends, leaving early, talking, and going online or texting during class time appalled student veterans who were accustomed to respecting those in a position of authority, such as faculty (Jones, 2017). Additionally, a lack of knowledge or awareness of world events and mis-conceptions about relationships with entities outside of the United States, held by traditional students, are a source of frustration for student veterans (Gregg et al., 2016; Vacchi & Berger, 2014).

Military service changes a person's worldview (Elliott et al., 2017). And many times, non-military students lack understanding about what service members have gone through during their time in the military (Graf et al., 2015; Kato et al., 2016). As a result, student veterans have reported difficulties interacting with younger, traditional students (Sportsman & Thomas, 2015). Student veterans in one study perceived that they lacked the "social skills need[ed] to relate to their peers" (Gregg et al., p. 6). Missing was a sense of connectedness from being around others who share similar experiences and values (Naphan & Elliott, 2015). The loss of camaraderie and difficulty making friends were associated with loneliness and isolation for student veterans (Jenner, 2017; Naphan & Elliott, 2015). Opportuni-ties to engage with other student veterans provided a source of support that could not be achieved by civilian students who were unable to relate to their military experiences. Additionally, making con-nections with other student veterans may promote academic success and positive reintegration to the college setting (Elnitsky et al., 2018). Naphan and Elliott (2015) cautioned that regardless of the degree of social support provided to veterans in higher education, they may still feel alone.

At times, student veterans have encountered bias about the military or serving in the military from civilian peers and faculty (Ackerman et al., 2009). Student veterans describe incidents when peers shared strong opinions about U.S. military participation in ongoing conflicts or asked whether they had ever killed anyone (Ackerman et al., 2009). The belief that all service members who deploy have posttraumatic stress disorder (PTSD) or express symptoms of PTSD are more misconceptions com-monly encountered by student veterans (Kato et al., 2016). Jenner (2017) cautioned that student veter-ans may actually encounter a stereotype threat created from compounding stereotypes such as race and veteran status. These stigmas and stereotypes are potential transitional barriers for student veterans and often result in a reluctance to disclose current or prior military service (Dyar, 2016; Kato et al., 2016). For student veterans, the transition to academia included learning how to respond to misinfor-mation and unsolicited opinions (Kato et al., 2016).

Physical and Psychological Challenges

Psychological injuries resulting from military service also impact the transition to higher education. Advances in technology and combat operations mean that the outcomes of service for those partici-pating in Operations Enduring Freedom (OEF) and Operation Iraqi Freedom (OIF) are vastly different than for those that served during previous eras including Korea or Vietnam. More sophisticated combat tactics, including improvised explosive devices, frequently cause devastating soft tissue and bone injuries resulting in disfigurements or requiring amputation (Church, 2009). Additionally, prolonged deployment tours requiring heavy equipment to perform job functions or maintain safety result in arthritis and chronic pain (Johnson et al., 2013). In one study, half of student veterans who reported service-related injuries were qualified to receive a disability rating from the VA (Elnitsky et al., 2018). In the classroom, these military-connected ailments and injuries may or may not be evident but certainly may influence learning. Planned and unplanned absences from class due to medical conditions or pain, attending medical appointments, and side effects of medication can interfere with academic performance (Church, 2009). Efforts to coordinate with disability services on campus are suggested (Church, 2009).

"Military service, especially service-related trauma, results in higher rates of mental health challenges and social and educational adjustment difficulties for veterans compared with their civilian peers" (Eakman et al., 2016, p. 2). Those veterans experiencing combat-related trauma endorsed more posttraumatic stress (PTS) symptoms (Barry et al., 2012). PTS was further associated with problem drinking, lower GPA, and decreased academic motivation (Barry et al., 2012). Traumatic brain injury (TBI) is an acquired injury resulting from an external force that causes temporary or permanent impairment of cognitive, physical, or psychological functioning (Dawodu, 2019). Between 2001 and 2013, more than 700,000 OIF/OEF veterans screened positive for TBI, qualifying to receive additional diagnostic services (Whiteneck et al., 2015). In those veterans who completed a comprehensive clinical evaluation, 61% were diagnosed with TBI with a majority classified as mild TBI (81%; Whiteneck et al., 2015). The predominant cause of diagnosed TBI were blast injuries (77%; Whiteneck et al., 2015). In student veterans, academic performance may be impacted by cognitive impairments resulting from TBI (ACE, n.d.). Difficulty concentrating, processing, and recalling information may be observed (ACE, n.d.). Academic stressors, changes in interpersonal relationships, sleep deprivation, and separation from trusted sources of support may further exacerbate symptoms in student veterans (ACE, n.d.).

According to the VA (n.d.), roughly one fifth, or 11% to 20%, of those who served in Iraq or Afghanistan reported experiencing symptoms of PTSD. The prevalence of student veterans who screen positive for PTSD and depression is high, although this does not always translate to a clinical diagnosis (Currier et al., 2016; Eakman et al., 2016; Schonfeld et al., 2015). In a national sample of student veterans ($N = 945$), 21% reported moderately severe levels of depression (Currier et al., 2016). In two single university studies, the rates of depression ranged from 46% to 69% (Eakman et al., 2016; Schonfeld et al., 2015). Similarly, rates of PTSD in the student veteran population are also frequently reported. Symptoms of PTSD were endorsed by 37% (Schonfeld et al., 2015) and 69% (Eakman et al., 2016) of student veterans who completed the Posttraumatic Stress Disorder Checklist-Civilian Version. Schonfeld et al. (2015) concluded that student veterans reporting difficulty adjusting to college life were more likely to have PTSD, depression, and other mental health disorders. However, for participants in one study, the overt manifestations of PTSD, such as hypervigilance and jumpiness, appeared to dissipate within 1 year (Kato et al., 2016). Graf et al. (2015) determined that veterans who were out of the military between 2 and 7 years were more likely to report classroom anxiety, difficulty concentrating, and emotional disturbances that interfered with educational endeavors. These issues were less prominent in those who left military service less than 2 years or more than 7 years before transitioning to higher education (Graf et al., 2015).

Several have investigated support and help-seeking behaviors in student veterans endorsing mental health needs (Currier et al., 2016; Eakman et al., 2016). Medications and professional counseling are widely reported treatment modalities for those with mental health issues. There is a reluctance to seek out these sources of support by service members due to the perception of appearing weak or the potential impact to their career (Vacchi, 2012). Investigating nontraditional sources of mental health support, Currier et al. (2016) determined that student veterans were 46% more likely to seek help from a religious counselor and 22% to 30% less likely to reach out to family or friends compared to nonveteran students. Utilization of campus disability services occurred more often in student veterans with a TBI compared to those veterans without a TBI (Elnitsky et al., 2018).

It has been suggested that higher education is ill-prepared to meet the mental and physical needs of student veterans (Eakman et al., 2016). Appreciating that either directly impacts the success or failure of these students means that greater efforts to meet student veterans where they are at is needed. Recommendations for faculty, staff, and administrators in higher education will be presented.

Work and Family Challenges

Student veterans are often juggling multiple, simultaneous demands in addition to their student role impacting their success in higher education. Jenner (2017) noted student veterans often do not describe their primary identity as being a student. As older students, it is not surprising that veterans are more likely to have family and work obligations (Dyar, 2016; Jenner, 2017). Attending classes and completing course requirements are often additional responsibilities for student veterans. As a result, student veterans are more likely to attend classes online, in the evening, or on weekends (ACE, 2014). In military service members returning from deployment, added stress may result from the expectation to resume family, work, and school responsibilities (Sportsman & Thomas, 2015). Flexible policies that appreciate concomitant responsibilities of student veterans are suggested. This is especially important for those still serving one weekend a month in the Reserves as they have less control over time during these trainings.

Administrative Challenges

Translating military training and experience into terms understood by civilian organizations is challenging. Veterans may not give themselves credit for what they bring to their new role. Perhaps, skills and training simply do not directly translate to marketable skills outside of the military or service members may forget to include transferable skills acquired early in their career. As a result, they may miss employment opportunities, administrative positions, and salaries in the civilian job market. Participants in Naphan and Elliott's (2015) study reported feeling demoralized that their training and accomplishments were not properly recognized in the civilian world.

In higher education, failure to translate the knowledge and skills brought from the military could prevent receiving transfer credit (Elliott et al., 2019; Jenner, 2017). In particular, medics and corpsman may be susceptible to circumstances whereby courses in which they maintain significant experience would need to be retaken to graduate. Efforts to formally acknowledge valuable knowledge and skills from military service are widely reported in the higher education literature. Suggestions include awarding college credit based on a review of official military transcripts (Allen et al., 2012; Sikes et al., 2018) and prior learning assessments (Allen et al., 2014; Bergman & Herd, 2017).

Of paramount importance is the need for student veterans to be able to navigate higher education. This requires a steadfast understanding of the various systems that impact student veterans. The trouble lies in the fact that information related to attaining a college degree may not be wholly and clearly communicated during transition preparation programs offered by the military (Jones, 2017). This results in student veterans who report feeling unprepared for higher education, frustrated with bureaucratic processes, and poorly supported (Jenner, 2017; Naphan & Elliott, 2015). They expect clear communication and to be oriented to university processes rather than being left to decipher an unfamiliar system alone.

Coordinated efforts to support student veterans and enhance their college education experience are needed. Norman et al. (2015) suggested this begins with employing staff with knowledge of both military and higher education to facilitate student veteran recruitment and the application process. Appreciating that some veterans may not self-disclose, it is important for student services offices to reach out to known veterans to provide an orientation to the academic environment, processes common to higher education including academic advising and direction for receiving assistance with education benefits (Naphan & Elliott, 2015; Vacchi, 2012). A single campus office capable of handling all veteran-related requirements and coordination with the VA is one viable solution for overcoming feelings of frustration and unpreparedness in student veterans. "A successful veterans' center should include academic advising, resources for counseling, financial aid, tutoring, mentoring, and other academic and social needs" (Sportsman & Thomas, 2015, p. 50). Assigning an advisor or mentor, who is also veteran, may help students make sense of the college culture, acclimate to the new environment, and overcome socialization issues more quickly as they can relate to the student in a way that civilians are not able to (McCormick et al., 2019). Consistently, research demonstrates that ineffective or inconsistent interactions and campus supports negatively impact student veteran success in college (DiRamio et al., 2008; Vacchi & Berger, 2014). Nationally, significant improvements in institutional commitment (dedicated offices) and academic/co-curricular support services for service members and veterans on college campuses are noted (McBain et al., 2012). Specific recommendations for enhancing veterans' services in schools of nursing are provided later in the chapter.

OVERVIEW OF VETERANS IN HIGHER EDUCATION

The influx of military service members and veterans into higher education has prompted the investigation of their experiences in academia. The result is an abundance of literature spanning multiple disciplines. Initially, literature focused on the transition from the military to academia and the associated challenges of acclimating to the academic environment. Over time, the literature has focused on translating military traits and skills to achieve success. This section provides a summary of this literature identifying three key areas: fitting in, repurposing military service, and identity reformation.

It is important to remember that military socialization and values are deeply embedded in the student veteran's identity and behaviors. These behaviors and values do not simply disappear when a veteran leaves military service. Often, student veterans will carry their military service into the classroom. Coll and Weiss (2015) asserted that veterans bring leadership, professionalism, diverse perspectives, teamwork, adaptability, work ethic, self-directedness, and a global awareness to their college education. As a result, veterans may perceive that they have a great deal to offer their peers and faculty (Graf et al., 2015). Findings from another study (Elliott et al., 2019) also offer support for these attributes. Nurse faculty participants in this study concurred perceiving that student veterans in the nursing classroom broadened the worldview of peers and provided opportunities for faculty to learn about military culture (Elliott et al., 2019).

Culminating the transition to higher education are several critical junctures necessitating veterans' re-examination of their position in civilian culture and higher education, military training and professional experience, and their identity as a veteran. Each are described in the sections that follow.

Fitting In

Adapting to the social and cultural norms of higher education is a priority for student veterans seeking to fit in (Gregg et al., 2016). Fitting in depends on an environment of support, acknowledging the student's background, and connecting with peers and faculty (Barry et al., 2014). When veterans leave the military, important support groups are often left behind (Kato et al., 2016). A connection to others sharing similar circumstances enhances social cohesion, the degree to which "members of a group like each other and feel emotionally close" (Naphan & Elliott, 2015, p. 43). Often these close-knit groups become family for those who are geographically separated from family. As a valuable aspect of military service, student veterans seek opportunities to re-establish social cohesion in the academic environment (Naphan & Elliott, 2015). However, the reality is that *[v]eterans suddenly find themselves as part of what may seem to be an undefined group where status or position is not determined by standardized advancement procedures or evaluation, and where dedication to compatriots rarely, if ever, approaches the level of "brotherhood" that permeates the military environment.*

(Sportsman & Thomas, 2015, p. 45)

Fitting in describes the process of integrating into a new culture (academia) and being accepted by group members. Smith et al. (2017) developed a survey to measure how well student veterans' function in college with measures for fitting in included. Student veterans scored significantly worse on fitting in as compared to civilian students (Smith et al., 2017). The perception of being different from peers and believing that civilians could not relate influences the ability to successfully fit in (Graf et al., 2015; Kato et al., 2016).

Research suggests that student veterans are at increased risk for social isolation stemming from difficulties connecting to civilian peers (DiRamio et al., 2008). A study by Whiteman et al. (2013) supported these conclusions noting that civilian students received greater peer emotional support than student veterans although emotional support did increase over time. Additionally, improved academic and mental health outcomes were associated with greater peer emotional support for both civilian student and student veterans (Whiteman et al., 2013). Participation in student activities for veterans and creating dedicated spaces for veterans on campus provide opportunities for peer emotional support and fitting into the campus community (Jenner, 2017).

Repurposing Skills

Many veterans pursue educational opportunities that do not match their work role in the military; that is, their military occupational specialty (Zoli et al., 2017). Routine training and ongoing education during military service provided a foundation for learning. This means that student veterans are accustomed to learning and maintain at least a basic understanding of how they learn most effectively. Yet the educational environment and teaching methods in academia are significantly different than those employed in the military creating uncertainty and stress for veterans. In the military, teaching frequently relies on an interactive, hands-on approach compared to traditional pedagogies in higher education. Success in higher education required veterans to learn and study in new ways, often falling back on skills brought from their military service (Patterson et al., 2019b).

Student veterans in one study identified "repurposing military traits and skills to support the student role" as vital to their academic success (Gregg et al., 2016). Some skills developed during military service easily carry over into higher education, namely organization, time management, and perseverance to complete difficult tasks (Zoli et al., 2017). According to student veterans, accountability and discipline are particularly valuable in college (Gregg et al., 2016). Norman et al. (2015) investigated the barriers and facilitators of student veterans' abilities to reach academic goals. Data revealed positive person factors which included discipline, organizational skills, perseverance, and motivation, while negative person factors included readiness to assimilate into campus life, physical/mental health, lack of skills to succeed, financial strain, and deployments for active duty and Reserve members (Norman et al., 2015). Faculty teaching in disciplines requiring a specific skillset can assist student veterans to make sense of what skills may be kept without change, those that should be repurposed, and those no longer needed (Elliott et al., 2019).

Other skills require modification to enhance usefulness in higher education. In the military, leadership, teamwork, and communication are essential skills needed to fulfill mission requirements. Service members are expected to collaborate with members of a team, tackle increasingly challenging leadership positions as time in the military and rank increase, and clearly communicate in a timely manner. However, blunt patterns of communication coupled with a take-charge attitude are often not well received by peers in the college classroom. Civilian students often dislike working in teams and certainly do not respond favorably to an authoritative leader who employs direct communication to ensure equal participation and assignment completion. Student veterans must take a step back, appreciating that academia is not the same environment with potentially dire consequences as that in the military. With assistance from mentors, faculty, and peers, veterans can learn to role-model teamwork allowing others the opportunity to lead rather than always taking charge. Patterns of communication should remain clear but less confrontational in tone and directness (Elliott et al., 2017).

Identity Reformation

Veterans undergo changes in identity during the transition out of the military into the civilian world and again when they enter higher education (Elliott et al., 2017; Sportsman & Thomas, 2015). Identity reformation results from the acknowledgment that previously held values, norms, and beliefs are not always useful or beneficial in the new role or environment. As student veterans become aware of these differences, there are conscious and unconscious efforts to adjust or modify elements of their military socialization to better align with social morays and role expectations in their new environment. It is not uncommon for veterans to temporarily experience a sense of grief or loss as they begin to let go of parts of their military identity (Elliott et al., 2017; Kato et al., 2016). According to Jenner (2017), intersecting identities require student veterans to "make sense of who they are, what they do, and their beliefs in their new context" (p. 29).

Faculty, administrators, and peers with previous military experience may be helpful in assisting student veterans struggling to make sense of their changing identity. Finding someone who understands the experience of transition can provide a sounding board for expressing thoughts and suggestions for moving beyond a state of stress and frustration. Tapping into campus resources directed toward student veterans enables student veterans to connect with others in the same or similar situation. Faculty are encouraged to assist students by providing clear expectations, constructive feedback, and sharing of observations.

Student Veterans' Perceptions of Higher Education

There are a number of published studies investigating student veterans' perceptions of higher education yielding useful insights about the academic environment and those in it (Graf et al., 2015). Repeatedly, student veterans report significant differences between the military and higher education cultures which influence their perceptions. In fact, participants in the study by Kato et al. (2016) reported that respect, earned from military service, is not acknowledged in the civilian world, particularly higher education. This loss of respect was deemed a great source of frustration for student veterans (Kato et al., 2016). While student veterans do not want to be treated differently than their peers (Patterson et al., 2019a; Vacchi, 2012), they do expect that their service is respected.

Traditional pedagogical approaches are not always effective for student veterans. In the military, training and education relied heavily on hands-on practice with instructor guidance. In some college classrooms, on the other hand, there is a focus on the dissemination of large volumes of new information using a lecture or "sage on the stage" approach. The adjustment to higher education may be supported or hindered by teaching pedagogies and classroom management (Sportsman & Thomas, 2015). Characteristics of a flipped classroom resonate with student veterans seeking to apply newly learned information in a practical way (Elliott et al., 2019). Data support that student veterans are not content to merely learn information; they want to understand its utility outside of the classroom. Student veterans become bored and frustrated when there is a lack of purpose to their education, when they perceive their time is wasted or could be better spent (Elliott et al., 2019).

Frustrating for student veterans were classes in which military stigma and bias were knowingly or unknowingly supported by faculty. Instances when participation in current military operations are brought into classroom discussions of an unrelated topic or when veterans are compelled to share aspects of their military service have been described in the literature (Dyar, 2016). Nursing faculty in one study reported their practice of asking veterans to share military experiences as a way to identify and connect the military ideals and traits that could enhance their student nurse practice (Elliott et al., 2019). Faculty are cautioned against such blanket practices as they have the potential to cause irritation and resentment (Dyar, 2016). Instead, student veterans should be permitted to self-disclose if and when they feel it is appropriate.

Faculty Perceptions of Teaching Student Veterans

Despite the increasing numbers of veterans in higher education and the plethora of research exploring their experiences, few publications have investigated faculty experience teaching student veterans. Qualitative reports of student veterans' transition to academia have yielded insight into teaching practices and interactions with student veterans; however, exploration of first-hand experiences is missing, creating a gap in our knowledge of student veterans. Two studies, one qualitative and one quantitative, have explored the experience of teaching veterans.

Research demonstrates that faculty lack general military knowledge, which is not surprising given that a small percentage of the U.S. population has served in the military or had family members who served in the military (Cox, 2019). Faculty teaching in nursing programs in the United States felt strongly that getting to know and understand student veterans' backgrounds was important to facilitating their success (Elliott et al., 2019). In return for serving our country, faculty commented that student veterans were worthy of the time and energy needed to improve their teaching practice and efforts to enhance learning transfer (Elliott et al., 2019). Additionally, faculty described challenges teaching this student population with one participant stressing the importance of delineating a student issue from a veteran issue (Elliott et al., 2019).

Teaching self-efficacy is also linked to faculty's lack of military knowledge (Barnard-Brak et al., 2011). A national survey of almost 600 college faculty, Barnard-Brak et al. (2011) concluded that faculty who maintain negative feelings about military service are less likely to set personal feelings aside and respect students' military service. Conversely, the researchers concluded that if faculty reported positive feelings about serving in the military, they were more likely to report increased self-efficacy teaching student veterans with symptoms of PTSD (Barnard-Brak et al., 2011).

VETERANS IN NURSING EDUCATION

All student veterans pursuing a career in nursing will be educated in a civilian nursing program (Cox, 2019). Yet efforts to understand the experiences of student veterans in nursing education are only beginning to emerge in the nursing literature. In fact, a recently published integrative review acknowledged this disparity noting that only 12 references related to student veterans in nursing education were located (Cox, 2019). This leaves the nursing education community to apply insights from general higher education research related to student veterans in a much different context. The risk is that the environment and expectations of nursing education are sufficiently different that nurse educators may, in fact, unintentionally fail to meet the unique needs of this student cohort. Dyar (2016) cautioned that research investigating student veterans in nursing programs is needed to avoid such scenarios. This section is dedicated to what is known about student veterans in nursing education, followed by a discussion of federal initiatives directed toward student veterans in the nursing classroom.

First Lady Michelle Obama and Dr. Jill Biden launched the *Joining Forces* initiative in 2012 to increase awareness, support, and resources for veterans, military service members, and their families (The White House: President Barack Obama, n.d.). Shortly thereafter, the American Association of Colleges of Nursing and the American Nurses Association pledged support for the *Joining Forces* campaign through efforts to improve veteran health by integrating veteran health content in nursing education, developing professional development related to veterans for nurses, and disseminating research related to key areas impacting veteran health (Saver, 2012). For the first time, professional nursing organizations recognized veteran health needs and the importance of nurses' involvement in promoting veteran health.

Student veterans have identified barriers which influence their ability to enter and matriculate in nursing education (D'Aoust et al., 2016; Dyar, 2016). Issues including a failure to receive academic credit for military skills and training, difficulty transferring previous college credits, low college GPAs in courses taken before military service, interruptions in program progression due to on-going military obligations (National Guard or Reserve), transitional stressors, and financial worries have been reported (D'Aoust et al., 2016). These barriers are similar to those reported in the general higher education literature related to student veterans (Ackerman et al., 2009; Gregg et al., 2016; Griffin & Gilbert, 2015; Jenner, 2017; Jones, 2017; Sportsman & Thomas, 2015; Vacchi, 2012). Dyar (2016) highlighted specific barriers contributing to transitional struggles including stigma, peer relationships, differences in education structures, and outside responsibilities. Although student veterans bring a valuable skillset to the nursing classroom, they described difficulties integrating into a culture that is significantly different than where they came from (Dyar, 2016). This was supported in another study whereby student veterans enrolled in accredited baccalaureate nursing programs acknowledged a need to learn a new culture but a lack of structure and understanding of academia created unforeseen challenges (Patterson et al., 2019b). A sense of perseverance prevailed as the student veterans appreciated another role which afforded a similar sense of purpose and meaning, like serving in the military (Patterson et al., 2019b).

Important to student veterans' success in nursing education is the ability to transfer knowledge and skills from their military service. Learning transfer is the ability to apply learning occurring in one context to a completely new or different context (Perkins & Salomon, 1992). Clinical laboratory experiences, simulation, and disaster preparedness using tabletop exercises have been reported in the nursing literature to facilitate transfer of learning (Evans, 2016; Johnston et al., 2017, 2019; Maginnis & Croxon, 2010). Data from group interviews with undergraduate baccalaureate nursing students, primary healthcare clinical site nurses, and clinical instructors revealed that the transfer of learning is influenced by student characteristics, educational design, the learning climate, and the clinical (workplace) environment (Botma & MacKenzie, 2016). Meyer et al. (2007) advocated for collaborative relationships between nursing education and practice settings to ensure learning is organized, relevant, timely, and student focused with adequate time afforded for practice and application of skills.

In some cases, student veterans enter nursing education with previous military healthcare experience as medics and corpsmen. In qualitative interviews investigating baccalaureate nursing students' perceptions of learning transfer, data revealed that student veterans did indeed learn and transfer military knowledge and skills to their nursing education (Patterson et al., 2019b). Differences between military and civilian healthcare systems and scopes of practice for healthcare providers means that nursing faculty must help student veterans to decipher the skills and traits that will be of value in their professional practice (Patterson et al., 2019b).

Veterans' Bachelor of Science Degree in Nursing

In 2013, the U.S. Department of Health and Human Services (DHHS) Health Resources and Services Administration (HRSA) began awarding cooperative agreements to schools of nursing to "increase enrollment, progression, and graduation of veterans from Bachelor of Science Degree in Nursing (BSN) programs" (DHHS, 2015). The aims of the Nurse Education, Practice, Quality and Retention— Veteran's Bachelor of Science Degree in Nursing (VBSN) Program were to reduce barriers for veterans seeking a career in nursing, develop career progression ladders that appreciate the unique needs of veterans, explore avenues for awarding academic credit for military service and training, improve

TABLE 12.1 VETERAN'S BACHELOR OF SCIENCE DEGREE IN NURSING GOALS

Goal 1	Create opportunities for veterans to advance in existing baccalaureate nursing programs
Goal 2	Implement policies to assess and measure competencies for which academic credit may be awarded
Goal 3	Address physical, emotional, and environmental issues that could impact learning, matriculation, degree completion, or employment in nursing after graduation
Goal 4	Support faculty development initiatives to increase knowledge and awareness of military culture and evidence-based teaching practices that meet student veterans learning needs
Goal 5	Collaborate with campus and community organizations to support veterans' transition to civilian life

VBSN, Veteran's Bachelor of Science Degree in Nursing.

SOURCE: Adapted from U.S. Department of Health and Human Services: Health Resources and Services Administration. (2014). *Nurse education, practice, quality and retention (NEPQR) program – Veteran's bachelor of science degree in nursing.* https://bhw.hrsa.gov/fundingopportunities/default.aspx?id=b72536b5-6cde-41dd-9fca-93fcefdf6f7d

employment opportunities for veterans, and facilitate solutions for addressing workforce shortages in nursing (HRSA, 2014). The anticipated goals of VBSN programs are outlined in Table 12.1.

The VBSN program is targeted to service members with healthcare experience—medics and corpsman. Since the inception of the program, a total of 31 schools of nursing have received grant monies to initiate or sustain a VBSN program (USDHHS, 2015). Commonalities across all VBSN programs include processes in place to award academic credit for military experience, dedicated efforts to educate faculty and staff about military and veteran culture, and enhanced support and resources for student veterans. Reporting and understanding the impact of the VBSN initiative is beginning to emerge in the literature. Currently, the published literature related to VBSN programs has focused on program initiation and lessons learned (D'Aoust et al., 2016; Sikes et al., 2018). One VBSN program recipient has reported student outcomes, with 76% completing the program and 98% of those students passing the National Council Licensing Exam on their first attempt (McNeal et al., 2019).

INSTITUTIONAL RECOMMENDATIONS FOR SUPPORTING STUDENT VETERANS

Several models and theories have been used to guide investigation of the student veteran experience in higher education (Elnitsky et al., 2018; Gilbert & Griffin, 2015; Naphan & Elliott, 2015; Vacchi et al., 2017; Van Dusen, 2017). One of the more commonly used is Schlossberg's Theory of Adult Transitions and later Schlossberg's 4S Transition Model (Anderson et al., 2012). Vacchi et al. (2017) argued Schlossberg's theory relies on traditional interpretation of transition that is not likely to capture the unique and complex experience of student veterans. Instead, appreciating the complexities associated with a veteran's transition to higher education and support needed to achieve success, Vacchi's Model for Student Veteran Support has been suggested (Vacchi & Berger, 2014). Four cornerstones including services, academic interaction, transition support, and support (peer and community) serve as a foundation to successful matriculation and degree completion (Vacchi & Berger, 2014). This model serves as a framework to outline recommendations for supporting student veterans in nursing education.

Research investigating student veterans' experiences transitioning into and effectively functioning within higher education have culminated in an array of institutional recommendations. It was important for leaders in higher education to recognize that the military often does not provide comprehensive information about higher education during briefings required of service members before exiting the military. Veterans, as a result, are left to navigate alone education benefits and the climate of higher education. The term *veteran friendly* emerged as a designation colleges and universities use to identify efforts to reduce or remove barriers impacting education goal attainment, streamline processes

TABLE 12.2 MULTILEVEL SUPPORT AT THE INSTITUTION LEVEL

Administrative support	Identification of student veterans Veteran office Knowledgeable staff Financial Channels of communication Recruitment practices and admission policies Maximize partnerships
Academic support	Recruitment of student veterans Admission policies and procedures Transcript review and awarding academic credit for military service Registration policies Withdrawal, incomplete, and readmission policies Academic advisors
Social support	Veteran space on campus Student veteran organization Representation of student veterans in student body Engaging student veterans in campus life
Individual support	Disability services Mental health services Career services

to ensure a smooth transition to college life, and inform veterans of available benefits and services (Lokken et al., 2009). However, a one-size-fits-all approach to meeting student veteran needs is not appropriate nor student-centered (Norman et al., 2015). Evidence suggests that student veterans need individualized support beyond merely processing education benefits provided by the VBA (Ackerman et al., 2009). Griffin and Gilbert (2015) asserted "institutions cannot assume that all veterans need the same support and resources; ... leaders must continue to examine within-group differences and seek to understand what individual students need based on their multiple identities" (p. 95). The ACE (2018) developed a *Toolkit for Veteran Friendly Institutions* to help colleges and universities develop programs and policies for military-connected students.

Creating a veteran-friendly campus involves providing administrative, academic, social, and individual student support. Strategies for providing each of these supports are broken down into sub-categories presented in Table 12.2 and discussed in the following sections.

Administrative Support

The ability of colleges and universities to fully meet student veteran needs relies on identification of veteran status. Graf et al. (2015) highlighted a "catch 22" situation exists when there is a reluctance to self-identify but an expectation to provide veteran-centered services when they are needed. Lack of knowledge about military culture, stigma, differences in age from other students, and significant differences in military and higher education cultures are several reasons why veterans may not report their service experience (Zoli et al., 2017). Generally, college administrators employ several methods for identifying student veterans including review of prior college transcripts, certification of VA education benefits, reliance on self-identification, or the Free Application for Federal Student Aid application (ACE, 2018). Regardless if one or a combination of methods are used, identification of student veterans should be a priority for administrators in higher education. To facilitate accurate self-disclosure ACE (2018) recommends asking all students, "Have you ever served in the U.S. Armed Forces?" rather than "Are you a veteran?" because some service members may not recognize themselves as a veteran. Ford et al. (2009) argued, "Identifying military students is critical to communicating effectively with them" (p. 67).

Veteran support offices are often created to provide a point of contact for student veterans on campus. A large majority of college campuses responding to a national survey (71%) report creating a dedicated office for veterans (McBain et al., 2012). Ideally, these support offices are centrally located, easily identified, staffed with knowledgeable employees, and are able to comprehensively meet the administrative needs of veterans. Employing a customer service approach, veteran's offices should include staff from the admissions office and student affairs, academic advisors, and counseling professionals (Gibbs et al., 2019). However, exploration of student veterans' perceptions of campus administrative support frequently reveals a fragmented system with ineffective communication and staff who are unwilling or unable to assist student veterans in a meaningful way (Jenner, 2017; Jones, 2017; Kato et al., 2016). For example, in order to receive Post-9/11 education benefits, all classes must be "certified" by a campus VA official each term, as directly required for graduation in the student's major (Jenner, 2017). The certification process takes a significant amount of time and knowledge of both military and higher education. In the past, student veterans were automatically dropped from classes when tuition payments were delayed from the VBA (Norman et al., 2015). Therefore, it is recommended that student veterans are afforded priority registration to facilitate a timely certification of registered classes (Vacchi, 2012). It is suggested that a single person, with military experience, be designated as the certifying official (ACE, 2018). Further, Vacchi (2012) recommended policies for withdrawing student veterans for missed tuition payments acknowledge the federal government's fiscal year and the impact on processing and payment of Post-9/11 education benefits each fall semester.

Griffin and Gilbert (2015) suggested explicit policies and procedures for disseminating veteran information, administering education benefits, and implementation of support services for veterans. Institutional facilitators and barriers to achieving academic goals were identified by student veterans (Norman et al., 2015). Positive institution factors included academic services tailored to veterans, veteran clubs, and the presence of veterans on campus (Norman et al., 2015). Conversely, frustration with academic processes including registration and advising, coordination of education benefits including GI Bill payments, and communication with campus and VA officials were identified as negative institution factors (Norman et al., 2015). Efforts to re-conceptualize antiquated or cumbersome bureaucratic processes, resulting in frustration and stress, are suggested by student veterans. A well-trained, knowledgeable, and supportive veterans' office can prevent unnecessary administrative burdens student veterans frequently encounter in higher education.

The cornerstone of effective administrative support for student veterans is clear and succinct communication. This begins with recruitment efforts employed by colleges and universities. While specific recruitment practices vary, creating a designated veteran recruiter position who can help veterans apply to college, access military education benefits or financial aid, and be familiar with military culture is recommended (ACE, 2018). Ongoing communication is imperative once a student veteran begins to integrate into campus life. Well informed staff and interdepartmental coordination of student veteran resources are appreciated. Kato et al. (2016) recommended someone with prior military service, a Veteran Service Officer, regularly communicate with student veterans on a personal level during their academic journey. Several also recommended a dedicated advisor within the school of nursing to facilitate more individualized support (D'Aoust et al., 2016; McNeal et al., 2019; Morrison-Beedy & Rossiter, 2018; Sikes et al., 2018). Ford et al. (2009) reported integrating an online newsletter which provided up to date information on class registration, certifying classes, and answered frequently asked questions.

Finally, college administrators should facilitate and support partnerships with community agencies and veterans' organizations (ACE, 2018). These partnerships allow institutions of higher learning to access veteran resources and supports that may not be available on campus (Coll & Weiss, 2015). It is also another way college communities can demonstrate their commitment to student veteran success. Examples of community, state, and national organizations are presented in Table 12.3. Gregg et al. (2016) suggested that these agencies may be able to support faculty and staff professional development, identify lesser known outreach programs, and provide remedial educational classes for veterans.

TABLE 12.3 NATIONAL VETERAN-AFFILIATED ORGANIZATIONS

Veterans Administration	www.va.gov
Student Veterans of America	www.studentveterans.org
Veterans Service Organizations	www.va.gov/ogc/apps/accreditation/index.asp www.va.gov/vso/VSO-Directory.pdf
VFW	www.vfw.org
American Legion	www.legion.org
USO	www.uso.org
American Veterans	www.amvet.org
American Veterans Alliance	www.wesupportvets.org
Bob Woodruff Family Foundation	www.bobwoodrufffoundation.org
Wounded Warrior Project	www.woundedwarriorproject.org
Hope for the Warriors	www.hopeforthewarriors.org
National Association for Black Veterans	www.nabvets.com
Disabled American Veterans	www.dav.org
Operation Homefront	www.operationhomefront.org
American Widow Project	www.americanwidowproject.org

USO, United Service Organization; VFW, Veterans of Foreign Wars.

Establishing partnerships on campus are also suggested (Coll & Weiss, 2015). Campus-based collaborative partnerships can enhance the student veteran experience by training and mentoring faculty and staff on military and veteran culture, creating a veteran-friendly environment, raising awareness, and engaging student veterans (Coll & Weiss, 2015). One way to create a welcoming environment for veterans on campus is to display positive symbols associated with the military and military service (Norman et al., 2015) or military appreciation programs for faculty, staff, and student veterans (Ford et al., 2009). Coll and Weiss (2015) suggested including student veterans, employees with prior military experience, and other interested stakeholders to generate new ideas for campus and community partnerships.

Academic Support

Academic support reduces transition-related stressors and retains student veterans in their respective programs of study. Across published research investigating student veterans in higher education, academic support consistently receives a great deal of attention. Clear admission and retention policies, awarding academic credit for military service and training, early registration practices, tracking veterans to graduation, access to mentors/tutors, and inclusive disability services are discussed (Coll & Weiss, 2015; Kato et al., 2016; Norman et al., 2015). Vacchi (2012) stressed the importance of directed efforts to "meet veterans at their level, assess their potential, and then include them in developing their academic plan" (p. 19).

As previously stated, veterans encounter difficulty translating military skills, training, and experience in a way understood by civilian entities, including higher education (Morrison-Beedy et al., 2015). ACE (2018) recommends an admission process that considers a veteran's professional and academic portfolio, official military transcripts, and college entrance exam scores. Student veterans expect colleges and universities to apply military experience toward academic goals by awarding college credit (ACE, 2018). Traditionally, military training and experiences are translated into a common language allowing civilian colleges and universities to better determine whether transfer credit may be awarded. Approximately 83% of colleges and universities participating in a national survey reported awarding academic credit for military training and 63% award credit for military experience (McBain et al., 2012). Unfortunately, inconsistent policies for awarding academic credit for military service are widely reported, creating frustration for student veterans (Vacchi, 2012).

Veterans with prior healthcare experience in the military may not be able to transfer credentials to civilian employment (Morrison-Beedy et al., 2015). Therefore, it is not uncommon for medics and corpsman to enter nursing education for the purpose of gaining these credentials. Efforts to fast-track these students to graduation and licensure by acknowledging previous healthcare and military experiences are widely reported. For example, they may receive credit for leadership courses, health assessment, and foundations courses if they successfully demonstrate clinical skills or pass a comprehensive exam covering course content (Morrison-Beedy et al., 2015; Sikes et al., 2018). Similarly, Bergman and Herd (2017) recommended using prior learning assessment to determine competence needed to award academic credit. It is suggested that "colleges should give every reasonable consideration to student veterans" while being careful not to award so much transfer credit that veterans are rushed to graduation (ACE, 2018; Vacchi, 2012, p. 19). Further, college administrators in one study felt that awarding credit may not always be in the best interest of the student veteran as gaps in information could impede success in upper level courses (Griffin & Gilbert, 2015).

Efforts to track student veterans over the continuum of their academic journey are recommended (Griffin & Gilbert, 2015; Kato et al., 2016). These begin with deliberate efforts to identify veterans as soon as possible. Each student veteran should have ready access to a mentor, ideally a faculty member with previous military experience. In schools of nursing with VBSN programs, advisors with knowledge of the military and nursing profession serve as a conduit between the student and the program (Morrison-Beedy et al., 2015). This mentor/liaison could serve as an academic advisor, initial point of contact for veteran-related issues, and an expert on veteran-related policies and campus resources (Elliott et al., 2019; Sikes et al., 2018).

Close monitoring of student veterans' academic performance is recommended (Cox, 2019). Informing and linking the student veteran to campus resources including the Office of Disability Services, tutoring services, or the writing center can promote student engagement and facilitate retention (ACE, 2018; Kato et al., 2016). Student veterans struggling academically may not seek help over fear of appearing weak or incompetent, a reluctance to acknowledge service-related disabilities as impacting academic performance, lack of knowledge of available academic accommodations, or that they are not entitled to services unless they have a disability rating from the VA (ACE, 2018; Coll & Weiss, 2015). Elnitsky et al. (2018) reported that few student veterans with traumatic injuries (TBI, PTSD, and chronic pain) used campus disability services. The authors further determined that disability services were accessed more often by student veterans with TBI. Participants in one study felt campus disability services were either lacking, difficult to use, or did not align with their perceived need (Norman et al., 2015). In response, ACE (2018) recommends faculty inform all students of available veteran and disability services in course syllabi. Further, student veterans recommend screening for PTSD and TBI in addition to re-evaluating disability services aligning with service connected issues more prevalent in Post-9/11 veterans.

Colleges and universities should strive to create flexible options for veterans to attain a college degree. Appreciating that student veterans are older and more likely to have outside work and family obligations, distance learning courses or clustering classes together to maximize time on campus are recommended. In addition, online classes allow military-connected students, who may be recalled to serve, to continue coursework and avoid educational delays (Ford et al., 2009).

Social Support

Student veteran organizations and dedicated spaces for veterans to connect are important sources of social support (Griffin & Gilbert, 2015; Kato et al., 2016). The most widely recognized veteran organization, SVA, has thousands of chapters at public and private colleges and universities around the United States. Despite an abundance of recommendations calling for colleges and universities to promote socialization efforts of student veterans on campus, Jenner (2017) noted that the impact of campus-based veteran organizations has yet to be investigated. What is known is that connecting to peers impacts the ability to acclimate and matriculate in higher education (Whiteman et al., 2013).

Congruent with other student organizations on college campuses, veteran organizations are organized by group members, adhere to university regulations, and often require a faculty advisor (Summerlot et al., 2009). Veteran student organizations may bring all student veterans on campus together in a single location (centralized) or hold smaller gatherings in individual schools or colleges (decentralized; Griffin & Gilbert, 2015). Regardless of structure, interacting with other veterans on campus increases comfort in the academic setting (Griffin & Gilbert, 2015). Although veterans report less peer emotional support compared to civilian students, there is evidence that both groups perceive greater support over time (Barry et al., 2013). Support received from peers is a protective factor associated with positive mental and physical health states (Barry et al., 2013; Eakman et al., 2016). An added, though unrelated, benefit of these organizations are representation from student veterans within the student body ensuring veteran-related issues and needs are sufficiently addressed (Griffin & Gilbert, 2015).

Creating space on campus for veterans to meet, interact, find support, and study is widely recommended (ACE, 2018; Cox, 2019; Kato et al., 2016). It is not uncommon for student veterans to report a lack of connection to peers or the campus community (Kraus et al., 2017). Not only will these spaces allow student veterans to connect with others who may be experiencing the same or similar struggles and feelings, they also help reduce social isolation (Cox, 2019). Kato et al. (2016) noted that engaging with other veterans may help disseminate veteran-related information and provide assistance navigating administrative processes on campus. For disabled student veterans, Kraus et al. (2017) noted that "incorporating intentional opportunities for collaboration in engagement opportunities would not only capitalize on some of their reported strengths but may also increase their sense of perceived gains" (p. 52). Developing resilience and successfully integrating into the campus community depends on social supports received by student veterans (Eakman et al., 2016; Whiteman et al., 2013).

Individual Student Support

In some respects, providing individual student support may be achieved through the administrative and academic recommendations provided earlier. However, appreciating that the achievement of academic goals may be impacted by service-related injuries and disabilities is crucial in highlighting the necessary recommendations for individualized services (Ford et al., 2009). In a national survey, 84% of responding colleges and universities provided counseling services for student veterans with PTSD, with fewer institutions having services available to veterans with physical and brain injuries (McBain et al., 2012). Campus counseling services must be prepared to respond to all student veteran issues (Kato et al., 2016), though Eakman et al. (2016) noted that college campuses are largely unprepared to handle OIF/OEF veterans' mental health needs. Unaddressed mental health issues are connected to lower GPAs, a lack of socialization, and attrition (Barry et al., 2012). In response, ACE (2018) recommended that a variety of options and mental health services be available to student veterans. A lack of trained staff is a limitation frequently reported (McBain et al., 2012). Partnering with the VA and community providers, using VA resources, and collaborating with local veterans' organizations are options for overcoming these limitations (ACE, 2018). Student veterans' preferences for receiving mental health services should be considered as they may not align with traditional treatment modalities (Currier et al., 2016). Coll and Weiss (2015) suggested that individualized support begin with assisting student veterans to identify "their personal strengths, interests, areas in need of growth, and goals" (p. 19). Overarching recommendations related to creating successful support programs and policies are outlined in Table 12.4.

TABLE 12.4 HOLISTIC RECOMMENDATIONS FOR SUPPORTING STUDENT VETERANS

Recommendation 1	Develop orientation programs to facilitate a smooth transition to academia
Recommendation 2	Appoint a single person, with prior military experience, to mentor and advise student veterans during their academic journey
Recommendation 3	Create a comprehensive office for veterans' services and support, staffed with employees who are up to date on VA education benefit policies as well as campus/community resources
Recommendation 4	Consider opportunities to validate military knowledge and skills guided by consistent policies
Recommendation 5	Proactively establish and refer student veterans to campus support resources (disability services, tutoring, writing center)
Recommendation 6	Garner support for veteran student organizations and meeting spaces on campus
Recommendation 7	Provide ongoing professional development for faculty and staff related to student veterans and military/veteran culture

FACULTY RECOMMENDATIONS FOR SUPPORTING STUDENT VETERANS

The higher education literature is robust with recommendations for faculty teaching student veterans. These recommendations are largely the result of the reported experiences of student veterans in academia and the collective analysis of student veterans reported by federal agencies. The lack of empirical support of the experiences teaching veterans as perceived by nursing faculty and the discussion of beneficial teaching and learning modalities for this population limits the scope and breadth of the following discussion. In large measure, the following recommendations are derived from published literature of student veterans in the collective college classroom. The three main areas of recommendations include faculty development, teaching and learning practices, and interacting with student veterans.

Faculty Development

As part of the HRSA grant for VBSN programs, nurse faculty are required to attend professional development programs related to understanding military culture and student veterans (Sikes et al., 2018). A national survey of public and private colleges and universities revealed 47% of military- and veteran-serving institutions provide opportunities for professional development for faculty and staff (McBain et al., 2012). Several programs for achieving this goal are described in the nursing literature (Allen et al., 2012; Gibbs et al., 2019; Morrison-Beedy et al., 2015; Morrison-Beedy & Rossiter, 2018). Additionally, several veteran-affiliated organizations have created online programs to facilitate a greater collective understanding of service members and veterans (Chargualaf, 2019).

The ACE (2018) advocates for staff and faculty training as one step toward creating *veteran-friendly* institutions. There exist no specific curricula guiding faculty development; rather, it appears to be the product of individual groups or institutional efforts and directives. Therefore, two examples reported in the literature will be highlighted. Carlson (2016) identified essential concepts needed to teach civilian nurses to provide quality patient care for veterans. It is argued that these same competencies could apply to faculty teaching student veterans. The four essential concepts are *military service* inclusive of military history, structure, rank, and culture; *military experiences* including sequelae of participation in wartime operations, the impact of service on self and family, and reintegration or transition challenges; *veteran experiences* encompassing the culture and community of veterans extending to issues impacting veterans; and finally *veteran affairs* consisting of the identification of local and federal resources available to the veteran population in the United States (Carlson, 2016). Morrison-Beedy and Rossiter (2018) asserted that faculty should participate in training that highlights characteristics of student veterans, adult learning theory, communication with veterans in the classroom, and recognition of the experiences of student veterans in academia. Ultimately, the responsibility to learn about and remain abreast of military and veteran initiatives belongs with the individual faculty member. Participants in Patterson et al. (2019a) study reaffirmed the importance of making time to learn about this cohort of students. Chargualaf (2019) advocates for ongoing professional development that is documented as part of the annual evaluation process.

Teaching and Learning Practices

Historically, dominant members of society directly influenced higher education (Coll & Weiss, 2015). A culture of institutional discrimination affected some minority students' and veterans' access to post-secondary education (Coll & Weiss, 2015). In the classroom, White female educators unilaterally applied teaching pedagogies to all student populations. As the student landscape continues to diversify, nurse educators must "teach to accommodate all learning styles … to account for students who have different experiences, learning, preferences, and capabilities" (ACE, 2018, p. 8). Sportsman and Thomas (2015) cautioned against lowering expectations while individualizing teaching and learning practices. Veterans expect to receive a quality education and are willing to work to be successful.

Military socialization influences veterans' needs and expectations in the college classroom. Like a military commander, the faculty member is a person of authority (Coll & Weiss, 2015). As such, faculty are expected to establish the class structure and rules, defining what is to be done and when (Coll & Weiss, 2015). Veterans take the student role seriously. Faculty should provide clear instructions, apply fair evaluation methods to all students, and offer timely constructive feedback (Coll & Weiss, 2015). It is recommended that feedback clearly identify shortcomings with faculty willing to assist the student veteran to problem solve to improve academic performance (ACE, 2018). Opportunities to interact with peers through collaborative learning and group work are preferred over individual activities and lecture (Coll & Weiss, 2015; Patterson et al., 2019b). Sportsman and Thomas (2015) asserted that hands-on learning in a group setting offers "more accurate data on which to base evaluations and future lessons" for student veterans (p. 51). Finally, understanding that veterans may not be comfortable turning their backs on a room, faculty are encouraged to accommodate seating preferences (ACE, 2018).

Creating an environment that is safe for learning is important for student veterans. Faculty should avoid interjecting their own biases and opinions related to military service and involvement in ongoing wars (Coll & Weiss, 2015; Vacchi, 2012). Role modeling behaviors that foster a "constructive learning environment" are encouraged (Coll & Weiss, 2015). Veterans should be encouraged to seek help and ask questions when needed (Gibbs et al., 2019). This may extend beyond the classroom itself as faculty assist student veterans to receive needed accommodations or access resources needed to be successful (Gibbs et al., 2019; Sportsman & Thomas, 2015).

Interacting With Veterans

As a diverse population of students with a unique cultural background, it is important for faculty to get to know them, individually and collectively. Recalling that veterans may feel reluctant to discuss their military service with those who have no military experience means that faculty members should take the initiative to ask about their military experiences (Gibbs et al., 2019). Having a sincere interest in student veterans helps to establish trust. "Speaking their language" helped faculty in one nursing program build rapport with student veterans (Allen et al., 2012). Gibbs et al. (2019) cautions faculty against "embellishing relatability" while connecting with student veterans as this can result in a loss of trust (p. 349). However, faculty must also maintain boundaries to avoid assuming roles for which they are not qualified; for example, mental health counselor.

Faculty are encouraged to make themselves available to student veterans. This may include overt gestures, such as communicating office hours, or less explicit strategies, such as displaying military symbols that alert student veterans to faculty who embrace and understand veterans (Elliott et al., 2019;

Gibbs et al., 2019). These actions demonstrate a "caring willingness to help and encourage these students" (Gibbs et al., 2019, p. 349). Faculty should seek to learn about student veterans' strengths and weaknesses that may be leveraged to enhance their education experience. It is important to create a safe space where veterans are comfortable sharing, know who their allies are, and where privacy and confidentiality are maintained.

Ascertaining information about issues student veterans perceive as impacting their academic success is also important (Gibbs et al., 2019). However, general pleasantry questions such as "are you doing okay?" are not likely to yield valuable and meaningful responses from student veterans (Sportsman & Thomas, 2015, p. 49). Nor should faculty put student veterans on the spot or pressure them to share their military experiences (Gibbs et al., 2019; Morrison-Beedy et al., 2015). Distinguishing a student issue from a veteran issue is vital to ensuring equal accommodations for all students (Coll & Weiss, 2015; Elliott et al., 2019). Helping veterans tap into and re-purpose their military traits and service experience may be a starting point (Elliott et al., 2019; Gibbs et al., 2019). As needed, faculty may recommend VA resources, such as academic readiness classes, to help student veterans' bridge the gap between military service and higher education (Norman et al., 2015). Faculty should know what resources are available to student veterans and how to access them (Gibbs et al., 2019). Cox (2019) states "a nursing faculty that becomes familiar with the uniqueness of this student population and proactively recognizes when they are challenged is a faculty who will best serve other students who may need to tap into resources before it is too late to academically succeed" (p. 398).

IMPLICATIONS FOR NURSING EDUCATION

Differences in life experiences, confidence, maturity, and academic challenges demonstrate the uniqueness of the student veteran population in higher education (Barry et al., 2014). As more veterans leave the military, the number of student veterans also increases. As such, university administrators and faculty have an obligation to understand this group of nontraditional students so that their needs are met in a meaningful way. Although there is limited empirical literature related to the student veteran experience in nursing education, findings from the higher education literature maintain clear implications for nursing education.

Admission policies should include an accurate evaluation of military service and training to facilitate awarding academic credit. Deliberate efforts to support student veterans in transition should include programs which identify "ways in which campus and military culture are similar and different and how to navigate their new environment" (Barry et al., 2014, p. 39). Likewise, nurse faculty must overcome a deficit in knowledge related to military and veteran culture. Schools of nursing should establish relationships with student veterans and maintain communication to ascertain their ongoing needs and challenges while enhancing strengths and reducing barriers to successful matriculation (Dyar, 2016).

FUTURE RESEARCH PRIORITIES

Nursing education has not kept pace in our understanding of student veterans in the nursing classroom. As such, nurse educators should endeavor to conduct research investigating veterans as students, nursing program outcomes specific to student veterans, and the integration of veteran health competencies into nursing curricula. More specifically, a better understanding of the actualization of the *Joining Forces* goals is needed to uncover best practices. Recipients of HRSA cooperative agreement grants should articulate methods used to achieve VBSN goals with a focus on program outcomes. A clear understanding of the predictors of student veteran success in nursing education, such as awarding academic credit for military experience, is also needed. Longitudinal studies of student veteran's academic journey from application to graduation are needed to properly address barriers and identify areas for improvement in nursing education. Only then will faculty know whether nursing education has sufficiently met student veteran academic needs and prepared graduates to address healthcare needs in the community.

CONCLUSIONS

More veterans are coming to college classrooms, so nursing programs and nurse educators must be prepared. Each veteran enters higher education with unique life experiences largely influenced by their military service. Significant progress has been made in understanding the lived experiences of veterans in transition out of the military into civilian life and into higher education. However, the nursing education literature is only beginning to investigate student veterans. Nursing faculty have more work to do.

Understanding the challenges reported by student veterans is a starting point. Appreciating that there is no one solution that will guarantee all student veterans achieve their academic goals is important. Nursing faculty are called to increase their understanding of military and veteran culture, make an effort to get to know student veterans enrolled in their classes/programs, examine teaching and learning practices to meet learning needs and expectations, communicate with student veterans, advocate for campus resources for student veterans, and match veterans to resources.

REFERENCES

The complete reference list for this chapter appears in the digital version of the chapter, accessible at https://connect.springerpub.com/content/book/978-0-8261-3597-1/chapter/ch12

ABBREVIATIONS

6MWT	Six-Minute Walk Test
AACN	American Association of Colleges of Nursing
AAN	American Academy of Nursing
ACE	American Council on Education
ACE.V	Advancing Care Excellence for Veterans
ADL	activity of daily living
AFHSB	Armed Forces Health Surveillance Branch
AIS	Asia Impairment Scale
ALS	amyotrophic lateral sclerosis
AMCC	Assessment of Military Cultural Competence
aMFLS	annual Military Family Lifestyle Survey
ANA	American Nurses Association
APNA	American Psychiatric Nurses Association
ARS	audience response system
ASVAB	Armed Services Vocational Aptitude Battery
AVF	all-volunteer force
BDRC	Birth Defect Research for Children
BMI	body mass index
BSN	Bachelor of Science in Nursing
C-TraC	Coordinated Transitional Care
CAF	Canadian Armed Forces
CAM	complementary and alternative medicine
CAPS	Counseling and Psychological Services
CARC	chemical agent resistant coating
CBO	Congressional Budget Office
CBOC	community-based outpatient clinic
CBT	cognitive-behavioral therapy
CCNE	Commission on Collegiate Nursing Education
CDC	Centers for Disease Control and Prevention
CE	continuing education
CIHS	Center for Integrated Health Solutions
CLC	community living center
CMI	chronic multisymptom illness
CMV	Center for Minority Veterans

CNL	clinical nurse leader
COACH	Caring for Older Adults and Caregivers at Home
CTE	chronic traumatic encephalopathy
DADT	Don't Ask, Don't Tell
DAI	Diffuse axonal injury
DAV	Disabled American Veterans
dBA	decibels
DCAS	Defense Casualty Analysis System
DEP	Delay Entry Program
DMZ	Demilitarized Zone
DNP	Doctor of Nursing Practice
DoD	U.S. Department of Defense
DU	depleted uranium
DVA	Department of Veteran Affairs
DVBIC	Defense and Veterans Brain Injury Center
EBP	evidence-based practice
ECHO	Extension for Community Healthcare Outcomes
EHR	electronic health record
ELNEC	End-of-Life Nursing Education Consortium
EOL	end of life
EVC	Enhancing Veterans' Care
EWI	Enterprise-Wide Initiatives
FDA	Food and Drug Administration
FRG	family readiness group
FtM	female to male
FUDD	female urinary diversion device
FY	fiscal year
GWI	Gulf War illness
GWOT	Global War on Terrorism
HMMWV	high mobility multipurpose wheeled vehicle
HPTAV	Health Professionals' Attitude Towards Veterans
HRSA	Health Resources and Services Administration
HSCR	Homelessness Screening Clinical Reminder
HUD	U.S. Department of Housing and Urban Development
HVRP	Homeless Veterans Reintegration Program
ICN	International Council of Nurses
IMPROVE	Integrated Management and Polypharmacy Review of Vulnerable Elders
IOM	Institute of Medicine
IPCP	Interprofessional Collaborative Practice
IPE	interprofessional education
IPEC	Interprofessional Education Collaborative
IPV	intimate partner violence
ISS	injury severity score
KSA	knowledge, skills, and attitudes
LATR	later-adulthood trauma reengagement
LORAN	long range navigation
MCCP	Military Culture Certificate Program
MEPS	Military Entrance Processing Station
MHS	Military Health System

MISSION	Maintaining Internal Systems and Strengthening Integrated Outside Networks
MNO	military nurse officer
MOS	military occupational specialty
MSEP	Military Spouse Employment Partnership
MSM	military service member
MSN	Master of Science in Nursing
MST	military sexual trauma
mTBI	mild traumatic brain injury
MtF	male to female
MVA	motor vehicular accident
MVF-CCM	Military and Veteran Family Cultural Competency Model
NAF	Naval Air Facility
NASEM	National Academies of Sciences, Engineering, and Medicine
NCA	National Cemetery Administration
NCLEX	National Council Licensing Exam
NCO	non-commissioned officer
NIDCD	The National Institute on Deafness and Other Communication Disorders
NLCHP	National Law Center on Homelessness and Poverty
NLN	National League for Nursing
NONPF	National Organization of Nurse Practitioner Faculties
NP	nurse practitioner
OCS	Officer Candidate School
OEF	Operation Enduring Freedom
OIF	Operation Iraqi Freedom
OND	Operation New Dawn
ORH	Office of Rural Health
OSA	obstructive sleep apnea
OST	Osteoporosis Self-Assessment Tool
PA	physician assistant
PACT	Patient Aligned Care Team
PB	pyridostigmine bromide
PCAFC	Program of Comprehensive Assistance for Family Caregivers
PCB	polychlorinated biphenyls
PCS	permanent change of station
PFT	physical fitness test
PIT	point-in-time
PLS	palletized load system
PM	particulate matter
PMC	private military contractor
PME	professional military education
POWER	Posts Working for Veterans Health
PPE	personal protective equipment
PSC	Polytrauma System of Care
PTSD	posttraumatic stress disorder
PVA	Paralyzed Veterans of America
QI	quality improvement
QSEN	Quality and Safety Education for Nurses
RC	Reserve and National Guard component
ROTC	Reserve Officer Training Corps

RTD	return to duty
RWB	Red, White, & Blue
SAMHSA	Substance Abuse and Mental Health Services Administration
SCAN	Specialty Care Access Network
SCI	spinal cord injury
SDOH	social determinants of health
SECO	Spouse Education and Career Opportunities
SHAD	Shipboard Hazard and Defense
SMART	Specific, Measurable, Attainable, Realistic, Time frame
SP	standardized patients
SSVF	Supportive Services for Veteran Families
STI	sexually transmitted infection
SUD	substance use disorder
SWL	satisfaction with life
SVA	Student Veterans of America
TBI	traumatic brain injury
TCLS	Transition to Civilian Life Scale
TDY	temporary duty
TEFSC	Toxic Embedded Fragment Surveillance Center
TUG	Timed Up and Go
UCMJ	Uniform Code of Military Justice
UN	United Nations
USAF	U. S. Air Force
USAHPC	U.S. Army Public Health Command
USDHHS	U.S. Department of Health & Human Services
UTI	urinary tract infection
VA	U.S. Department of Veterans Affairs
VA FARMS	VA Farming and Recovery Mental Health Services
VAHCS	Veterans Affairs Health Care System
VAMC	Veterans Affairs Medical Centers
VANA	Veterans Affairs Nursing Academy
VANAP	Veteran Affairs Nursing Academic Partnership
VASH	Veteran Affairs Supportive Housing
VBA	Veterans Benefits Administration
VBSN	Veteran's Bachelor of Science Degree in Nursing
VCP	VA Community Partnerships
VCUNE	Veteran Competencies for Undergraduate Nursing Education
VFW	Veterans of Foreign Wars
VHA	Veterans Health Administration
VHIE	Veterans Health Information Exchange
VISN	Veterans Integrated Service Network
VLER	Virtual Lifetime Electronic Record
VRHRC	Veterans Rural Health Resource Center
VSO	Veterans Service Organization
VVA	Vietnam Veterans of America
WHV	We Honor Veterans
WO	warrant officer
WV	West Virginia
WW II	World War II

INDEX

Printed in the United States
by Baker & Taylor Publisher Services